Respiratory
Pharmacology and
Pharmacotherapy

Series Editors:

Dr. David Raeburn
Discovery Biology
Rhône-Poulenc Rorer Ltd
Dagenham Research Centre
Dagenham
Essex RM10 7XS
England

Dr. Mark A. Giembycz
Department of Thoracic Medicine
National Heart and Lung Institute
Imperial College of Science, Technology and Medicine
London SW3 6LY
England

Autoimmune Aspects of
Lung Disease

Edited by
D. A. Isenberg
S. G. Spiro

Springer Basel AG

Editors:

Professor David A. Isenberg
Centre for Rheumatology/
Bloomsbury Rheumatology Unit
Department of Medicine
University College London
40-50 Tottenham Court Road
London W1P 9PG
UK

Dr. Stephen G. Spiro
University College London Hospitals
Department of Thoracic Medicine
Middlesex Hospital
Mortimer Street
London W1M 8AA
UK

Library of Congress Cataloging-in-Publication Data
A CIP catalogue record for this book is available from the library of Congress,
Washington D.C., USA

Deutsche Bibliothek Cataloging-in-Publication Data

Autoimmune aspects of lung disease / ed. by D. A. Isenberg ; S. G. Spiro –
Basel ; Boston : Berlin : Birkhäuser, 1998
  (Respiratory pharmacology and pharmacotherapy)
    ISBN 978-3-0348-9830-0   ISBN 978-3-0348-8926-1 (eBook)
    DOI 10.1007/978-3-0348-8926-1

© 1998 Springer Basel AG
Originally published by Birkhäuser Verlag Basel Switzerland in 1998
Softcover reprint of the hardcover 1st edition 1998
Printed on acid-free paper produced from chlorine-free pulp. TCF ∞

Cover design: Markus Etterich

ISBN 978-3-0348-9830-0

9 8 7 6 5 4 3 2 1

Contents

Contents

List of Contributors

Carlo Agostini, Department of Clinical and Experimental Medicine, Padua University School of Medicine, Padua Hospital, 35128 Padua, Italy

Robert M. Bernstein, Rheumatology Department, Manchester Royal Infirmary, Manchester M13 NWL, UK

Helen Booth, Centre for Cardiopulmonary Biochemistry and Respiratory Medicine, University College London Medical School and Royal Free Hospital School of Medicine, London WC1E 6JJ, UK

Graham H. Bothamley, Department of Respiratory Medicine, Homerton Hospital, London E9 6SR, UK

James R. Catterall, Respiratory Department, Bristol Royal Infirmary, Bristol BS2 8HW, UK

Jan Willem Cohen Tervaert, Department of Clinical Immunology, University Hospital, 9713 GZ Groningen, The Netherlands

Beratha S. Devi, Centre for Rheumatology/Bloomsbury Rheumatology Unit, Department of Medicine, University College London, London W1P 9PG, UK

David A. Isenberg, Centre for Rheumatology/Bloomsbury Rheumatology Unit, Department of Medicine, University College London, London W1P 9PG, UK

Geoffrey J. Laurent, Centre for Cardiopulmonary Biochemistry and Respiratory Medicine, University College London Medical School and Royal Free Hospital School of Medicine, London WC1E 6JJ, UK

Peter D. Phelan, Department of Paediatrics, Royal Children's Hospital, Parkville, Victoria 3052, Australia

Angela Rapti, Department of Thoracic Medicine, University College London Hospitals, London WC1E 6AH, UK

Douglas S. Robinson, Department of Allergy and Clinical Immunology, Imperial College School of Medicine at the National Heart and Lung Institute, London SW3 6LY, UK

Graham A.W. Rook, Department of Bacteriology, University College London Medical School, London W1P 6DB, UK

Rosaria Sancetta, Department of Clinical and Experimental Medicine, Padua University School of Medicine, Padua Hospital, 35128 Padua, Italy

Gianpietro Semenzato, Department of Clinical and Experimental Medicine, Padua University School of Medicine, Padua Hospital, 35128 Padua, Italy

Tariq Sethi, Respiratory Medicine Unit, Department of Medicine (RIE), University of Edinburgh Royal Infirmary, Edinburgh EH3 9YW, UK

Penny Shaw, Department of Imaging, University College London Hospitals, London WC1E 6AH, UK

Edward A. Sheffield, Respiratory Department, Bristol Royal Infirmary, Bristol BS2 8HW, UK

Stephen G. Spiro, Department of Thoracic Medicine, University College London Hospitals, London WC1E 6AH, UK

Monica A. Spiteri, Department of Respiratory Medicine, North Staffordshire
    Hospital Trust/Keele University, Stoke-on-Trent, Staffordshire ST4 6QG,
    UK
Coen A. Stegeman, Department of Clinical Nephrology, University Hospital,
    9713 GZ Groningen, The Netherlands
Wim Timens, Department of Clinical Pathology, University Hospital, 9713
    GZ Groningen, The Netherlands
Tjip van der Werf, Department of Clinical Pulmonology, University Hospital,
    9713 GZ Groningen, The Netherlands

Autoimmune Aspects of Lung Disease
ed. by D. A. Isenberg and S. G. Spiro
© 1998 Birkhäuser Verlag Basel/Switzerland

CHAPTER 1
The Lung and the Immune System

James R. Catterall and Edward A. Sheffield

Respiratory Department, Bristol Royal Infirmary, Bristol, UK

1. Introduction

The lungs are in a uniquely vulnerable position in that they are constantly exposed to a wide range of inhaled foreign particles, including microbial pathogens, allergens and environmental toxins. They also have the largest blood supply of any organ, and this also is capable of delivering harmful substances. The need to balance protection from these hazards against the requirements for maximum surface area for gas exchange has been achieved by a highly flexible combination of defence mechanisms. Abnormalities of this system contribute to the pathogenesis of many respiratory disorders.

Inhaled particles which pass through the larynx are initially exposed to mechanical and physical defences such as the cough reflex and the muco-ciliary escalator. They are also met by a range of innate phagocytic and chemical defences, including macrophages, neutrophils, complement, lysozyme and transferrin, some of which contribute to the inflammatory response. However, the enormous flexibility of the immune system, both in terms of its specificity and in the magnitude and variety of its response, lies in the acquired, antigen-specific, response, at the heart of which lie the lymphocytes. These cells recognise foreign antigen and store the information in their memory. When antigen persists or reappears in the respiratory tract, the lymphocytes home to the lungs, where they proliferate and differentiate into effector or regulatory cells. These in turn contribute to the removal of antigen, usually with the assistance of other cells.

Recent studies have helped to elucidate some of the basic mechanisms involved in these responses. The mechanisms by which pulmonary lymphocytes are recruited from the circulation, the ways in which lymphocytes interact with other cells in the lungs, and the processes involved in regulation of the pulmonary immune response are beginning to be understood at the molecular level. These insights into normal immune responses not only help us to understand the pathogenesis of many respiratory diseases but also offer the prospect of therapeutic intervention in a range of pulmonary conditions with are associated with local or generalised abnormalities of the immune system.

2. Structural Basis of the Pulmonary Immune Response

As in other organs, the lymphoid tissue consists of antigen-presenting cells, memory cells (lymphocytes) and effector cells (including lymphocytes), which are organised into a number of separate functional compartments.

2.1. Lymph Nodes

The pulmonary lymph nodes lie in the paratracheal region and adjacent to major bronchi. They receive lymphatic drainage both from the mucosa of the airways and from the lung parenchyma. They are similar in structure to lymph nodes at other sites and contain antigen-presenting cells and a wide range of lymphocytes, creating an environment that is conducive to antigen presentation. Detailed kinetic studies involving localisation and quantitation of both antigen-specific plasma cells and immunoglobulin-specific mRNA have pinpointed lymph nodes as the sites at which antigen-specific IgE and IgG responses to inhaled soluble protein antigen are initiated [1, 2].

2.2. Bronchus-Associated Lymphoid Tissue

Bronchus-associated lymphoid tissue (BALT) consists of lymphoid tissue which appears to be an intrinsic part of the airway mucosa and of the lymphoid tissue in the peripheral lung [3]. It is characterised by the local production of dimeric IgA and by its relationships with mucosal tissue in other organs. Although there is controversy about the existence of BALT in normal human lung, it has been well studied in animals and has been found in the human lung in abnormal conditions such as chronic pneumonia, autoimmune disease, immunodeficiency and sudden infant death syndrome [4].

BALT does not develop until after birth and appears to depend on a local mucosal response to inhaled antigen. As in lymph nodes, antigen-presenting cells are present, and there are T lymphocyte- and B lymphocyte-dominant areas. Unlike in lymph nodes, however, there do not appear to be T lymphocyte-dependent areas, since neonatal thymectomy does not alter the overall morphology, and also BALT does not contain afferent lymphatics. Another difference from lymph nodes is that BALT contains a modified epithelial cell called the M cell (microfold cell) which is particularly effective at transporting insoluble antigen by endocytosis and delivering it to underlying lymphoid tissue without processing it or otherwise behaving as an antigen-presenting cell [5, 6]. This cell has received attention because of its potential to act as a portal of entry for vaccines to the mucosal lymphoid compartment [7].

BALT is part of a collection of similar lymphoid tissues which are found, for example, in the gastrointestinal tract and nasopharynx. The collective term "mucosal associated lymphoid tissue (MALT)" is used to include all these tissues. An important feature of the concept of MALT is that there is recirculation of lymphocytes away from and back to the mucosa of origin. As well as this lymphocytic homing, there is also circulation of lymphocytes between the mucosal surfaces of different organs, for example between the lung and the gastrointestinal tract (see below).

2.3. Lung Parenchyma

In the alveoli and interstitium of the normal lung, immune cells are relatively sparse. However, during invasion by micro-organisms or other foreign antigen the numbers can increase dramatically as lymphocytes and other cells migrate from the circulation [8, 9]. In contrast to BALT and lymph nodes, in which the lymphocytes are a mixture of naive and memory cells, and also in contrast to peripheral blood, the great majority of lymphocytes in the alveoli and interstitium are of memory type [10], having already been primed by antigen. Memory cells can be distinguished from naive cells by monoclonal antibodies to different isoforms of the CD45 common

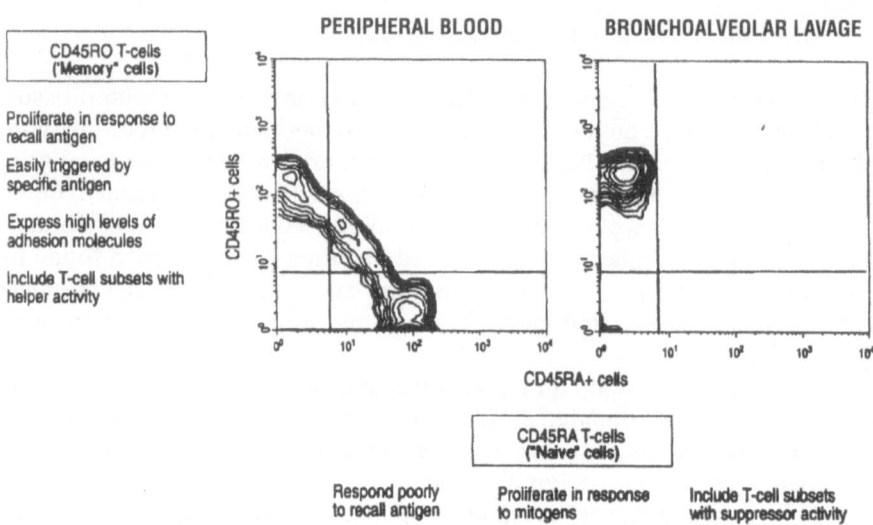

Figure 1. Flow cytometric analysis of CD45RO+ and CD45RA+ T-cell subpopulations in peripheral blood and BAL fluid. All lymphocytes retrieved from the BAL of this representative healthy subject are represented by CD45RO+ T-cells that express high levels of adhesion receptors and show functional capabilities of memory cells. After [12].

leukocyte antigen. Naive lymphocytes express a high molecular weight isoform designated CD45RA, whilst memory cells express the CD45RO antigen (Figure 1).

Immunological events in the alveoli are often studied by analysis of bronchoalveolar lavage (BAL) fluid [11]. In the normal non-smoking adult, more than 90% of cells in BAL fluid are alveolar macrophages, and 5–10% are lymphocytes. Of the lymphocytes, 75–90% are T-cells, fewer than 5% are B-cells and the remainder include natural killer (NK) cells. Most of the T-cells express the $\alpha\beta$ T-cell receptor (TCR) in association with either CD4 or CD8 determinants. As in blood, there are approximately twice as many CD4 helper cells as CD8 cytotoxic/suppressor cells [12].

A small number of the T lymphocytes in BAL fluid are of TCR $\gamma\delta$ type. These cells can respond to an antigen which has not been processed by an antigen-presenting cell, probably by mechanisms similar to the way antibodies recognise antigen. The function of $\gamma\delta$ cells is not known, though they are mainly found in the mucosa, and there is evidence from animal studies that they can regulate the pattern of cytokine production in response to inhaled antigen [13]. Most $\gamma\delta$ cells are negative for CD4 and CD8 determinants; however, $\gamma\delta$ cells which co-express the CD8 determinant have been found in the BAL fluid of human immunodeficiency virus (HIV-1) infected patients. Although the role of these cells is also uncertain, it has been suggested that TCR $\gamma\delta$ cells might play a role in the pulmonary immune system of some patients with acquired immunodeficiency syndrome (AIDS), perhaps by the recognition of sets of HIV-1 antigens different from those recognised by TCR $\alpha\beta$ cells [14].

3. Lymphocyte Circulation

A crucial step in the immune process is the compartmentalisation of circulating lymphocytes to lung tissue. This applies both to naive lymphocytes, which need to be available to make initial contact with antigen, and to memory cells, which may subsequently be required for antigen which persists or reappears in the lung.

3.1. Homing Molecules

The localisation of lymphocytes to lung tissue involves the interaction between surface homing molecules on the lymphocytes with receptors on endothelial cells, known as vascular addressins. The site of localisation in BALT and other organised lymphoid tissue has been identified as the high endothelial venule. The process is independent of antigen, though there is evidence that the presence of antigen increases the rate of migration and accumulation of lymphocytes [15].

Recent studies have demonstrated that L-selectin, the β-2 integrin LFA-1 (lymphocyte function antigen-1) and the β-1 integrin VLA-4 (very late antigen-4) are involved in the homing of circulating lymphocytes to pulmonary endothelium [9, 16]. It is likely, as with other leucocytes adhering to pulmonary endothelium [17, 18], and as with lymphocytes adhering to endothelial monolayers [19], that selectins cause rolling and initial tethering of leucocytes to endothelium, and that integrins lead to firm adhesion [16]. However, there is evidence that selectins may not always be necessary for lymphocyte adhesion [20]. As with other adhesion molecules, including those in pulmonary tissue [8, 21], it is also very likely that expression of these adhesion molecules and their receptors is regulated by cytokines. Once the lymphocytes have passed through the endothelium, adhesion molecules are involved in the localisation of lymphocytes to other tissues. For example, $\alpha E\beta7$ integrin has been implicated in the adhesion of lymphocytes to pulmonary epithelial tissue [22, 23].

Different lymphocytes have different receptors. Naive lymphocytes express homing receptors for mucosal tissue and lymph nodes. This explains the ability of populations of normal lymphocytes (predominantly comprising naive cells) to recirculate more or less uniformly through lymph nodes in different organs. Memory lymphocytes tend to home to specific organs and/or specific tissues [15, 24–26]. For example, some memory lymphocytes, unlike naive lymphocytes, have the ability to localise selectively within the pulmonary parenchyma [10], whereas other memory lymphocytes home only to mucosal tissue [15].

3.2. Some Pulmonary Lymphocytes Are Derived from the Intestine

Animal studies of acute bacterial pulmonary infection have shown that survival can be improved, and clearance of bacteria from the lungs enhanced, by prior immunisation with the same organism [15, 27]. This is associated with increased numbers of lymphocytes in BAL fluid [28], with evidence of increased migration of both IgA-containing B-cells [29, 30] and antigen-specific T-cells [15] from the intestine to the lung.

Thus there is evidence of recirculation of lymphocytes between mucosal tissue in different organs. Once a lymphocyte has been primed at one mucosal site (e.g. Peyer's patches in the intestinal mucosa), it can home not only to that site but to mucosal associated lymphoid tissue at other sites. It is believed that different mucosal tissues contain similar vascular addressins, and that lymphocytes which have been primed in mucosal tissue have similar homing molcules irrespective of the organ in which priming took place. For example, *in vitro* studies have shown that lymphocytes from Peyer's patches will bind to BALT [31].

As well as having potential implications for pulmonary immunity in general, these findings have led to studies of oral vaccines for protection against lung infection [32, 33]. Not only would oral immunisation be a more convenient route of vaccination than parenteral administration, but animal studies have suggested that the mucosal immune system may be less susceptible to age-related dysfunction that the systemic system. Thus, murine splenic immune responses to different antigens, including pneumococcal antigens, have been shown to decline with age, whilst mucosal responses have remained constant [34, 25].

4. Sequence of Events in the Pulmonary Immune Response

Most pulmonary antigens are protein-based and dependent on T lymphocytes for an immune response. However, some bacteria which cause respiratory disease possess polysaccharide antigens which can generate an immune response without the involvement of T lymphocytes. An important clinical example is the capsule of *Streptococcus pneumoniae*. T-dependent antigens have two disadvantages as immunogens compared with T-independent antigens, namely their inability to elicit a memory booster response and their ineffectiveness in children under 2 years of age. These features may help to explain the high incidence of pneumococcal disease, particularly in the young. However, T-independent antigens can be converted into T-dependent ones by conjugation to a protein carrier as in the vaccine against *Haemophilus influenzae* type B and experimental vaccines against *Streptococcus pneumoniae* [33].

4.1. Antigen-Presenting Cells

T-cells can only respond to exogenous antigen if the antigen is presented by an accessory cell. Accessory cells process the antigen and present it to the lymphocyte in a partially degraded form on their surface, in association with a class II major histocompatibility complex (MHC) antigen.

Although antigen-presenting activity in the lung has classically been associated with alveolar macrophages, recent attention has focused on dendritic cells and the closely related Langerhans' cells. The former are widely distributed in the normal lung; the latter lie in the airway mucosa, where they form a dense interconnecting network between the epithelial cells. Both cell types have long cytoplasmic processes which maximise the surface area for exposure to antigen and lymphocytes, both are able to migrate to lymph nodes, where their antigen-presenting ability is probably augmented by increased exposure to cytokines, and both can adapt to the antigenic and inflammatory environment [36, 37]. Smoking causes dendritic cell hyperplasia and altered function of dendritic cells [38], while corticosteroids reduce dendritic cell numbers in the respiratory tract by modulating either the response to cytokines or the expression of adhesion molecules [39].

Dendritic cells and Langerhans' cells are probably the most important cells in the initial presentation of antigen to lymphocytes, for they are superior to other cells in their ability to prime naive T-cells [40]. However, once lymphocytes have been primed, they can respond to antigen presented by a number of different cells. Pulmonary cells which have a constitutive ability to present antigen are the alveolar and tissue macrophages, and B lymphocytes. However, antigen-presenting ability can also be induced. Thus in some conditions even cells that are not usually capable of presenting antigen – endothelial cells, epithelial cells, type II alveolar cells and fibroblasts – attain the ability to act as antigen-presenting cells [41].

The strong ability of dendritic cells to activate lymphocyte antigen presentation lies not so much in their production of cytokines as in their expression of surface molecules which aid adhesion of lymphocytes and which act as costimulatory [41–43] molecules (see below). In *in vitro* studies the difference between blood monocytes and pulmonary dendritic cells in their ability to stimulate lymphocyte proliferation could not be explained by differences in levels of cytokine production, whereas monoclonal blocking antibodies against a number of integrin components on dendritic cells caused significant reduction in lymphocyte proliferation [41].

4.2. Antigen Recognition

Most pulmonary T-cells possess either CD4 or CD8 antigens. Thus their interactions with antigen are MHC-restricted. As well as influencing which type of T-cell a particular antigen will activate (CD4 or CD8), this MHC restriction affects which epitopes from the invading organism or foreign antigen are involved in the immune response. For example, during influenza vaccination it was found that the epitopes of the influenza A haemagglutinin molecules selected by the lymphocytes from different individuals were precisely defined by HLA in spite of differences in age, nationality and previous exposure to influenza A visuses, and that lymphocytes from individuals with identical HLA-DR alleles selected identical epitopes [44].

4.3. Lymphocyte Activation

Activation of T-cells depends not only on the recognition of antigen by the T-cell receptor but also on a number of other interactions between the surface molecules on the lymphocytes and the antigen-presenting cells (Table 1). These are (1) adhesion of the antigen-presenting cell to the lymphocytes by surface molecules, including β-1 and β-2 integrins [41], (2) interactions between MHC class I and CD8 antigens, or between MHC class II and CD4 antigens, resulting in cytotoxic/suppressor activity or helper cell activity, respectively, and (3) additional (costimulatory) signals resulting from the interaction of other surface molecules on the antigen-presenting cells and lymphocytes. The importance of costimulatory signals in this and other interactions between cells of the immune system has been recognised only recently. In the activation of both CD4 and CD8 T lymphocytes by antigen-presenting cells, costimulatory signals are provided by the B-7 molecules CD86 and CD80 on antigen-presenting cells, and their respective ligands CD28 and CTLA4 on lymphocytes [45]. Regulation of surface molecules is likely to be important in the control of immune responses and may also have therapeutic potential. For example, there is a low expression of B-7 molecules on some tumour cells, and this can be upregulated by altering the cytokine environment of the cell [46].

4.4. Cytokines

Many of the effects of lymphocytes are mediated by lymphokines. These are hormone-like peptides or glycopeptides which, in collaboration with cytokines produced by other cells, and with adhesion molecules and costimulatory molecules on cell surfaces, exert a wide range of stimulatory and suppressive effects on other cells which take part in the immune process. In vitro studies of individual cytokines have enabled different biological activities to be assigned to each cytokine (Table 2). The in vivo effects, however, are dependent on many interactive factors, including the presence of other cytokines which may act synergistically or antagonistically, the density of cytokine receptors on the interacting cells and the presence of

Table 1. A selection of adhesion and costimulatory molecules discussed in text

Class	Cell expression	Ligand	Function
L-Selectin	Leucocytes	Cell surface carbohydrates	Leucocyte rolling/tethering
E-Selectin	Endothelium	Cell surface carbohydrates	Leucocyte rolling/tethering
P-Selectin	Platelets, endothelium	Cell surface carbohydrates	Leucocyte rolling/tethering
Integrin (name)			
$\alpha 4\beta 1$ (VLA-4)	Lymphocytes, monocytes	VCAM-1, fibronectin	Mononuclear cell migration, B- and T-cell adhesion
$\alpha L\beta 2$ (LFA-1)	Lymphocytes, monocytes macrophages, neutrophils	ICAM-1	Inflammatory cell and lymphocyte adhesion
$\alpha 4\beta 7$	Mucosal lymphocytes	E-cadherin	Binds to pulmonary epithelium

Table 1 (continued)

Class	Cell expression	Ligand	Function
Immunoglobulin superfamily			
CD4	T-helper cells, monocytes	MHC class II	MHC II-restricted responses
CD8	Cytotoxic/suppressor cells	MHC class I	MHC I-restricted responses
ICAM-1	Monocytes, endothelium Induced on B, T, dendritic, epithelial cells	LFA-1, Mac-1, CD43	Adhesion of inflammatory cells to endothelium
VCAM-1	Activated endothelium, macrophages, dendritic cells	VLA-4, $\alpha 4\beta 7$	Lymphocyte/ monocyte/eosinophil endothelial adhesion
B7 (CD80)	B-cells, dendritic cells	CTLA-4	T- and B-cell interaction
B7-2 (CD86)	Activated B-cells, monocytes	CD28	T- and B-cell interaction
CD28	T-cells, activated B-cells	B7	T- and B-cell interaction
Other adhesion molecules			
CD40	CD40-ligand on activated T-cells	B-cells, dendritic cells, epithelial cells	T- and B-cell interaction
Other costimulatory molecules			
Fas	T-cells, NK cells	Fas-ligand	Immunoregulation Apoptosis

Table 2. Cytokines: Summary of sources and biological activities

Cytokine	Source	Target	Action
IL-1	Macrophages, B cells, endothelium, fibroblasts	T-cells, B-cells, macrophages, endothelium, fibroblasts	Lymphocyte activation macrophage stimulation, leukocyte adhesion
IL-2	T-cells	T-cells	T-cell proliferation
IL-3	Th2 cells	Stem cells	Colony stimulating activity
IL-4	Th2 cells, basophils	B and T-cells	B-cell growth factor, isotype switching
IL-5	Th2 cells	B-cells	B-cell differentiation, IgA production
IL-6	T, B-cells, fibroblasts	B-cells, hepatocytes	B-cell differentiation Enhances T cell activation
IL-7	Marrow stromal cells	Pre-B cells, T-cells	T- and B-cell proliferation
IL-8	Monocytes, macrophages, T-cells, endothelium	Neutrophils, basophils	Pro-inflammatory Neutrophil chemotaxis
IL-10	T-cells	Th1 cells	Inhibits cytokine production and Th1 cells
IL-12	Monocytes, NK cells	T-cells	Induction of Th1 cells
IL-13	Activated T-cells	Monocytes, B-cells	Blocks IL-12 synthesis
IL-15	Monocytes	T-cells, activated B-cells	Proliferation
TNF-α	Macrophages, lymphocytes, mast cells	Macrophages, granulocytes, tissue cells	Activates macrophages, neutrophils, NK cells Inflammatory cell adhesion
TNF-β	T-cells	Macrophages, granulocytes, tissue cells	Activates macrophages, neutrophils, NK cells Inflammatory cell adhesion
Interferon-α	Leucocytes	Tissue cells	HLA-1 induction, antiviral
Interferon-β	T-cells	Th1 cells	HLA-1,2 induction
Interferon-γ	T-cells, NK cells	Th2 cells	Macrophage activation

cytokine inhibitors. Attempts to clarify the roles of individual cytokines in animal models of pulmonary infection or aeroallergen exposure have included the abrogation of lymphokine activity by blocking antibodies and the use of transgenic mice which do not express the gene for a particular cytokine. Additional information has been obtained by following the kinetics of lymphokine production and relating them to biological events.

4.5. Th_1 and Th_2 Lymphocytes

Some insight into the relationships between different lymphokines, and therefore the possible functions of the lymphokines, has recently come from the identification of two distinct clones of T-helper cells, Th_1 and Th_2, with different patterns of lymphokine production. These were originally identified in mice but have now been found in human lungs [47–49]. Th_1 cells secrete interleukin-2 (IL-2) and γ-interferon, whereas Th_2 cells secrete IL-4, IL-5, IL-6 and IL-10. Both subsets produce IL-3, granulocyte-monocyte colony-stimulating factor (GM-CSF) and tumour necrosis factor-α (TNF-α). The functions of the different subsets are reflected in their different cytokine profiles. Thus Th_1 cells tend to activate macrophages. In contrast, Th_2 cells tend to increase production of eosinophils and mast cells, and enhance production of antibody, including IgE. Furthermore, the two patterns of cytokine production, once established, tend to inhibit each other. Gamma-interferon produced by Th_1 cells inhibits the proliferation of Th_2 cells, whereas IL-10 produced by Th_2 cells suppresses the proliferative activity of Th_1 cells. Associated with these two subsets are Th_0 cells, which are capable of secreting a wide range of cytokines.

Although the cytokine networks that control the commitment of Th_0 cells to Th_1 or Th_2 activity are not fully understood, there is increasing evidence that IL-4 is implicated. For example, in mouse models of eosinophilic airway inflammation induced by exposure to inhaled allergen, transgenic mice with deletion of the IL-4 gene had markedly reduced evidence of Th_2 activity [50, 51].

4.6. Effector Cells

With the exception of cytotoxic T-cells, activated T lymphocytes exert their effects on foreign material by involving other cells. This includes activation of B lymphocytes to produce immunoglobulins, recruitment and activation of phagocytic cells, and involvement of mast cells and eosinophils. The functions of these cells will be reviewed only briefly here, and the discussion will be limited mainly to their effector and related roles. It should be noted, however, that these cells also have immunoregulatory properties that are mediated by cytokines and surface molecules which interact with lymphocytes and other cells.

4.6.1. B-cells: Most mature B-cells are found in the follicles of lymphoid tissue surrounding the airway. They secrete predominantly IgA in a dimeric form, in contrast to the monomeric form which exists in serum. IgA enhances phagocytosis of antigen opsonised by IgG, and Fc receptors for IgA are expressed on neutrophils by the influence of inflammatory mediators [52]. The ability to destroy IgA1 by secretion of IgA protease is a recognised virulence factor among airway pathogens [53].

Pulmonary B-cells also secrete small amounts of IgM and IgG, though IgG is also derived by transudation from serum, particularly in the lower respiratory tract. The ratio of IgA to IgG decreases from the main airway to the periphery. IgE is found in only very low concentrations in the non-allergic state and appears to be derived from the circulation. The low concentration of IgE in lung washings is probably due to extensive binding to mast cells.

T-dependent activation of B-cells depends not only on the specific interaction between the T-cell receptor and the antigen-MHC II complex but also involves IL-6 and other cytokines, and interactions between surface molecules on the cells. The most potent activating signal comes from the interaction between CD40 antigen on the B-cells with CD40 ligand expressed on the activated T lymphocyte [45]. T-cells also influence the type of immunoglobulin that is produced. Transforming growth factor-β (TGF-β) produced by T lymphocytes causes B lymphocytes to switch to IgA production [54], whereas IL-4 favours the production of IgE [55].

4.6.2. Cytotoxic lymphocytes: Cytotoxic viruses are thought to be involved in the elimination of viruses. In the normal lung, they are present in only small numbers; most are non-MHC-restricted and exhibit natural killer (NK) activity. However, CD8$^+$ cells increase in number during HIV infection, chronic pulmonary allograft rejection and in some forms of interstitial lung disease. Both MHC and non-MHC-restricted lymphocytes are able to lyse cells containing viruses or certain tumours, with or without antibody, a process which involves interaction between the surface molecule Fas on the target cell and with Fas-ligand on the lymphocyte [56]. CD8$^+$ cells also secrete IL-2 and interferon-γ.

The factors which control cytotoxic lymphocyte activity in the lungs remain incompletely understood. However, it has been shown that alveolar macrophages exert a suppressive effect on NK cells. In contrast, IL-2 can stimulate NK cell activity in BAL fluid.

4.6.3. Pulmonary macrophages: Pulmonary macrophages differ in their functional capabilities, depending on their location. Alveolar macrophages are predominantly effector cells which phagocytose and kill inhaled micro-organisms by oxidative and non-oxidative mechanisms [57]. Similarly, intravascular macrophages are also highly phagocytic and are believed to remove foreign material which enters the lung via the bloodstream. In contrast, interstitial macrophages have poor phagocytic capability and are better adapted for antigen presentation.

Immune stimulation of alveolar macrophages is brought about largely by interferon-γ, secreted by activated lymphocytes [58]. This cell-mediated response to pathogens and foreign antigens increases phagocytic and microbicidal activity of the macrophages, enabling, for example, intra-cellular organisms to be killed. However, if the macrophage is unable to eliminate an infecting organism or antigenic material and if lymphokine stimulation continues, granuloma formation occurs, as in tuberculosis. On the other hand, if interferon-γ is not secreted by pulmonary lymphocytes, as in AIDS, the intracellular organisms proliferate.

Among the products secreted by activated macrophages are neutrophil chemotaxins, including IL-8, and macrophage inhibitory protein (MIP)-1α, which attracts monocytes and CD8$^+$ lymphocytes to the lungs. There is recent evidence that IL-13 can inhibit MIP-1α from alveolar macrophages and thus inhibit macrophage-mediated inflammation in the lungs [59].

4.6.4. Neutrophils: Neutrophils are important in defence against bacterial and fungal infections. If an associated immune response against the patho-gen is present, the function of neutrophils is enhanced [60, 61]. Neutro-phils, like macrophages, kill micro-organisms by both oxidative and non-oxidative mechanisms.

As with lymphocytes, neutrophils are selectively recruited to the lungs by selectins and integrins, and their respective ligands, P and E selectins, and the integrin ICAM-1 (intercellular adhesion molecule-1) have been most implicated in neutrophil recruitment. These are upregulated by TNF-α released from alveolar macrophages [8, 21] and by interferon-γ released from T lymphocytes [8, 62]. Alveolar macrophages also secrete neutrophil chemotaxins, including IL-8 and leukotriene-B4 (LTB-4), whilst CD4$^+$ cells secrete GM-CSF, which promotes microbial killing by neutrophils. In contrast, a number of other peptides and lipids in BAL fluid have been shown to inhibit neutrophil function and may have a moderating role [63].

4.6.5. Mast cells: Mast cells are present on the respiratory tract mucosa and in the pulmonary interstitium. They have polyclonal IgE firmly attach-ed to their surface and numerous histamine-containing granules in their cytoplasm. Cross-linking of surface IgE molecules by antigen causes release of histamine and other mediators, leading to immediate hypersensitivity responses and the accumulation of inflammatory cells including eosino-phils. Studies in animals have also shown that mast cells and eosinophils are increased during helminth infections [64]. Recent evidence suggests that the rapid release of IL-5 by mast cells following IgE-mediated activa-tion may have a primary role in inducing airway eosinophilia [65].

Mast cells in the mucosa proliferate under the influence of T lympho-cyte-derived IL-3 and IL-4, whereas connective tissue mast cells require fibroblast-derived stem cell factor to differentiate. Mucosal mast cells are often found in the same sites as T-cells, and often share common adhesion receptors with them. Also, during parasitic infection of mast cell numbers is dependent on T-cells. These findings suggest that mucosal mast cells and T-cells may collaborate. However, *in vitro* studies with human mast cells have demonstrated no convincing effect of T-cell derived cytokines on IgE-mediated release of histamine and other mediators [64, 66].

4.6.6. Eosinophils: Like mast cells, eosinophils have a high density of FcεR I receptors, and degranulate when surface-bound IgE is cross-linked by antigen. However, they do not feature in the normal lung. Eosinophils are attracted to the lung during helminth infections in animals, and they are also present in a number of lung diseases, notably asthma. They secrete a large number of substances that are toxic to helminths and other micro-organisms, as well as tumour cells.

As with other leucocytes, recruitment and activation of eosinophils involves adhesion molecules, chemoattractant cytokines and activating cytokines. Although many molecules have been shown to affect eosinophils, some are of particular interest. Specifically, the interaction between the integrin VLA-4 and its ligand ICAM-1, which is upregulated by the Th_2 cytokine IL-4, affects eosinophils (as well as basophils, lymphocytes, monocytes and dendritic cells) but not neutrophils [9, 67], and the Th_2 cytokine IL-5 is a relatively specific growth and activation factor for eosinophils [65, 68]. Selective expression of these molecules may help to explain the tendency for eosinophils rather than neutrophils to accumulate in the lung during some immune processes.

5. Regulation of the Pulmonary Immune Response

In view of the constant entry of foreign substances into the lungs, it is perhaps surprising that there is not a greater immune response at all times. The above account also does not explain how the immune system avoids attacking the lung tissue itself, nor does it fully account for differences in response between individuals or the choice of one effector mechanism in preference to another. These basic questions regarding the limitation and direction of the lungs' immune response to antigens cannot be answered fully, but partial answers lie in a number of different regulatory mechanisms, some local and some generalised.

5.1. Immunoregulation by Alveolar Macrophages

Although alveolar macrophages can act as antigen-presenting cells or effector cells and secrete immunoregulatory cytokines, there is evidence that their net effect on the pulmonary immune response is negative. Thus they may prevent pulmonary lymphocytes from over-reacting to the many foreign antigens which reach the lungs.

There are a number of lines of evidence for these negative effects. First, lymphocytes obtained by BAL are less responsive than T lymphocytes from other sites [69]. Second, laboratory animals which have been depleted of alveolar macrophages show increased antigen presenting-activity by pulmonary dendritic cells [70], increased cloning efficiency of T lymphocytes obtained by BAL [69], and increased secondary immune responses to antigen [71, 72]. And third, in most studies, though not all, T lymphocytes have become less responsive when incubated with alveolar macrophages [72, 73]. However, inhibition by alveolar macrophages is very selective and affects only specific areas of lymphocyte function. For example, when T lymphocytes were stimulated in the presence of alveolar macrophages, although they produced cytokines such as IL-2 and interferon-γ, and expressed IL-2 receptors, they were unable to proliferate. This finding suggests that alveolar macrophages limit the magnitude of each immune response by preventing local clonal expansion of the activated cells [72, 74].

A number of possible mechanisms by which alveolar macrophages may exert these inhibitory effects have been identified, including secretion of prostaglandin E2 and hydrogen peroxide [75], a relative paucity of adhesion and costimulatory molecules [76], release of the IL-1 receptor antagonist [77] and production of the inhibitory cytokine IL-10 [41]. Furthermore, alveolar macrophages may not act alone in the alveolar milieu, since surfactant has also been shown to inhibit lymphocyte proliferation and effector function [78].

5.2. Immunological Tolerance

The mechanisms by which lymphocytes tolerate self-antigen are the subject of recent reviews [79, 80]. Advances in this field have been aided by the development of transgenic mice in which most of the T-cells or B-cells are directed against a single antigen, enabling the development and fate of these cells to be followed *in vivo*.

One mechanism of immune tolerance is clonal deletion, in which lymphocytes which react with self-antigen are deleted early in their development, before they reach the circulation. There is evidence that immature lymphocytes are more susceptible to this negative selection than mature cells, and that MHC molecules are involved. Immature lymphocytes which bind strongly to epitopes on the surface of cells (reflecting lymphocyte binding not only to MHC molecules but also to epitopes from self-antigen) are deleted, whereas those which bind only lightly (reflecting binding of class I or class II MHC molecules to the lymphocytes but not binding of self-antigen) are retained. Thus the lymphocytes which are retained, and which circulate to other organs, are those which fail to respond to self-antigen. The cells which are deleted undergo apoptosis, partly mediated by Fas/Fas-ligand interactions [56].

However, not all lymphocytes with receptors for self-antigen are deleted in the thymus or bone marrow. Some circulate but do not function immunologically, either because of clonal anergy (in which the cells are rendered unable to react to self-antigen) or clonal ignorance (in which the cells are able to react to self-antigen but do not). It has been suggested that clonal anergy may involve similar mechanisms to clonal deletion, with recently released lymphocytes being particularly susceptible to negative selection [81]. Furthermore, there is evidence that anergic B-cells have a shortened life, suggesting that anergy and deletion may form a spectrum [82]. Clonal ignorance can occur when self-antigen is inaccessible to circulating lymphocytes or when a T-lymphocyte receptor has very little affinity for self-antigen or when the self-antigen is present in only very low concentrations. There is also evidence that both anergy and ignorance can be influenced by the level of expression of costimulatory molecules [79].

5.3. Immune Deviation

A selective form of immune tolerance, more correctly known as immune deviation, occurs when only part of the immune system fails to respond to antigen. An example is the IgE response to inhaled antigen which only occurs in atopic individuals. "Normal" (non-atopic) individuals develop tolerance; the atopic do not.

In animals this type of tolerance can be induced by exposing the naive animal to repeated low doses of aerosolised proteins [83, 84]. The process appears to be mediated by antigen-specific CD8 "suppressor" cells that are initially activated in lymph nodes draining the large conducting airways. By secreting interferon-γ these cells suppress the development of antigen-specific Th_2 cells and promote the development of Th_1 cells, thus providing long-term protection against potentially pathogenic Th_2 responses [72, 82, 85].

In human subjects, initial exposure to inhaled antigen is likely to take place in childhood, especially the neonatal period, a time when there is considerable variation in the maturity of the immune system between individuals. Evidence from a variety of sources [86–89] suggests that the speed of development of T-cell-mediated immunity in the neonatal period may play a key role in the normal development of immune deviation in the lungs and thus influence whether an individual exhibits this form of tolerance [72, 85]. However, environmental factors are also likely to affect the outcome. The recent observation that positive tuberculin responses in children who have been vaccinated with Bacillus Calmette-Guerin (BCG) predict lower serum IgE and lower Th_1 type cytokine profiles, as well as a lower incidence of asthma, are consistent with the view that childhood infection may skew immune responses towards tolerance of specific antigen by Th_2 cells [90] and thus towards a "normal" or non-atopic response.

These observations are consistent with the view that pulmonary immune responses are greatly influenced by events that occur in early childhood. Although the studies to date have concentrated on Th_2- and IgE-mediated responses, it is possible that other pulmonary immune responses will be similarly affected by imprinting early in life.

References

1. Sedgwick JD, Holt PG (1986) Induction of IgE secreting cells in the lymphatic drainage of the lungs of rats following passive antigen inhalation. *Int Arch Allergy Appl Immunol* 79: 329–331.
2. McMenamin C, Gim B, Holt PG (1992) The distribution of IgE-plasma cells in lymphoid and non-lymphoid tissues of high-IgE-reponder rats: Differential localization of antigen-specific and "bystander" components of the IgE response to inhaled antigen. *Immunology* 77: 592–596.
3. Sminia T (1996) A review of the mucosal immune system: Development, structure and function of the lower and upper respiratory tract. *Eur Respir Rev* 6: 128–141.
4. Pabst R (1992) Is BALT a major component of the human lung immune system? *Immunol Today* 13: 119–122.
5. Sminia T, Van der Brugge-Gamelkoorn GJ, Jeunissen SHM (1989) Structure and function of bronchus-associated lymphoid tissue (BALT). *Crit Rev Immunol* 9: 119–150.
6. Pankow W, Wichert P (1988) M cells in the immune system of the lung. *Respiration* 54: 209–219.
7. Kagnoff MF (1996) Mucosal immunology: New frontiers. *Immunol Today* 17: 57–59.
8. Kang B, Manderscheid BD, Huang YT, Crapo JD, Chang L (1996) Contrasting response of lung parenchymal cells to instikked TNF-α and IFN-γ. The inducibilty of specific cell ICAM-1 *in vivo*. *Am J Resp Cell Mol Biol* 15: 540–550.
9. Richards IM, Kolbasa KP, Hatfield CA, Winterrowd GE, Vonderfecht SL, Fidler SF, Griffin RL, Brashler JR, Krzesicki RF, Sly LM, et al. (1996) Role of very late activation antigen-4 in the antigen-induced accumulation of eosinophils and lymphocytes in the lungs and airway lumen of sensitized brown Norway rats. *Am J Resp Cell Mol Biol* 15: 172–183.
10. Saltini C, Kirby M, Trapnell BC, Tamura N, Crystal RG (1990) Biased accumulation of T-lymphocytes with "memory-type" CD45 leucocyte common-antigen gene expression on the epithelial surface of the human lung. *J Exp Med* 171: 1123–1140.
11. Klech H, Pohl W (1989) Technical recommendations and guidelines for bronchoalveolar lavage (BAL). *Eur Resp J* 2: 561–585.
12. Agostini C, Chilosi M, Zambello R, Trentin L, Semenzato G (1993) Pulmonary immune cells in health and disease: Lymphocytes. *Eur Respir J* 6: 1378–1401.
13. McMenamin C, Pimm C, McKersey M, Holt PG (1994) Regulation of CD4+ TH-2-dependent IgE responses to inhaled antigen in mice by antigen-specific γ/δ T-cells. *Science* 265: 1859–1861.
14. Agostini C, Zambello R, Trentin L, Cerutti A, Bulian P, Crivellaro C, Cipriani A, Semenzato G (1994) $\gamma\delta$ T-cell receptor subsets in the lung of patients with HIV-1 infection. *Cell Imunol* 153: 194–205.
15. Dunkley M, Pabst R, Cripps A (1995) An important role for intestinally derived T cells in respiratory disease. *Immunol Today* 16: 231–236.
16. Li X, Abdi K, Rawn J, Mackay CR, Mentzer R (1996) LFA-1 and L-selectin regulation of recirculating lymphocyte tethering and rolling on lung microvascular endothelium. *Am J Respir Cell Mol Biol* 14: 394–398.
17. Symon FA, Wardlaw AJ (1996) Selectins and their counter receptors: A bitter sweet attraction. *Thorax* 51: 1155–1157.

18. Pilewski JM, Albelda SM (1995) Cell adhesion molecules in asthma: Homing, activation and airway remodelling. *Am J Resp Cell Mol Biol* 12: 1–3.
19. Luscinskas FW, Ding H, Lichman AH (1995) P-selectin and vascular cell molecule 1 mediate rolling and arrest, repectively, of CD4+ T lymphocytes on tumour necrosis factor α-activated vascular endothelium under flow. *J Exp Med* 181: 1179–1186.
20. Berlin C, Bargatze RF, Campbell JJ, von Andrian UH, Szabo MC, Hasslen SR, et al. (1995) α-4 integrins mediate lymphocyte attachment and rolling under physiologic flow. *Cell* 80: 413–422.
21. Mulligan MS, Vaporciyan AA, Miyasaka M, Tamatani T, Ward P (1993) Tumour necrosis factor alpha regulates *in vivo* intrapulmonary expression of ICAM-1. *Am J Pathol* 142: 1739–1749.
22. Cepek KL, Parker CM, Madara JL, Brenner MB (1993) Integrin αEβ7 mediates adhesion of T lymphocytes to epithelial cells. *J Immunol* 150: 3459–3470.
23. Rihs S, Walker C, Virchow J Jr, Boer C, Kroegel C, Giri SN, Braun RK (1996) Differential expression of αEβ7 integrins on bronchoalveolar lavage T lymphocyte subsets: Regulation by α4β1-integrin crosslinking and TNF-β. *Am J Respir Cell Mol Biol* 15:600–610.
24. Springer TA (1994) Traffic signals for lymphocyte recirculation and leukocyte emigration: The multistep paradigma. *Cell* 76: 301–314.
25. Mackay CR (1993) Homing of naive, memory and effector lymphocytes. *Curr Opin Immunol* 5: 423–427.
26. Picker LJ (1994) Control of lymphocyte homing. *Curr Opin Immunol* 6: 394–406.
27. Dunkley ML, Cripps AW, Clancy RL (1994) A role for CD4+ T-cells from orally immunized rats in enhanced clearance of *Pseudomonas aeruginosa* from the lung. *Immunology* 83: 362–369.
28. Delventhal S, Hensel A, Petzoldt K, Pabst R (1992) Cellular changes in the bronchoalveolar lavage (BAL) of pigs, following immunization by the enteral or respiratory route. *Clin Exp Immunol* 90: 223–227.
29. Scicchitano R, Stanisz A, Ernst P, Bienenstock J (1988) In: Husband AJ (ed.). *Migration and Homing of Lymphoid Cells*, vol. 2. CRC Press, Boca Raton, 1–34.
30. Weisz-Carrington P, Grimes Jr SR, Lamm ME (1987) Gut-associated lymphoid tissue as a source of an IgA immune response in respiratory tissues after oral immunization and intrabronchial challenge. *Cell Immunol* 106: 132–138.
31. Van der Brugge-Gamelkoorn, Kraal G (1985) The specificity of the high endothelial venule in bronchus-associated lymphoid tissue (BALT). *J Immunol* 134: 3746–3750.
32. Healy B (1993) Mucosal immunity, vaccine development's new frontier. *JAMA* 269: 1612.
33. Perry FE, Catterall JR (1994) The pneumococcus: Host-organism interactions and their implications for immunotherapy and immunoprophylaxis. *Thorax* 49: 946–950.
34. Szewczuk MR, Campbell RJ, Jung LK (1981) Lack of age-associated immune dysfunction in mucosal associated lymph nodes. *J Immunol* 126:2200–2204.
35. Garg M, Subbarao B (1992) Immune responses of systemic and mucosal lymphoid organs to Pnu-Immune vaccine as a function of age and the efficacy of monophosphoryl lipid A as an adjuvant. *Infect Immun* 60: 2329–2336.
36. McWilliam AS, Nelson D, Thomas JA, Holt PG (1994) Rapid dendritic cell recruitment is a hallmark of the acute inflammatory response at mucosal surfaces. *J Exp Med* 179: 1331–1336.
37. Schon-Hegrad MA, Oliver J, McMenamin PG, Holt PG (1991) Studies on the density, distribution and surface phenotype of intraepithelial class II major histocompatibility complex antigen (Ia)-bearing dendritic cells (DC) in the conducting airways. *J Exp Med* 173: 1345–1356.
38. Soler P, Moreau A, Basset F, Hance AJ (1989) Cigarette smoking-induced changes in the number and differentiated state of pulmonary dendritic cells/Langerhans' cells. *Am Rev Respir Dis* 139: 1112–1117.
39. Nelson D, McWilliam AS, Haining S, Holt PG (1995) Down-modulation of airway intra-epithelial dendritic cell populations following local and systemic exposure to steroids. *Am J Resp Crit Care Med* 151: 475–481.
40. Steinman RM (1991) The dendritic cell system and its role in immunogenicity. *Annu Rev Immunol* 9: 271–296.
41. Nicod LP (1996) Role of antigen-presenting cells in lung immunity. *Eur Respir Rev* 6: 142–150.

42. Nicod LP, El Habre F (1992) Adhesion molecules on human lung dendritic cells and their role for T-cell activation. *Am J Respir Cell Mol Biol* 7: 207–213.
43. Nicod LP, Galve-de-Rochemonteix G, Dayer JM (1990) Dissociation between allogeneic T-cell stimulation and interleukin-1 or tumor necrosis factor production by human lung dendritic cells. *Am J Resp Cell Mol Biol* 2: 515–522.
44. Gelder CM (1996) Human CD4+ T-cell recognition of influenza A haemaglutinin is precisely defined by HLA-DR. *Thorax* 61 (Suppl 3): A2.
45. Janeway CA Jr, Bottomly K (1994) Signals and signs for lymphocyte responses. *Cell* 76: 275–285.
46. Gajewski TF, Fallarino F, Uyttenhove C, Boon T (1996) Tumor rejection requires a CTLA-4 ligand provided by the host or expressed on the tumor: Superiority of B7-1 over B7-2 for active tumor immunization. *J Immunol* 156: 2909–2917.
47. Mosmann TR, Coffman RL (1989) Th1 and Th2 cells: Different patterns of lymphokine secretion lead to different functional properties. *Annu Rev Immunol* 7: 145–168.
48. Robinson DS, Hamid Q, Ying S, Tsicopoulos A, Barkens J, Bentley AM, Corrigan C, Durham SR, Kay AB (1992) Predominant Th2-like bronchoalveolar T-lymphocyte population in atopic asthma. *N Engl J Med* 326: 298–304.
49. Gerblich AA, Campbell AE, Schuyler MR (1984) Changes in T-lymphocyte subpopulations after antigenic bronchial provocation in asthmatics. *N Eng J Med* 310: 1349–1352.
50. Coyle AJ, LeGross G, Bertrand C, Tsuyuki S, Heusser CH, Kopf M et al. (1995) Interleukin-4 is required for the induction of lung Th$_2$ mucosal immunity. *Am J Respir Cell Mol Biol* 13: 54–59.
51. Ahija A, Oh N, Chao W, Spragg RG, Smith RM (1996) Inhibition of the human neutrophil respiratory burst by nature and synthetic surfactant. *Am J Resp Cell Mol Biol* 14: 496–503.
52. Hostoffer RW, Krukovets I, Berger M (1993) Increased Fc alpha R expression and IgA mediated function on neutrophils induced by chemoattractants. *J Immunol* 150: 4532–4540.
53. Mulks MH, Kornfield SW, Plaut AG (1980) Specific proteolysis of human IgA by *Streptococcus pneumoniae* and *Haemophilus inflenzae*. *J Infect Dis* 141: 450–456.
54. Van Vlassetaer P, Punnonen J, de Vries JE (1992) Transforming growth factor-beta directs IgA switching in human B cells. *J Immunol* 148: 2062–2067.
55. Paul WE (1991) Interleukin-4: A prototype immunoregulatory cytokine. *Blood* 77: 1859–1870.
56. Nagata S, Golstein P (1995) The Fas death factor. *Science* 267: 1449–1456.
57. Catterall JR, Sharma SD, Remington JS (1986) Oxygen independent intracellular killing by alveolar macrophages. *J Exp Med* 163: 1113–1131.
58. Black CB, Catterall JR, Remington JS (1987) *In vivo* and *in vitro* activation of alveolar macrophages by recombinant gamma-interferon. *J Immunol* 138: 491–495.
59. Berkman N, John M, Roesems G, Jose P, Barnes PJ, Chung KF (1996) Interleukin 13 inhibits macrophages. *Am J Respir Cell Mol Biol* 15: 382–389.
60. Zhang JH, Ferrante A, Arrigo A-P, Dayer J-M (1992) Neutrophil stimulation and priming by direct contact with human T lymphocytes. *J Immunol* 148: 177–181.
61. Buret A, Dunkley ML, Clancy RL, Cripps AW (1993) Effector mechanisms of intestinally induced immunity to *Pseudomonas aeruginosa* in the rat lung: Role of neutrophils and leukotriene B4. *Infect Immun* 61: 671–679.
62. Pierangeli SS, Sonnenfeld G (1993) Treatment of murine macrophages with murine interferon-gamma and tumour necrosis factor-alpha. *Clin Exp Immunol* 93: 165–171.
63. Allen J, Cooper J Jr, Culbreth RR (1996) Characterization of a neutrophil inhibitor peptide harvested from human bronchial lavage: Homology to influenza A nucleoprotein. *Am J Resp Cell Mol Biol* 15: 207–215.
64. Warner JA, Kroegel C (1994) Pulmonary immune cells in health and disease: Mast cells and basophils. *Eur Respir J* 7: 1326–1341.
65. Jaffe JS, Claum MC, Raible DG, Post TJ, Dimitry E, Govindaro D, Wang Y, Schulman ES (1995) Human lung mast cell IL-5 gene and protein expression: Temporal analysis of upregulation following IgE mediated activation. *Am J Resp Cell Mol Biol* 13: 665–675.
66. Smith TJ, Weiss JH (1996) Mucosal T-cells and mast cells share common adhesion receptors. *Immunol Today* 17: 60–63.

67. Ohkawara Y, Yamauchi K, Maruyama N, Hoshi H, Ohno M, Homma Y (1995) *In situ* expression of the cell adhesion molecules in bronchial tissues from asthmatics with airflow limitation: *In vivo* evidence of VCAM-1/VLA-4 interaction in selective eosinophil infiltration. *Am J Resp Cell Mol Biol* 12: 4–12.
68. Lopez AF, Sanderson CJ, Gamble R, Campbell HD, Young IG, Vadas AM (1988) Recombinant human interleukin 5 is a suitable activator of human eosinophil function. *J Exp Med* 167: 219–224.
69. Strickland DH, Thepen T, Kees UR, Kraal G, Holt PG (1993) Regulation of T-cell function by pulmonary alveolar macrophages. *Immunology* 80: 266–272.
70. Holt PG, Oliver J, Bilyk N, McMenamin C, McManamin PG, Kraal G, Thepen T (1993) Downregulation of the antigen-presenting cell function(s) of pulmonary dendritic cells *in vivo* by resident alveolar macrophages. *J Exp Med* 177: 397–407.
71. Thepen T, McMenamin C, Oliver J, Kraal G, Holt PG (1992) Regulation of IgE production in presensitised animals: *In vivo* elimination of alveolar macrophages preferentially increases IgE responses to inhaled allergen. *Clin Exp Allergy* 22: 1107–1114.
72. Holt PG (1996) Current concepts in pulmonary immunology: Regulation of primary and secondary T-cell responses to inhaled antigens. *Eur Respir Rev* 6: 128–135.
73. Holt PG (1993) Regulation of antigen presenting functions(s) in lung and airway tissues. *Eur Respir J* 6: 120–129.
74. Holt PG, Oliver J, McMenamin C, Schon-Hegrad MA (1992) Studies on the surface phenotype and functions of dendritic cells in parenchymal lung tissue of the rat. *Immunol* 75: 582–587.
75. Metzger ZVI, Hoffeld JT, Oppenheim JJ (1990) Macrophage-mediated suppression. *J Immunol* 124: 983–988.
76. Chelen CJ, Fang Y, Freeman GJ, Secrist H, Marshall JD, Hwant PT, Frankel LR, Dekruyff RH, Umetru DT (1995) Human alveolar macrophages present antigen ineffectively due to defective expression of B7 co-stimulatory cell surface molecules. *J Clin Invest* 95: 1415–1421.
77. Nicod LP, Galve-de-Rochemonteix G, Dayer JM (1994) Modulation of IL-1 receptor antagonist of TNF-soluble receptors produced by alveolar macrophages and blood monocytes. *Ann NY Acad Sci* 725: 323–330.
78. Wilsher ML, Hughes DA, Haslam PL (1988) Immunoregulatory properties of pulmonary surfactant: Influence of variations in the phospholipid profile. *Clin Exp Immunol* 73: 117–122.
79. Nossal GJV (1994) Negative selection of lymphocytes. *Cell* 76: 229–239.
80. Goodnow CC (1992) Transgenic mice and analysis of B-cell tolerance. *Ann Rev Immunol* 10: 489–518.
81. Hammerling GJ, Schonrich G, Ferber I, Arnold B (1993) Peripheral tolerance as a muti-step mechanism. *Immunol Rev* 133: 93–104.
82. Fulcher DA, Basten A (1994) Reduced lifespan of anergic self-reactive B cells in a double transgenic model. *J Exp Med* 179: 125–134.
83. Holt PG, Batty JE, Turner KJ (1981) Inhibition of specific IgE responses in mice by pre-exposure to inhaled antigen. *Immunology* 42: 409–497.
84. Turner KJ, Plozza T, Holt PG (1985) Cell-cycle dependent fluctuations in IgE secretion in a human myeloma line. *Clin Immunol Immunopathol* 36: 212–216.
85. Holt PG, Sly PD (1997) Allergic respiratory disease: Strategic targets for primary prevention during childhood. *Thorax* 52: 1–4.
86. Rinas U, Horneff G, Wahn V (1993) Interferon-γ production by cord-blood mononuclear cells is reduced in newborns with a family history of atopic disease and is independent from cord blood IgE-levels. *Ped Allergy Immunol* 4: 60–64.
87. Tang MLK, Kemp AS, Thorburn J, Hill DJ (1993) Reduced interferon-γ secretion in neonates and subsequent atopy. *Lancet* 4: 60–64.
88. Warner JA, Miles EA, Jones AC, Quint DJ, Colwell BM, Warner JO (1994) Is deficiency of interferon-gamma production by allergen triggered cord blood-cells a predictor of atopic asthma? *Clin Exp Allergy* 24: 423–430.
89. Holt PG (1995) Postnatal maturation of immune competence during infancy and early childhood. *Ped Allergy Immunol* 6: 59–70.
90. Shirakawa T, Ehemoto T, Shimazu S, Hopkin JM (1997) The inverse association between tuberculin responses and atopic disorder. *Science* 275: 77–79.

Autoimmune Aspects of Lung Disease
ed. by D. A. Isenberg and S. G. Spiro
© 1998 Birkhäuser Verlag Basel/Switzerland

CHAPTER 2
The Respiratory System in Rheumatic Diseases

Angela Rapti[1], Beratha S. Devi[2], Stephen G. Spiro[1]
and David A. Isenberg[2]

[1] *Department of Thoracic Medicine, University College London Hospitals, and*
[2] *Centre for Rheumatology/Bloomsbury Rheumatology Unit, Department of Medicine,*
   University College London, London, UK

1. Introduction

The lung and its contiguous structures are commonly involved in several of the rheumatic diseases (Table 1), either by direct manifestation of disease or as a secondary effect from infection or complications of therapy. In this chapter, we detail the various pulmonary manifestations of the major rheumatological conditions. The common symptoms of pulmonary diseases and how frequently they are implicated in rheumatic disorders are reviewed. In addition, radiology and physiology of the lung, diagnostic procedures and therapeutic options are discussed.

Table 1. Respiratory associations of the rheumatic disorders

Disease	Airways	Parenchyma		Vessels	Wall/muscles
		Lung	Pleura	Pulmonary	Chest
Rheumatoid arthritis	bronchiectasis, obliterative bronchiolitis	pneumonia, fibrosing alveolitis, nodules	pleurisy effusion empyema	hypertension	
Systemic lupus erythematosus		pneumonia fibrosing alveolitis, atelectasis	pleurisy effusion	hypertension shrinking lungs with high diaphragm	
Systemic sclerosis	bronchiectasis	fibrosing alveolitis, aspiration pneumonia		hypertension	"encased chest"
Sjögren's syndrome	bronchitis	fibrosing alveolitis lymphoma			
Dermatomyositis polymyositis		aspiration pneumonia, fibrosing alveolitis			myopathy
Ankylosing spondylitis fixation		upper lobe fibrosis			costo-vertebral joint
Behçet's syndrome		haemorrhage		aneurysm	
Relapsing polychondritis	upper airway narrowing				
Pulmonary vasculitides		nodules			

1.2. Respiratory Symptoms

The most common respiratory symptoms in patients with rheumatic disease and pulmonary involvement are non-specific and include cough, breathlessness and chest pain and can be the result of involvement of airways, lung parenchyma, pleura, chest wall or pulmonary vessels.

1.3. Tissue Involvement

1.3.1. Airway narrowing: Major airways involvement is rare but may be observed in some patients with rheumatoid arthritis (RA) in association with Sjögren's syndrome, and in isolated cases of cricoarytenoid joint involvement. Synovitis of the cricoarytenoid joint in these patients may cause supraglottic narrowing and also hoarseness and breathlessness. Small airways obstruction may also be seen in patients with RA, but this is not always directly related to RA. It is associated with Sjögren's syndrome, and smoking is a major confounding factor [1]. Narrowing of the large airways occurs in relapsing polychondritis [2] due to inflammatory swelling during the active stage of the disease and destruction of tracheal or bronchial cartilages with the formation of fibrous tissue and associated scarring. The airway narrowing may be localised to the larynx, to a narrow segment of the trachea or more distally along the cartilage-containing airways. Narrowing of the airways usually complicated by secondary infection is due to inadequate clearance of secretions which itself is due in part to diminished effectiveness of coughing. However, patients with polychondritis and respiratory tract involvement usually present with hoarseness, dyspnoea, cough and shortness of breath. Plain X-ray or computed tomography (CT) of the trachea and main bronchi help to determine the extent of the disease. When airways obstruction becomes very severe, resting ventilation may be compromised, and hypercapnia can develop. Tracheostomy is sometimes necessary for severe disease limited to the larynx and the immediately adjacent trachea. Full functional radiographic assessment including CT scanning is essential before embarking on this. It is not known whether corticosteroids can help, but this appears unlikely.

1.3.2. Bronchiectasis: An association between bronchiectasis and RA has been reported [3]. The prevalence of this complication in patients with RA, may be 10 times higher than in patients with osteoarthritis [4].

Bronchiectasis may antedate or postdate the appearance of arthritic symptoms but does not affect the severity of disease or the frequency of other extra-articular manifestations. In a recent study [5], the arthritis developed first in 18 of 23 patients ultimately diagnosed to have RA and bronchiectasis; most were women with seropositive nodular disease; productive cough, haemoptysis and dyspnoea were the most common respiratory symptoms. Bronchiectasis may be a common sequel of fibrotic interstitial lung disease. As the fibrosis matures, cicatrisation occurs with traction on the adjacent bronchi and consequent ectasia of the airways. The cause of this complication is unclear. According to some [6], RA or its treatment increases the incidence of infection, which may progress to bronchiectasis. Recently HLA DQB1*0601 was found to be associated with bronchiectasis in British patients with RA, and the frequencies of human leucocyte antigen (HLA) DQB1*0301, DQB1*0201 and DQA1*0501 were greater in patients with RA and bronchiectasis than in those with RA alone [7].

1.3.3. Obliterative bronchiolitis: Obliterative bronchiolitis (OB) develops either as part of the rheumatological disease or as a complication of treatment. OB was reported in patients with RA treated with D-penicillamine [8] or intramuscular gold [9], although a link between the treatment and this complication has never been satisfactorily established. The clinical presentation of OB is usually acute with cough, shortness of breath and other non-specific respiratory complaints. Chest radiographs show hyperinflation or, less commonly, patchy interstitial infiltrates. Pulmonary function tests generally show airways obstruction, without a decrease in carbon monoxide single-breath gas transfer factor (TLco). A minority of patients may have a restrictive pattern of spirometry or a mixed obstructive and restrictive pattern. Pathologically the small airways (<2 mm diameter) are narrowed or obliterated by this chronic inflammatory process with fibrotic scar formation. Two separate but overlapping groups have been described: cases with acute and chronic cellular bronchiolitis with less conspicuous scarring and cases showing constrictive bronchiolitis, with histology varying from fibrotic and inflammatory lesions to complete obliteration of the small airways [10]. The prognosis for patients with OB is poor, as there is little evidence of spontaneous recovery. Treatment with steroids sometimes in conjunction with azathioprine or cyclophosphamide has been reported to have some efficacy [11], but has no real impact on survival.

1.3.4. Parenchymal disease: Parenchymal involvement is not uncommon and often difficult to clarify, especially as the clinical and radiographic appearances are often non-specific. Associated conditions include fibrosing alveolitis, acute lupus pneumonia, sometimes with alveolar haemorrhage, pulmonary infections, drug-induced pneumonitis and bronchiolitis obliterans organising pneumonia (BOOP).

Fibrosing alveolitis can develop in association with almost all of the rheumatic disorders (Table 1). Its prevalence varies according to the diagnostic criteria chosen. Chest radiography suggests the presence of fibrosing alveolitis in approximately 5 to 10% of patients with RA, systemic lupus erythematosus (SLE) or dermatomyositis. The prevalence is greater, 40–64%, when lung function or histological findings are included [12, 13]. In 90% of patients with RA, joint disease precedes fibrosing alveolitis, and it is more common in men aged 50–69 years with seropositive nodular disease [14]. Fibrosing alveolitis may develop as a consequence of acute lupus pneumonitis or as an independent manifestation of SLE, after years of active disease [15]. The clinical, physiological, radiological and histopathological features are similar to those of idiopathic (cryptogenic) pulmonary fibrosis.

The clinical features include dry cough, dyspnoea, chest pain, bilateral inspiratory basal crackles and, late in the disease, hypoxaemia and cyanosis. The evolution of fibrosing alveolitis in patients with rheumatic diseases is no different from that of cryptogenic pulmonary fibrosis. Progession is variable but usually slow or stable, although rapid deterioration can occur. The radiological and physiological features are described below. Histopathological changes include thickening of the alveolar walls, oedema, infiltration with mononuclear cells and alveolar cell hyperplasia, followed by fibrosis of the alveolar wall and chronic inflammatory cell infiltration [16]. The differential diagnosis (Table 2) must include drug-induced pneumonitis (gold, cyclophosphamide, methotrexate), pneumonia (common in patients with a chronic disease, particularly if on corticosteroids and/or other immunosuppressive drugs), left ventricular failure, and opportunistic infections associated with a primary autoimmune rheumatic disorder or the consequence of its therapy. The pathogenesis of fibrosing alveolitis is uncertain, but the alveolitis may develop as a reaction to immune complexes deposited in the pulmonary capillaries. It is related to both RA-associated and independent factors [17, 18]. Tobacco usage and certain phenotypes of alpha 1-antitrypsin are RA-independent factors. RA-associated factors include certain HLA genes and the production of inflammatory mediators. The development of RA and its severity is associated with HLA-DRB1 antigens. The susceptibility to pulmonary involvement may be associated with HLA-B40. The production of proinflammatory cytokines by alveolar macrophages, in particular tumour necrosis factor-alpha (TNF-alpha) has been implicated in the pathogenesis of rheumatoid pulmonary fibrosis [18], concomitant with its probable role in the development of rheumatoid synovitis.

Table 2. Differential diagnosis of interstitial lung disease

Fibrosing alveolitis
Sarcoidosis
Infections (TB-fungus-*Pneumocystis carinii*)
Rheumatoid lung
Pneumoconiosis
Malignancy (alveolar cell carcinoma, lymphoma)
Pulmonary haemorrhage
Histiocytosis X
Drug-induced
Haemosiderosis

1.3.5. Acute lupus pneumonitis and alveolar haemorrhage: Acute lupus pneumonitis and alveolar haemorrhage are both uncommon life-threatening events that occur in fewer than 2% of patients with SLE [19]. They result from an acute injury to the alveolar capillary unit. Pneumonitis is characterised by the acute onset of dyspnoea, productive cough, fever, hypoxaemia and patchy alveolar infiltrates on the chest radiograph without evidence of underlying infection. These findings were the initial manifestation of SLE in 6 of 12 patients in one study [20]. Improvement with corticosteroid therapy supports the diagnosis, but the mortality rate is about 50%. In half of the patients surviving the acute illness, the chest radiograph clears completely. In the other half, the disease progresses to chronic interstitial pneumonitis with hypoxaemia, restrictive pulmonary function and decreased TLco [21].

The alveolar haemorrhage syndrome has a similar presentation to acute lupus pneumonitis, although some patients may present with haemoptysis and anaemia. In others there is no haemoptysis despite extensive alveolar shadowing on the chest radiograph. A fall in the haematocrit and diffuse alveolar infiltrates on the chest radiograph support the diagnosis, and sputum or bronchoalveolar lavage (BAL) specimens will contain iron-laden macrophages. Lung biopsy specimens show hyaline membranes, interstitial oedema, acute alveolitis and lymphocytic interstitial pneumonitis. Deposition of immune complexes in the alveolar walls and blood vessels as well as complement activation have been suggested as pathogenic mechanisms. Despite treatment with corticosteroids, immunosuppressive drugs and plasmapheresis, the mortality rate is high, ranging from 50 to 90% [22]. However, a recent series [23] of patients with SLE and pulmonary haemorrhage suggested that early diagnosis combined with aggressive immunosuppression may improve the prognosis.

1.3.6. Bronchiolitis obliterans organising pneumonia (BOOP): This condition has been associated with several autoimmune rheumatic disorders, especially RA, SLE and dermatomyositis. It is known as cryptogenic organising pneumonia, organising pneumonia or obliterative bronchiolitis. The latter term has generated confusion, as it is quite distinct from the clinical and histological picture of "obliterative bronchiolitis" which affects the small airways only, and the chest radiograph remains normal (see above). The term "BOOP", used for a specific type of interstitial pneumonia of unknown aetiology, refers to a clinical and pathological picture that affects both men and women equally in the general population. The clinical picture is non-specific with cough, dyspnoea and pulmonary crackles. It presents with a febrile flulike syndrome in 30% of cases, and the disease duration is usually less than 3 months [24]. The chest radiography shows patches of dense consolidation which can fluctuate, apparently spontaneously. Because the clinical profile of BOOP is non-specific, infection must be excluded, especially as the chest radiograph shows peripheral patches of consolidation or linear shadows, indistinguishable from bacterial pneumonia. If the disease progresses, an open lung biopsy should be performed, and treatment with steroids considered if the diagnosis of BOOP is confirmed. There are two histological groups of bronchiolitis: proliferative bronchiolitis associated with the clinical picture of BOOP and constrictive bronchiolitis associated with the clinical picture of OB, i.e. airways involvement only [10]. Proliferative bronchiolitis is a non-specific reaction characterised by an intraluminal exudate that includes fibroblasts, a matrix of mucopolysaccharides and inflammatory infiltrates, predominantly in the alveolar channels and distal alveoli (organised pneumonia) rather than in the bronchioli. Constrictive bronchiolitis displays just bronchiolar damage ranging from an inflammatory infiltrate to progressive concentric fibrosis and sometimes total occlusion. These changes may be associated with hyperplasia of smooth muscle, bronchiolectasis, and fibrosis of bronchiolar walls and remains confined of these structures. Confirmation of the clinical diagnosis of BOOP is made by histology showing proliferative bronchiolitis that may be idiopathic, or associated with other conditions; i.e. autoimmune rheumatic diseases, toxin exposure and infections. BOOP can also occur as a secondary process in malignancy, aspiration, eosinophilic pneumonia, and distal to airway obstruction.

2. Pleural Disease

2.1. Pleural Effusion

This is the most common manifestation of lung disease in patients with RA or SLE, occurring in 30 to 70% of patients at some stage during the course of the disease. Pleural effusion can be massive, although it is usually small and bilateral and may resolve completely, recur or persist for many months. The most frequent presenting symptoms and signs are pleuritic pain, dyspnoea, cough and fever. In patients with RA, the pleural effusion is often asymptomatic, possibly because the level of physical activity is limited by joint disease. It is more common in men in their 40s and 50s, and frequently occurs during periods of active arthritis, especially in patients with subcutaneous nodules. Occasionally it may occur concurrently with pulmonary nodules or interstitial lung disease. The pleural fluid is typically an exudate. Low levels of glucose (<20 mg/dl) and complement and high levels of lactate dehydrogenase (>100 U/l) are frequently recorded. Rheumatoid factor may be present, but it is non-specific [25]. Pericarditis is present in approximately 10% of patients with RA. In patients with SLE the glucose concentration and pH of the pleural fluid are within the normal range. The finding of lupus cells in the fluid is diagnostic [26]. Low complement levels, including total haemolytic complement activity as well as Cl, C4 and C3 component, also support the diagnosis [26]. The characteristic cytological pattern of rheumatoid pleuritis is the presence of elongated macrophages, giant multinucleated macrophages and cellular debris in the pleural fluid [27]. Pleural aspiration is advisable to exclude malignancy or infection. Ultrasound guidance is useful when attempting to aspirate a small or loculated effusion.

2.2. Empyema

Empyema is relatively common in patients with RA and is usually secondary to long periods of corticosteroid therapy, but is seen less often in other autoimmune rheumatic diseases. Breathlessness, fever, malaise and weight loss are the common symptoms, and the diagnosis is established on aspiration of purulent fluid, which should be cultured for aerobic and anaerobic organisms. Tuberculosis is also a cause to be considered. Treatment includes intercostal tube drainage and appropriate antibiotics. Recently instilling a thrombolytic drug such as streptokinase into the pleural cavity via an intercostal tube has been useful in facilitating drainage, as empyemas are frequently loculated. This process can be repeated daily, and it is remarkably effective in breaking down the pleural adhesions. Occasionally decortication may be necessary when the infection has resolved, particularly if a thick residual pleural cortex causes excessive restriction to the underlying lung. This procedure should ideally be performed at least 6 weeks after all infection has resolved, thus allowing the underlying lung to heal and recover, which facilitates the surgical procedure.

2.3. Chest Wall/Muscular Disease

Breathlessness can result from the patient's inability to ventilate the lungs adequately. Reduction in chest wall expansion occurs in advanced systemic sclerosis and in ankylosing spondylitis. Chest pain and restricted costovertebral mobility is a prominent feature of ankylosing spondylitis. Some investigators have suggested that this restrictive change impairs apical ventilation, resulting in increased atelectasis, chronic infection and apical fibrosis. However, a recent study [28] showed that deposition of inhaled particles in the apical segments was not increased in patients with ankylosing spondylitis when compared with controls. Lung function tests show restrictive changes with decreased forced vital capacity (FVC). The presence of kyphosis contributes to respiratory inadequacy, and the extent of respiratory failure is related to the severity of kyphosis.

The term "shrinking lung" is used to describe a rare association in some patients with SLE who present with unexplained dyspnoea, restrictive lung function and elevated diaphragms on chest radiographs. The role of diaphragm function in this syndrome is controversial. Gibson et al. [29]

reported dysfunction of the diaphragm in four of five patients with SLE and "shrinking lung syndrome". Laroche et al. [30] in a similar study found diaphragmatic dysfunction in only 3 of their 12 patients. It has also been suggested that weakness of respiratory muscles reflecting lupus-related myopathy, from long-term corticosteroid therapy or phrenic nerve palsy, may be relevant [15, 31]. Pleural adhesions, diaphragmatic fibrosis or scarring may also play a role. Very rarely patients may suffer from muscle weakness due to an association of myasthenia gravis with SLE. These patients respond to anticholinesterase drugs. Optimal treatment is still unclear. However, an improvement has been demonstrated in both symptoms and lung function with corticosteroid therapy [32].

In patients with dermatomyositis, the involvement of pharyngeal muscles, or a depressed cough reflex from respiratory muscle weakness, can lead to recurrent episodes of aspiration pneumonitis which can lead to death. The muscle weakness can also be severe enough to require mechanical ventilation.

3. Pulmonary Vessels

3.1. Hypertension

Severe pulmonary arterial hypertension with resultant cor pulmonale may occur as an isolated phenomenon (primary pulmonary hypertension) or in association with autoimmune rheumatic disease. It is associated more commonly with scleroderma, so-called mixed connective tissue disease (MCTD), and rarely with rheumatoid arthritis or SLE. In patients with scleroderma the respiratory symptoms are associated more with vascular disease than with interstitial fibrosis, and marked pulmonary hypertension develops in some patients independently of radiological or pathological evidence of interstitial lung disease [33]. In others pulmonary hypertension develops as a complication of interstitial fibrosis late in the course of the disease. The prognosis for patients with isolated pulmonary hypertension is poor, most dying within 3 years of diagnosis.

Pulmonary vascular pathology with progressive pulmonary hypertension and cor pulmonale is the most serious complication of MCTD. Cardiac involvement is usually absent, or it is restricted to echocardiographic abnormalities. Some, however, have heart block, supraventricular arrythmias or cardiomegaly. In addition, palpitations and congestive heart failure may develop which can further compromise the pulmonary vasculature. Pulmonary hypertension in SLE may be secondary to progressive pulmonary fibrosis, which causes lung destruction and hypoxaemia, or it may be due to the primary pulmonary vascular involvement of SLE [34]. The most common clinical symptoms are dyspnoea, chest pain and chronic dry cough. Simonson et al. [35] found that 5 of 36 patients with SLE and pulmonary arterial pressures higher than 30 mm Hg in the absence of cardiac dysfunction. Raynaud's phenomenon was present in 75% of the patients, and women make up more than 90% of cases. Serological tests show a high incidence of antiribonucleoprotein antibodies, rheumatoid factor and anti-phospholipid antibodies [36]. The pathogenesis of pulmonary hyperten-sion in SLE is unknown, although thrombosis related to the presence of anticardiolipin antibody, vasculitis, as well as platelet aggregation and Raynaud's phenomenon have been implicated [37]. How Raynaud's pheno-menon relates to the pathogenesis of any of these disorders is uncertain, unless one postulates a state of generalised vascular hyper-responsiveness. Prognosis is poor, and a reduction in pulmonary function despite treatment is usual.

3.2. Pulmonary Vasculitis

Pulmonary vascular disease constitutes one of the most severe manifesta-tions of Behçet's syndrome. The clinical presentation includes haemopty-sis in more than 70% of the patients, dyspnoea, cough and chest pain. The vasculitis may occur at any point in the course of the disease and is com-plicated by thrombosis, pulmonary infarction and haemorrhage. The underlying histological lesion in the lung is a non-specific vasculitis affect-ing vessels of any calibre. Sometimes the inflammatory process may extend to the adjacent areas, with bronchial artery erosion and subsequent massive haemoptysis, which is usually fatal [38]. With time the inflammatory in-filtrates in the arterial wall may destroy the elastic intima and lead to the formation of an aneurysm. Chest radiographs usually show peripheral infil-trates, often bilateral in segmental distribution due to pulmonary infarction. Ventilation-perfusion scans in these patients reveal multiple and usually bilateral perfusion defects with normal or near-normal ventilation scans. These changes mirror those seen in primary pulmonary embolic disease.

CT of the chest may demonstrate pulmonary vascular disease and aneurysm formation, often containing thrombus. Pulmonary angiography offers definitive proof of the vascular disease.

3.3. Thromboembolic Disease

The association of anticardiolipin antibodies or lupus anticoagulant and thromboembolic disease (the antiphospholipid-antibody syndrome) has been investigated extensively. The key lesion is a non-inflammatory throm-botic occlusion of small or large vessels – arterial, venous or both. The in-cidence of thrombophlebitis in SLE is reported to be 10%, and pulmonary embolism has been reported in 5% of patients with SLE [39]. The optimal treatment of these patients is unclear, but some authorities recommend anticoagulation for varying periods. However, some cases of pulmonary infarction responding to plasmapheresis and corticosteroids have been reported [21]. Serum anticardiolipin antibody levels may also be reduced with immunosuppression [40]. Preventing thrombosis in the antiphospho-lipid-antibody syndrome is important, but there is no consensus about the duration or extent of prophylactic antithrombotic treatment. Long-term anticoagulation therapy with warfarin or equivalent appears advisable in these patients [41].

3.4. Rarer Causes of Dyspnoea

Acute reversible hypoxaemia not associated with parenchymal lung disease has been described during acute episodes of SLE. In a recent study [42] hypoxaemia was found in 6 of 22 patients with SLE and acute dyspnoea. All patients responded within 72 h to corticosteroid therapy. The investigators suggested that the syndrome may be related to elevations in plasma levels of complement degradation products.

Other rare cases which have been described include fulminant lupus pneumonitis and pulmonary amyloidosis [43], pericardial tamponade and lupus pneumonitis [44], and acute pulmonary oedema as the initial presentation of SLE [45]. Pneumothorax has also been described in SLE and in rheumatoid arthritis [46]. In patients with RA it is often secondary to cavitating pulmonary nodules which have ruptured into the pleural space [47]. Recent literature has focussed on the increased association of lymphoproliferative malignancies with Sjögren's syndrome and RA. In Sjögren's syndrome pathological changes range from benign lymphocytic pneumonitis and benign pseudolymphoma to the malignant infiltration of true lymphoma. The latter is found most often in women who have had Sjögren's syndrome for 15 years or more and have no associated autoimmune rheumatic disease [48, 49].

4. Radiology

Parenchymal lung disease is a well-known radiological feature of systemic autoimmune diseases. There are many different appearances on the chest radiograph of these patients; the most common are the following:

4.1. Pulmonary Rheumatoid Nodules

Rheumatoid nodules occur in patients with RA and are usually located in the periphery of the right middle or both upper lobes. They range from a few millimetres to several centimetres in diameter, and may be single or

Table 3. Differential diagnosis of pulmonary nodules

Infections	*Immunological*
Tuberculosis	Rheumatoid
Nocardia	Wegener's granulomatosis
Fungus	Sarcoidosis
Septic emboli	Amyloidosis
Neoplastic	*Benign Lesions*
Bronchial carcinoma	Hamartoma
Lymphoma	Tracheobronchial papillomas
Metastases	Pulmonary arteriovenous fistula

multiple, increase in size, remain static or disappear. Central cavitation occurs in about half of the nodules, but calcification is rare. The most frequent complications include spontaneous pneumothorax, empyema and bronchopleural fistulas [50]. Pulmonary nodules are usually found in patients who have subcutaneous nodules and positive serology for rheumatoid factor. Small nodules are not evident on a chest radiography, but their identification is increased with CT. There is a considerable differential diagnosis of pulmonary nodules which are summarised in Table 3. In 1953 Caplan [51] described multiple bilateral pulmonary nodules on chest films of coalminers with pneumoconiosis and RA. Rheumatoid nodules are the most common histological finding in tissue samples obtained at lung biopsy in patients with RA. Although the pathogenesis of the nodules is unknown, vasculitis caused by immune complex deposition has been implicated.

4.2. Bronchiectasis

The characteristic chest X-ray appearance of bronchiectasis includes ring shadows due to dilated bronchi: peribronchial thickening causing "tramlines" due to a widened lumen and the thickened bronchial walls. In a recent study [5] the most common radiographic abnormalities in patients with RA and bronchiectasis were bibasilar diffusely increased interstitial markings and focal infiltrates. High-resolution computed tomography (HRCT) is the method of choice for detecting bronchiectasis. The hallmark of the disease is dilatation of the airway, with its diameter greater than that of the accompanying artery (signet-ring sign). Recent studies based on HRCT [52, 53] have reported a higher incidence of bronchiectasis (25%) in patients with RA than have earlier studies.

4.3. Interstitial Lung Disease

Pulmonary fibrosis can be associated with almost all autoimmune rheumatic diseases. The classic radiological presentation is of reticular shadowing with progression to a reticulonodular and honeycomb pattern, similar to the changes seen in idiopathic pulmonary fibrosis. Tpyically, the lung bases are affected early and the apices in more advanced disease [50, 54]. In patients with scleroderma, disseminated pulmonary calcification or pleural thickening may also be seen on chest radiographs [55]. The most common findings on HRCT in patients with rheumatic disease and pulmonary fibrosis are a ground-glass appearance, interlobular septal and intralobular interstitial thickening with a predominance in lower and middle zones, honeycombing and micronodules mainly in the upper zones [53, 56]. However, recent reports [57, 58] have focussed on the role of HRCT in the imaging of systemic autoimmune rheumatic diseases, and have suggested that neither the nature nor the distribution of HRCT findings in this group of disorders is reliably specific for a particular disease.

The ability of HRCT to show centrilobular and panacinar emphysema has been suggested to be very helpful in distinguishing between interstitial and airway involvement in patients with RA and mixed fibrosis and emphysema [59]. HRCT is also a very important non-invasive tool in the evaluation of pulmonary fibrosis, because HRCT patterns such as a ground-glass appearance, which suggests active inflammation, or a honeycomb pattern, which implies irreversible fibrosis, have been shown to correlate with histological findings on open lung biopsy and to response to treatment [60]. Moreover, HRCT has been successful in detecting mediastinal lymphadenopathy and asymptomatic oesophageal involvement in patients with scleroderma [61].

4.4. Acute Lupus Pneumonitis and Alveolar Haemorrhage

The radiographic findings are not specific. In acute lupus pneumonitis the chest film usually shows bilateral patchy alveolar infiltrates that appear to migrate over a period of time. Cardiomegaly and pleural thickening or small effusions can also be present [62]. In alveolar haemorrhage the most frequent abnormalities on the chest radiograph are bilateral perihilar infiltrates or a diffuse alveolar filling pattern.

4.5. Shrinking Lung Syndrome

The shrinking lung syndrome is characterised by "small lungs" on full inspiration with the diaphragms elevated. Associated findings include atelectatic shadowing above the diaphragm as a consequence of the basal hypoventilation [50, 62]. Apparent mediastinal widening may be present, but only as a consequence of the volume loss and not due to mediastinal disease.

4.6. Obliterative Bronchiolitis

Hyperinflated lungs or, less commonly, patchy interstitial infiltrates may occur in some patients with OB, unless there is emphysema as an independent feature in a patient with a rheumatic disease. However, in most of the cases the chest radiograph is normal.

4.7. Bronchiolitis Obliterans Organising Pneumonia

The idiopathic BOOP and secondary forms of proliferative bronchiolitis have similar radiographic appearances. Both are characterised by peripheral patches of consolidation or linear shadows on the chest radiograph [63]. The CT appearance of patchy, lobular areas of hyperlucency, with or without bronchiectasis, in association with areas of consolidation is reasonably characteristic of BOOP (see also Chapter 5).

4.8. Pulmonary Hypertension

In patients with SLE and pulmonary hypertension, chest radiographs may show cardiomegaly with prominent pulmonary arteries and clear lung fields. The appearance on pulmonary angiograms is a symmetrical dilation of the central pulmonary artery trunk associated with pruning of the peripheral blood vessels [62].

5. Lung Function

Lung function tests are not specifically diagnostic, but can be very useful in confirmation of the pattern and extent of an abnormality. Also, once the level of lung function has been established, serial tests can be used to evaluate disease progression or the response to treatment.

5.1. Lung Volumes

Measurement of lung volumes provides evidence of abnormalities in the airways, lung parenchyma, respiratory muscles, and compliance of the lungs or chest wall. The most important subdivisions of lung volume are:

- Tidal volume (VT), the volume of air moved in or out in each breath, usually from functional residual capacity
- Total lung capacity (TLC), the volume of air in the lungs after a maximal inspiration
- Functional residual capacity (FRC), the lung volume at the end of a normal relaxed expiration

Sub-divisions of lung volume

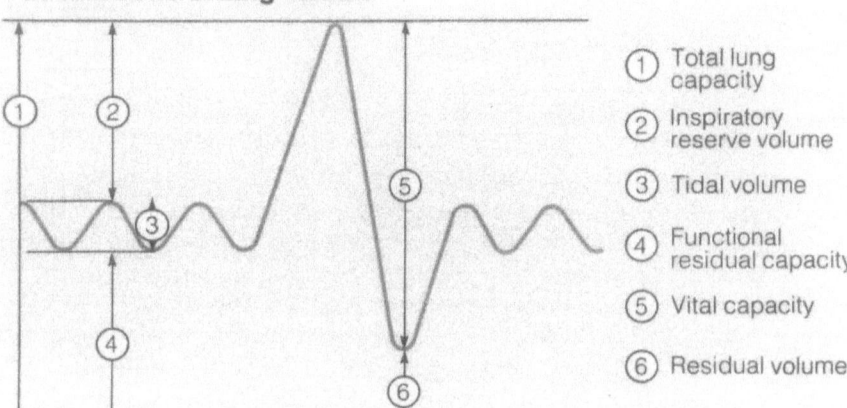

Figure 1. Sub-divisions of lung volume. (Reproduced from [63 a], with permission.)

- Residual volume (RV), the volume of air which remains in the lungs after a maximum expiration. The lung volume subdivisions are shown in Figure 1.

5.2. Tests

Assessment of lung function includes spirometry, peak expiratory flow, flow-volume curves, plethysmography and diffusing capacity tests.

5.2.1. Spirometry: The spirogram records a forced expiratory manoeuvre from total lung capacity after a full inspiration, out to residual volume, i.e. the forced vital capacity (FVC). The maximum volume expired in the first second of the FVC manoeuvre is the FEV1. The FEV1/FVC ratio expressed as a percentage should be greater than 80% but falls with normal ageing to 65% at 70 years. The obstructive pattern, characteristic of airways obstruction, with a greater reduction in FEV1 than in FVC, will produce an FEV1/FVC ratio below 65%. Diseases affecting the lung parenchyma cause a restrictive pattern and a reduced FEV1 and FVC, but relative preservation of the FEV1/FVC ratio. Typical obstructive and restrictive patterns of spirometry are shown in Figure 2. In patients with neuromuscular disorders the pattern of spirometry is also restrictive because of chest wall and muscle weakness. However, the FEV1/FVC ratio is not always increased, as the elastic recoil pressures within the lung remain normal in contrast to parenchymal diseases.

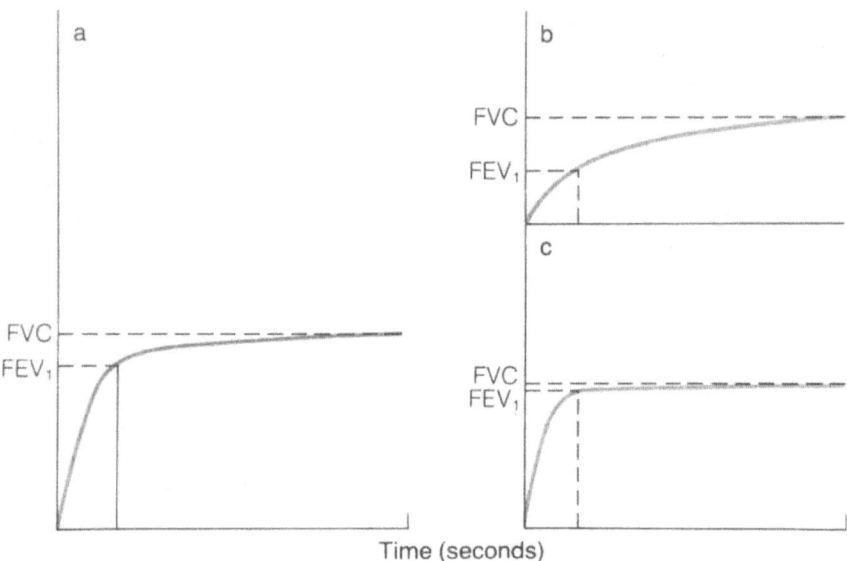

Figure 2. Spirogram (a). Normal (b), obstructive (c) and restrictive patterns are shown. (Reproduced from [63 a], with permission.)

5.2.2. Peak expiratory flow: This measues the maximum expiratory flow (PEF) rate over the first 10 milliseconds of a forced expiratory manoeuvre from TLC. PEF is an effort-dependent test and is unreliable if the patient is not giving maximum effort. The most common cause of a reduction in PEF is airways obstruction (e.g. asthma, chronic obstructive pulmonary disease); however, it is also seen in the presence of narrowing of the upper airways (e.g. by tumour or tracheal dysplasia) or by vocal cord palsy. It is of little value in restrictive lung diseases, as the airways remain normal.

5.2.3. Flow-volume curves: The envelope produced by forced expiratory flow from TLC to RV and then back in again to TLC is called the flow-volume curve. This provides a sensitive measure of both peak flow and expiratory flows at various lung volumes. Flows along subsections of the vital capacity (VC) are measured at 25 and 50% above the RV (V25 : V50) and represent flow in the small airways (<2 mm), and are early and sensitive measures of dysfunction (see Figure 3). In obliterative bronchiolitis flow at V50 and V25 is greatly reduced in comparison to FEV1 and PEF, as the disease predominantly affects the small airways. The typical curves for volume-dependent airways obstruction (asthma, chronic obstructive bronchitis) and pressure-dependent collapse (emphysema) are shown in Figure 3, b and c.

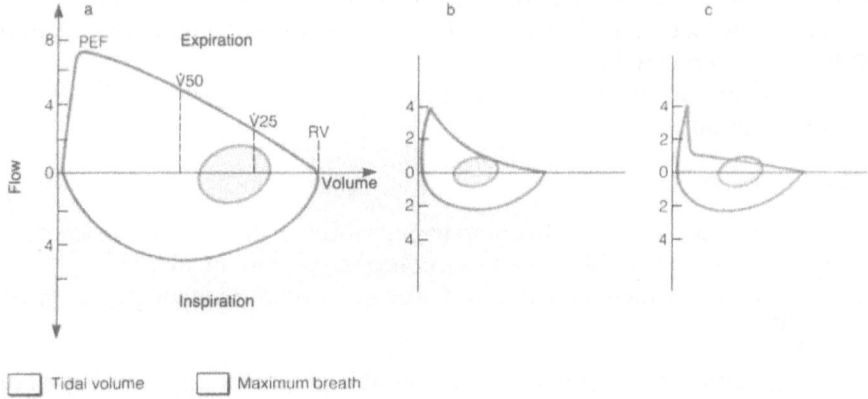

Figure 3. Flow-volume loops demonstrating (a) normal pattern, (b) volume-dependend airway narrowing (as seen in asthma, chronic bronchitis and obliterative bronchiolitis), (c) pressure-dependent airway collapse (typical of emphysema). (Reproduced from [63 a], with permission.)

5.2.4. Plethysmography: This procedure measures all gas within the lung, including non-ventilated areas such as cysts, bullae and pneumothoraces, and from the lung volume at which the test was done, TLC, RV and FRC are calculated. In parenchymal diseases all lung volumes are reduced, typically producing a restrictive ventilatory defect. In patients with muscle weakness lung volumes are also reduced, especially TLC and VC; FRC and RV are less affected. Plethysmography is also used to measure airways resistance.

5.2.5. Respiratory muscle function: Muscle weakness mimics a restrictive ventilatory defect. However, this restrictive pattern is not diagnostic, as it fails to differentiate between muscle weakness and reduced lung volumes due to parenchymal disease. Peak inspiratory and peak expiratory maximal mouth pressures (PImax, PEmax) are the best simple tests of respiratory muscle strength. Here a subject initially breathes in as hard as possible from RV against a closed shutter for PImax. PEmax is obtained by blowing maximally against an occlusion at TLC. The method is very reproducible. Any condition affecting muscle power (e.g. diaphragmatic weakness or paralysis, primary muscle diseases) results in reduced values of PImax and PEmax.

5.2.6. Diffusing capacity (TLco): The magnitude of carbon monoxide gas transfer (TLco) depends on the volume of the pulmonary capillary bed and the quality of matching between ventilation and perfusion within the lungs. TLco is reduced when:

● the alveolar capillaries are reduced in number (e.g. emphysema, fibrosis, pulmonary vascular disease);

- there is increased ventilation-perfusion mismatch (e.g. pneumonia, pulmonary infection and infiltrations, and sometimes pulmonary oedema);
- haemoglobin is reduced;
- patients are heavy smokers and therefore have a high level of carboxyhaemoglobin.

TLco increases when:

- there is acute alveolar haemorrhage, which increases the amount of haemoglobin available to carbon monoxide within the alveoli;
- polycythaemia increases the quantity of available haemoglobin in the capillaries.

The most common pulmonary function abnormalities associated with all rheumatic diseases are a restrictive pattern with a reduction of both FVC and TLC, and normal flow rates [64, 65]. An obstructive pattern with a reduction of FEV1 and FEV1/FVC ratio may be seen in patients with RA complicated by bronchiectasis or OB. Upper airways obstruction in patients with RA or polychondritis causes a considerable reduction in PEF and a (but less marked) reduction of FEV1 with a characteristic flow volume curve (see Figure 4). The shape of the curve depends on whether the obstruction is fixed (tracheal stricture, vocal cord palsy) or varies its effect on the upper airway.The effect on airflow depends on whether the lesion is in the extra- or intrathoracic airway (e.g. a tracheal tumour, relapsing polychondritis) (see Figure 4).

A decreased TLco is usually the earliest abnormality of function in infiltrative complications and may be present prior to any radiographic change [66, 67]. Abramson et al. [42] reported reduced lung volumes, decreased TLco and hypoxaemia in 6 of 22 patients with SLE with normal chest radiographs and dyspnoea. A reduction in oxygen consumption on exercise was also found in 25 patients with SLE, some of whom had no respiratory symptoms at rest, but a reduction of lung volumes and TLco was found in 15 of those who were breathless on exertion [68].

Respiratory muscle dysfunction may be a cause of hypoxaemia and reduced lung volumes in patients with SLE or dermatomyositis. Reduced respiratory muscle strength during maximal voluntary efforts, and a shallow pattern of breathing during tests of maximal voluntary ventilation, occur in patients with SLE and shrinking lung syndrome [30]. Scano et al. [69] have shown that in patients with SLE minor inspiratory muscle weakness may accompany an increased respiratory drive and contribute to a qualitatively abnormal ventilatory response to carbon dioxide stimulation. Schwarz [70] reported that respiratory muscle dysfunction can lead to respiratory failure in up to 10% of patients with dermatomyositis. Most of these patients had subclinical respiratory muscle dysfunction which led to tachypnoea and dyspnoea during exercise. They may also be predisposed to hypostatic pneumonia due to failure to generate an adequate cough if the weakness is severe.

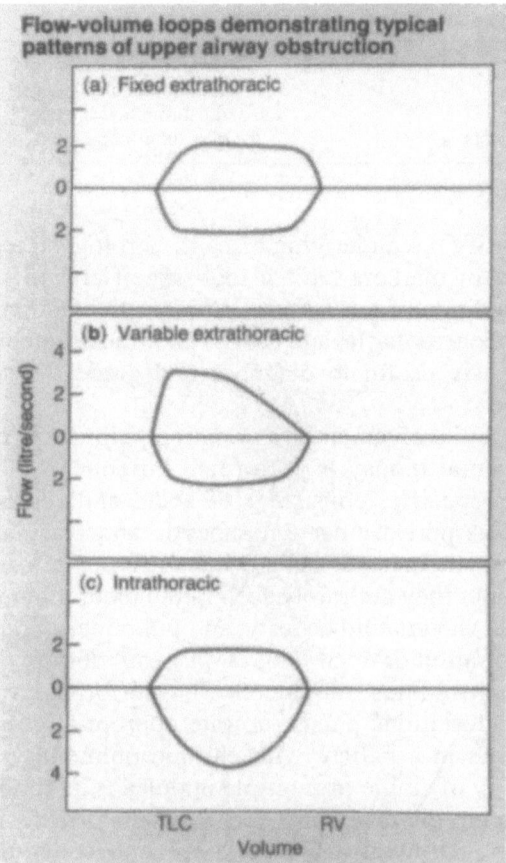

Figure 4. Flow-volume loops demonstrating typical patterns of upper-airway obstruction, caused by (a) a fixed tracheal lesion, e. g. sterosis; (b) variable flow with an extrathoracic lesion and
(c) an intrathoracic upper airway lesion. The site of the lesion determines the flow pattern.
(Reproduced from [63 a], with permission.)

Attempts have also been made to associate pulmonary function abnormalities with specific serological patterns. Groen et al. [71] found an
increased prevalence of anti-U1RNP and scleroderma traits in 28 patients
with SLE and a reduction of lung volumes and TLco. They also found a
decreased number of capillary loops in these patients and suggested that
microvascular changes seen in scleroderma may be factors in SLE lung
involvement.

6. Diagnostic Procedures

Many patients with a rheumatic disease present with respiratory symptoms
as the initial problem. In these patients a careful clinical evaluation is

Table 4. Diagnostic procedures in rheumatic lung disorders

Serological tests	Pleural aspiration/biopsy
Chest radiographs	Bronchoalveolar lavage
CT scans	Transbronchial biopsy
Pulmonary function tests	Open lung biopsy

necessary to identify the underlying disease. Serological tests can be helpful, because certain markers have a high specificity to some rheumatic diseases. Chest radiographs, CT scans, pulmonary function testing, pleural aspiration, bronchoalveolar lavage (BAL) and transbronchial or open lung biopsy are variously useful to diagnose and grade the severity of lung disease (Table 4).

Although pleural involvement is a common pulmonary manifestation in SLE and RA, pleural biopsy is performed infrequently. The histological findings are non-specific, consisting of acute and organising fibrinous pleuritis as well as perivascular lymphocytic and plasmacytic infiltrates [19, 21]. Lupus erythematosus cells occur in serous effusions only in patients with SLE, but they are rarely seen in the pleural biopsy tissue [72].

In patients with rheumatoid arthritis and pulmonary nodules, a percutaneous needle aspiration or open lung biopsy can identify the nature of the nodules. These procedures should only be performed when clinical or radiological manifestations persist despite appropriate treatment, or new shadowing appears in a patient with chronic pulmonary involvement or when the aetiology of single or multiple nodules is in doubt [73].

The real problem in diagnosis occurs when diffuse interstitial lung disease is present. Although fibre-optic bronchoscopy and BAL may be useful, transbronchial and open lung biopsy have a more important role in the diagnosis. The findings in BAL are non-specific, consisting of an increased percentage of lymphocytes or neutrophils. T-cells predominate in lymphocytic alveolitis with an increase in CD4 cells and CD4:CD8 ratio. In contrast, neutrophilic alveolitis is associated with a decreased CD4:CD8 ratio [74, 75]. A recent study [76] reported an increase in CD8$^+$ T-cells and CD56+/CD16+/CD3-NK cells in BAL of SLE patients, but the authors failed to show any association between these cells and general activity of the disease. According to these reports, the usefulness of BAL in the diagnosis of rheumatic diseases is poor. The role of BAL is more important in patients with SLE and alveolar haemorrhage in which the presence of haemosiderin-laden macrophages is diagnostic, or in patients complicated by infections (e.g. *Pneumocystis carinii*).

Transbronchial biopsy during bronchoscopy and open lung biopsy remain the main diagnostic methods in patients with interstitial lung disease. Although safer than open lung biopsy, transbronchial biopsy, is much less reliable in chronic interstitial lung diseases and is diagnostic in only 30 to 50% of patients [77]. It is useful for excluding opportunistic infections in patients with diffuse interstitial infiltrates, and can make the diagnosis in those complicated by BOOP, if the clinical and radiological features are compatible [21].

Open lung biopsy remains the best method of obtaining adequate lung tissue for histopathological analysis. Koh and Boey [78], found that the diagnosis made after open lung biopsy was different from the clinical impression in 5 of 12 patients (42%). Other investigators [79], have demonstrated that neither needle nor transbronchial biopsy achieved the diagnostic accuracy of open lung biopsy. The larger samples obtained allow a more accurate diagnosis and staging of disease activity (e.g. active inflammation vs fibrosis). Newer techniques of videoscopic surgery for diagnostic lung biopsy are also being performed, with similar diagnostic accuracy to a minithoracotomy and biopsy. Bensard et al. [80] compared video-thoracoscopic lung biopsy (VTLB, 22 patients) with open lung biopsy (OLB, 21 patients), and found the diagnostic accuracy of VTLB was 95% vs 100% for OLB, with fewer complications (9% in VTLB vs 19% in OLB).

Another method to identify early lung involvement in patients with rheumatic disorders is the clearance of 99m DTPA. Fanti et al. [81], for example, found an increase in pulmonary epithelial permeability in 16 asymptomatic patients with scleroderma using Tc-DTPA. This technique may be useful in early detection of pulmonary involvement in rheumatic diseases.

7. Treatment

The treatment of interstitial fibrosis in rheumatic diseases is based on corticosteroids and other immunosuppressive drugs. High daily doses of corticosteroids only benefit some patients. In others, high doses may suppress the disease, but reactivation occurs when doses are tapered [82].

In general, if the clinical presentation calls for aggressive therapy, treatment should start with pulses of methylprednisolone and the lowest possible daily dose of oral prednisone to maintain any improvement.

The most common immunosuppressive drugs used as a single therapy or in combination with corticosteroids are azathioprine, cyclophosphamide and methotrexate. A recent study [83] showed significant improvement in lung function and respiratory symptoms in two patients with lupus pneumonitis following several courses of intravenous pulses of cyclophosphamide. Plasmapheresis alone [22] or in combination with cyclophosphamide [84] has also resulted in an improvement in patients whose rheumatic disease was complicated by lung disease. However, pulse cyclophosphamide therapy is associated with substantial side effects. The risk of fatal opportunistic infections of the respiratory and central nervous system in patients with SLE has been emphasised [83]. The efficacy of azathioprine with prednisone in the treatment of cryptogenic pulmonary fibrosis has been reported, and both the fequency and risk of side effects are lower than those of cyclophosphamide. Raghu et al. [85] reported 27 patients with cryptogenic pulmonary fibrosis, randomised to prednisone alone or prednisone plus azathioprine, and they noted no significant toxicity, with a survival advantage for azathioprine/prednisone during a 9-year follow-up period.

The role of methotrexate in the treatment of interstitial lung disease in patients with rheumatic disease is not proven, and controlled studies in these patients are very difficult. Moreover, methotrexate-induced pneumonitis is a well-recognised, potentially life-threatening complication [86].

Corticosteroid therapy is effective in about 50% of patients with polymyositis or dermatomyositis and interstitial lung disease. Failure to respond to therapy is a serious sign, since the overall mortality rate in these patients is 40%, and 20% of the deaths are due to pulmonary disease [87]. The effectiveness of other immunosuppressive agents for lung involvement is unknown. In general, corticosteroids are the treatment of choice, and other immunosuppressive agents should be used for their steroid-sparing effect as much as for any independent effectiveness. Azathioprine is probably the drug of choice, with the best side-effect profile, and should be used to keept the corticosteroid maintenance dose at 10–7.5 mg daily.

In patients with systemic sclerosis corticosteroid therapy has little effect on the lung. Occasional improvement in TLco following D-penicillamine therapy has been reported [88, 89]. However, Steen et al. [90] showed that cyclophosphamide had a better effect on pulmonary function than did high-dose prednisone, D-penicillamine or other immunosuppressive drugs. In a 12-month trial of gamma-interferon therapy, a significant improvement was observed in skin involvement and arterial oxygen tensions [91]. Successful therapy of interstitial fibrosis depends upon commencing treatment early in the disease. Many studies [50, 91] have shown that independent of the actual drug, the only factor which predicted improvement was the initiation of prompt, early treatment. This is consistent with the belief that reversible inflammation is the dominant early feature and irreversible fibrosis occurs in late-stage disease.

Small pleural effusions in patients with SLE or RA usually resolve spontaneously. Large or persistent effusions can be treated with non-steroid anti-inflammatory drugs or low doses of corticosteroids [50]. Intrapleural corticosteroids have been tried without long-term efficacy in most cases. When extensive pleural thickening causes restrictive lung function, surgical decortication is sometimes necessary.

The treatment of pulmonary hypertension, particularly in patients with scleroderma or SLE, is complex. Early in the disease, before the changes in the vessels have become irreversible, vasodilator therapy (calcium channel-blocking agents) is helpful. Anticoagulation can be tried in patients with SLE when antiphospholipid antibody is present [36, 92, 93].

Chlorambucil or cyclophosphamide may be useful in Sjögren's syndrome and pseudolymphoma [94]. If all else fails, it may be possible to consider heart/lung transplantation for patients who fail to respond to any of the above measures.

8. Pulmonary Infections

Patients with autoimmune rheumatic diseases are prone to the development of infectious complications. Presumed immunodeficiency mechanisms associated with the disease itself appear to be primarily responsible [95], although treatment with corticosteroids and other immunosuppressive drugs may increase the risk. In patients with SLE, many parts of the immune system may be abnormal, including the antibacterial activity of the alveolar macrophages, defects of the Fc receptor function and diminished clearance of immune complexes [96]. Patients with RA have a predisposition to pleuropulmonary infection, and deaths due to respiratory infection are four times more frequent than expected. The drugs used to treat rheumatic diseases also adversely affect the immune system. The many side effects of corticosteroids have been described by Cupps and Fauci [97]. Cyclophosphamide affects virtually all the components of the cellular immune response but has a predilection for B lymphocytes.

Azathioprine inhibits both humoral and cellular immunity and suppresses T and B lymphocytes. Methotrexate interferes with transport of carbon fragments required for thymidine synthesis; DNA synthesis and cellular proliferation are inhibited [98].

Although various bacterial, viral and opportunistic infections have been associated with rheumatic diseases, certain infections occur more often than others. Herpes zoster occurs at a rate of 16 episodes per 1000 SLE patients a year [99]. Reports of salmonella bacteraemia, pneumococcal sepsis and Gram-negative polyarticular septic arthritis suggest an important role for defective reticuloendothelial function in the pathogenesis of these particular infectious complications.

A brief description of the important non-tuberculous infections is found in Chapter 5.

9. Drug-Induced Pulmonary Reactions

Many of the disease-modifying drugs used in autoimmune rheumatic disorders cause pulmonary complications (Table 5). They mimic either the pulmonary reaction to the diseases themselves or other causes of pulmonary damage.

There are no specific clinical features, laboratory findings or radiographic patterns to suggest a drug-induced disorder. The most common

Table 5. Clinical manifestations of drug-induced pulmonary disease

Pneumonitis	Bronchospasm
Methotrexate	Salicylate
Gold	NSAIDs
D-Penicillamine	Gold
Cyclophosphamide	D-Penicillamine
Clorambucil	Sulphasalsazine
Azathioprine	
Sulphasalazine	Non-cardiogenic pulmonary oedema
Non-steroidal anti-inflammatory	Methotrexate
drugs (NSAIDs)	Cyclophosphamide
	Salicylate
Fibrosis	NSAIDs
Methotrexate	Colchicine
Cyclophosphamide	
Clorambucil	Pulmonary/renal syndromes
Azathioprine	D-Penicillamine
Sulphasalazine	

Adapted from [98].

radiographic abnormalities include increased interstitial markings, reticulo-nodular shadows and alveolar infiltrates, often bilateral and in the lower zones. Pulmonary function tests tend to show a restrictive defect with a reduced TLco, unless the drug causes a problem that only affects the airways.

A diagnosis of drug-induced lung disease should be made after exclusion of other potential causes of the problem, including infection and direct lung involvement by the primary disease. Lung biopsy may demonstrate characteristic changes of drug-induced illness and exclude infection. Mononuclear cell infiltrates are common, and epithelial abnormalities include proliferation of both type I and type II pneumonocytes, with some dysplastic changes.

Broncholitis, giant cell and granuloma formation, and an eosinophilic infiltration may develop in those with an acute hypersensitivity drug reaction. D-Penicillamine is associated with the development of acute pulmonary/renal syndromes similar to Goodpasture's syndrome. Patients usually present with dyspnoea, chest pain and haemoptysis. The renal abnormalities are detected on urinalysis with haematuria, proteinuria and red cell casts. The mechanism by which D-penicillamine induces this reaction is unknown, but could be a result of drug-induced immune complex deposition.

Histological and immunological information is too scanty to be certain whether pulmonary infiltrates occur in the absence of haemorrhage or whether they represent capillary damage of the same immunopathogenesis but in a milder form [100].

Treatment with methotrexate (MTX) can cause severe pulmonary complications. Among the non-infectious adverse effects, interstitial pneumonitis and drug-induced asthma have been reported. A slowly progressive restrictive pattern and a deterioration of gas exchange may develop. However, Beyeler et al. [101] found no abnormality in lung function in 96 patients with RA treated with MTX. MTX pneumonitis is uncommon but potentially life-threatening. In a recent study [102], 4 to 130 patients with RA, treated with MTX, developed pneumonitis. The clinical presentation was non-specific, but the acute or subacute onset of a non-productive cough, dyspnoea, fever and rales is characteristic. Histological changes are also non-specific; however, massive lymphocytic interstitial infiltrate and granuloma formation have been reported, and their presence is helpful in differentiating MTX pneumonitis from rheumatic lung disease [103]. The mechanism of MTX pneumonitis is unknown. No correlations have been observed with disease duration, duration of MTX treatment, weekly dose or cumulative dose [104]. There is no consensus whether pre-existing lung disease in rheumatic patients predisposes to MTX pneumonitis; although an abnormal chest radiography before treatment may predispose to this form of pneumonitis [105].

Another drug-induced complication which may lead to death if the drug is continued is bronchospasm. It is very important to identify patients who develop bronchospasm in relation to salicylates or non-steroidal anti-inflammatory drugs. This reaction may be seen early in treatment and sometimes even after a single dose.

Pleuritis and pleural effusions are rare complications of antirheumatic drug therapy. Pleural effusions are usually part of an associated pneumonitis, but may develop as a separate problem.

References

1. Kelly CA (1993) Rheumatoid arthritis: Classical lung disease. *Balliere's Clin Rheum* 7: 1–16.
2. Lakhampl S, Lie J, Conn D, Martin W (1987) Pulmonary disease in polymyositis/dermatomyositis: A clinical and pathological analysis of 65 cases. *Ann Rheum Dis* 46: 26–29.
3. Solanki T, Neville E (1992) Bronchiectasis and rheumatoid disease. Is there any association? *Br J Rheum* 31: 691–693.
4. Walker WC (1967) Pulmonary infections and rheumatoid arthritis. *Q J Med* 142: 239–251.
5. Shadick NA, Fanta CH, Weinblatt ME, O'Donnell W, Coblyn JS (1994) Bronchiectasis: A late feature of severe rheumatoid arthritis. *Mecicine* 73: 161–170.
6. Banji A, Cooke N (1985) Rheumatoid arthritis and chronic bronchial suppurations. *Scand J Rheum* 14: 15–21.
7. Hillarby MC, McMahon MJ, Grennan DM, Cooper RG, Clarkson RWE, Davies EJ (1993) HLA associations in subjects with rheumatoid arthritis and bronchiectasis but not with other pulmonary complications of rheumatoid disease. *Br J Rheum* 32: 794–797.
8. Stein HB, Chalmers A, Schroeder ML, Dillon A (1984) Selected adverse reactions of D-penicillamine. *Clin Invest Med* 7: 73–76.
9. Holness L, Tenebaum J, Cooper NBE, Grossman RF (1995) Fatal bronchiolitis obliterans associated with chrysotherapy. *Ann Rheum Dis* 42: 593–596.
10. Colby TV, Myers JL (1992) Clinical and histological spectrum of bronchiolitis obliterans, including bronchiolitis obliterans organising pneumonia. *Semin Resp Med* 13: 119–123.

11. Fort JG, Scovern H, Abruzzo JL (1988) Intravenous cyclophosphamide and methylpred-nisolone for the treatment of bronchiolitis obliterans and interstitial fibrosis associated with chrysotherapy. *J Rheum* 15: 850–854.
12. Roschmann RA, Rothenberg RJ (1987) Pulmonary fibrosis in rheumatoid arthritis: A review of clinical features and therapy. *Semin Arthr Rheum* 16: 174–185.
13. Salmeron G, Greenberg SD, Lidsky MD (1981) Polymyositis and diffuse interstitial lung disease: A review of the pulmonary histopathologic findings. *Arch Intern Med* 141: 1005–1010.
14. Bacon PA (1993) Extra-articular rheumatoid arthritis. In: McCarty DJ, Koopman WJ (eds). *Arthritis and allied conditions*, 20th ed. Philadelphia: Lea and Febiger, 811–840.
15. Fishback N, Koss MN (1995) Pulmonary involvement in systemic lupus erythematosus. *Current Opin Pulm Med* 1: 368–375.
16. Quismorio FP (1988) Clinical and pathologic features of lung involvement in systemic lupus erythematosus. *Semin Resp Med* 9: 297–304.
17. Kolarz G, Scherak O, Popp W, Rischka L, Thumb N, Wottawa A, Zwich H (1993) Broncho-alveolar lavage in rheumatoid arthritis. *Br J Rheum* 32: 556–561.
18. Rochester CL, Elias J (1993) Cytokines and cytokine networking in the pathogenesis of interstitial and fibrotic lung disorders. *Semin Respir Med* 1389–1416.
19. Mulherin D, Breshnihan B (1993) Systemic lupus erythematosus. *Bailliere's Clin Rheum* 7: 31–57.
20. Matthay RA, Schwarz MT, Petty TL (1975) Pulmonary manifestations of systemic lupus erythematosus: Review of twelve cases of acute lupus pneumonitis. *Medicine* 54: 397–409.
21. Orens JB, Martinez FJ, Lynch JP (1994) Pleuropulmonary manifestations of systemic lupus erythematosus. *Rheum Dis Clin North Am* 20: 159–193.
22. Erickson RW, Franklin WA, Emlen W (1994) Treatment of hemorrhagic lupus pneumo-nitis with plasmapheresis. *Sem Arthritis Rheum* 24: 114–123.
23. Schwab EP, Schumacher HR, Freundlich B, Callegari PE (1993) Pulmonary alveolar hemorrhage in systemic lupus erythematosus. *Sem Arthritis Rheum* 23: 8–15.
24. Epler G (1992) Bronchiolitis obliterans organising pneumonia: Definition and clinical features. *Chest* 102 (Suppl.): 2s–6s.
25. Hunder GG, McDuffie FC, Hepper NG (1972) Pleural fluid complement in systemic lupus erythematosus and rheumatoid arthritis. *Ann Intern Med* 76: 357–363.
26. Good JT, King TE, Antony VB, Sahn SA (1983) Lupus pleuritis: Clinical features and pleural fluid characteristics with special reference to pleural fluid antinuclear antibodies. *Chest* 84: 714–718.
27. Nosanchuk JS, Naylor B (1968) A unique cytologic picture in pleural fluid from patients with rheumatoid arthritis. *Am J Clin Pathol* 17: 330–335.
28. Farquhar DR, Chamberlain MJ, McCain GA, Morgan WK (1989) Clearance of inhaled particles in ankylosing spondylitis. *Ann Rheum Dis* 48: 974–977.
29. Gibson JG, Edmonds JP, Hughes GRV (1977) Diaphragm function and lung involvement in systemic lupus erythematosus. *Am J Med* 63: 926–932.
30. Laroche CM, Mulvey DA, Hawkins PN, Walport MJ, Strickland B, Moxham J, Green M (1989) Diaphragm strength in the shrinking lung syndrome of systemic lupus erythema-tosus. *Q J Med* 265: 429–439.
31. Wilcox PG, Stein HB, Clarke SD, Pare PD, Pardy RL (1988) Phrenic nerve function in patients with diaphragmatic weakness and systemic lupus erythematosus. *Chest* 93: 352–358.
32. Walz-Leblanc BA, Urowitz MB, Gladman DD, Hanly PJ (1992) "The shrinking lung syndrome" in systemic lupus erythematosus – improvement with corticosteroid therapy. *J Rheum* 19: 1970–1972.
33. Owens GR, Follansbee WP (1987) Cardiopulmonary manifestations of systemic sclerosis. *Chest* 91: 118–127.
34. Segal AM, Reardon EV (1990) Systemic lupus erythematosus. In: Cannon GW, Zimmer-man G (eds). *The lung in rheumatic diseases*. New York: Marcel Dekker, 261–278.
35. Simonson JS, Schiller NB, Petri M, Hellman DB (1989) Pulmonary hypertension in systemic lupus erythematosus. *J Rheum* 16: 918–925.
36. Asherson RA, Oakley CM (1986) Pulmonary hypertension and systemic lupus erythem-atosus. *J Rheum* 13: 1–5.

37. Luchi ME, Asherson RA, Lahita RG (1992) Primary idiopathic pulmonary hypertension complicated by pulmonary arterial thrombosis. *Arthritis Rheum* 35: 700–705.
38. Moutsopoulos HM (1991) Behçet's syndrome. In: Isselbacher KJ, *Harrison Principles of Internal Medicine*, 12th ed. New York: McGraw-Hill, 145–156.
39. Peck B, Hoffman GS, Frank WA (1978) Thrombophlebitis in systemic lupus erythematosus. *JAMA* 240: 1728–1730.
40. Alarcon-Segovia D, Deleze M, Oria CV, Sanchez-Guerrero J, Gomez-Pacheco L, Cabiedes J, Fernandez L, Ponce de Leon S (1989) Antiphospholipid antibodies and the antiphospholipid syndrome in systemic lupus erythematosus. *Medicine* 68: 353–365.
41. Khamashta MA, Cuadrado MJ, Mujic F, Taub NA, Hunt BJ, Hughes GRV (1995) The management of thrombosis in the antiphospholipid-antibody syndrome. *N Engl J Med* 332: 993–997.
42. Abramson SB, Dobro J, Eberle MA, Benton M, Reibman J, Epstein H et al. (1991) Acute reversible hypoxemia in systemic lupus erythematosus. *Ann Intern Med* 114: 941–947.
43. Chan CN, Li E, Lai FM, Pang JA (1989) An unusual case of systemic lupus erythematosus with isolated hypoglossal nerve palsy, fulminant acute pneumonitis and pulmonary amyloidosis. *Ann Rheum Dis* 48: 236–239.
44. Inase N, Enomoto N, Sakaino H, Shigai T (1989) Systemic lupus erythematosus presenting with pericardial tamponade and lupus pneumonitis. *Jpn J Med* 28: 362–365.
45. Freter S, Davidman M, Bercovitch D, Brisson M (1994) Acute pulmonary edema as the initial hospital presentation of systemic lupus erythematosus. *Arch Intern Med* 154: 453–456.
46. Masuda A, Tsushima T, Shizume K, Mochizuki T, Isono K, Demura H et al. (1990) Recurrent pneumothoraces and mediastinal emphysema in systemic lupus erythematosus. *J Rheum* 17: 544–548.
47. Chauhan MS, Tewari SC, Prakash MJ, Dandona PK, Jayaswal R (1989) Necrobiotic pulmonary nodule leading to pyopneumothorax in a case of rheumatoid arthritis – a rare clinical presentation. *India J Chest Dis Allied Sci* 31: 217–220.
48. Boulware DW, Weissman DN, Dool NJ (1985) Pulmonary manifestations of the rheumatic diseases. *Clin Rev Allergy* 3: 249–267.
49. Isaacson P, Spencer J (1994) Autoimmunity and malignancy. In: Isenberg DA, Horsfill AC (eds) *Autoimmune diseases: focus on Sjögren's syndrome*. Oxford: Bios Scientific Publishers, 189–204.
50. Byrd SL, Case BA, Boulware DW (1993) Pulmonary manifestations of rheumatic disease. *Postgrad Med* 93: 149–166.
51. Caplan A (1953) Certain unusual radiological appearances in the chest of coal-miners suffering from rheumatoid arthritis. *Thorax* 8: 29–37.
52. Hassan WU, Keaney NP, Holland CD, Kelly CA (1995) High-resolution computed tomography of the lung in lifelong non-smoking patients with rheumatoid arthritis. *Ann Rheum Dis* 54: 308–310.
53. Muller-Leisse C, Bussmann A, Mayer O, Genth E, Gunther RW (1994) High-resolution computed tomography (HRCT) of the lung in collagenoses: A prospective study of 73 patients. *Rofo Forschr Geb Rontgenstr Neuen Bildgeb Verfahr* 161: 12–18.
54. Boumpas DT, Austin HA, Fessler BJ, Balow JE, Klippel JH, Lockshin MD (1995) Systemic lupus erythematosus: Emerging concepts. Part 1. Renal, neuropsychiatric, cardiovascular, pulmonary and haematologic disease. *Ann Intern Med* 122: 940–950.
55. Matthay RA, Schwarz MI, Petty TL (1977) Pleuropulmonary manifestations of connective tissue diseases. *Clin Notes Resp Dis* 16: 3–9.
56. Bankier AA, Kiener HP, Wiesmayr MN, Fleischmann D, Kontrus M, Herold CJ, Graninger W, Hubsch P (1995) Discrete lung involvement in systemic lupus erythematosus: CT assessment. *Radiol* 196: 835–840.
57. Grenier P, Valeyre D, Cluzel P, Brauner MW, Lenoir S, Chastang C (1991) Chronic diffuse interstitial lung disease: Diagnostic value of chest radiography and high resolution CT. *Radiol* 179: 123–132.
58. Meziane MA (1992) High-resolution computed tomography scaning in the assessment of interstitial lung diseases. *J Thorac Imag* 7: 13–25.
59. McDonagh J, Greaves M, Wright AR, Heycock C, Owen JP, Kelly C (1994) High-resolution computed tomography of the lungs in patients with rheumatoid arthritis and interstitial lung disease. *Br J Rheum* 33: 118–122.

60. Wells A, Hansell DM, Rubens MB, Cullinan P, Black CM, Dubois RM (1993) The predictive value of appearances on thin section computed tomography in fibrosing alveolitis. *Am Rev Resp Dis* 148: 1076–1082.
61. Bhalla M, Silver RM, Shepard JA, McLoud TC (1993) Chest CT in patients with scleroderma: Prevalence of asymptomatic oesophageal dilatation and mediastinal lymphadenopathy. *Arthritis J Roentgenol* 161: 269–272.
62. Mukerji B, Alpert MA, Hardin JG (1993) When the lungs are involved by connective tissue disease. *Postgrad Med* 94: 147–158.
63. Gammon RB, Bridges TA, al-Nezir H, Alexander CB, Kennedy JI (1992) Bronchiolitis obliterans organizing pneumonia associated with systemic lupus erythematosus. *Chest* 102: 1171–1174.
63a. Roberts and Spiro SG (1991) *Med International* 88:3661–3668.
64. Frank ST, Weg JG, Harkleroad LE, Fitch RF (1973) Pulmonary dysfunction in rheumatoid disease. *Chest* 63: 27–34.
65. Arroliga AC, Podell DN, Matthay RA (1992) Pulmonary manifestations of scleroderma. *J Thorac Imag* 7: 30–45.
66. Huang CT, Hennigar GR, Lyons HA (1965) Pulmonary dysfunction in systemic lupus erythematosus. *N Engl J Med* 272: 288–293.
67. Andonopoulos AP, Constantopoulos SH, Galanopoulos V, Drosos AA, Acritidis NC, Moutsopoulos HM (1988) Pulmonary function of nonsmoking patients with systemic lupus erythematosus. *Chest* 94: 312–315.
68. Hellman DB, Kirsch CM, Whiting-O'Keefe Q, Simonson J, Schiller NB, Petri M, Gramsu G, Gold W (1995) Dyspnoea in ambulatory patients with SLE prevalence, severity and correlation with incremental exercise testing. *J Rheum* 22: 455–461.
69. Scano G, Goti P, Duanti R, Misuri G, Emmi L, Rosi E (1995) Control of breathing in a subset of patients with systemic lupus erythematosus. *Chest* 108: 759–766.
70. Schwarz MI (1993) Pulmonary manifestations of the collagen-vascular diseases. In: Bone RA, Dantzker DR, George RB, Matthay RA, Reynolds HY (eds). *Pulmonary and critical care medicine*, vol. 2. St. Louis: Mosby, 1–16.
71. Groen H, der Borg EJ, Postma DS, Wouda AA, Van der Mark TW, Kallenberg CGM (1992) Pulmonary function in systemic lupus erythematosus in related to distinct clinical, serologic and nailfold capillary patterns. *Am J Med* 93: 619–627.
72. Naylor B (1992) Cytological aspects of pleural peritoneal and pericardial fluids from patients with systemic lupus erythematosus. *Cytopathology* 3: 1–8.
73. Hakala M, Paakko P, Huhti E, Tarkka M, Sutinen S (1990) Open lung biopsy of patients with rheumatoid arthritis. *Clin Rheum* 9: 452–460.
74. Wallaert B, Dugas M, Dansin E, Perez T, Marquette CH, Ramon P, Tonnel AB, Voisin C (1990) Subclinical alveolitis in immunological systemic disorders: Transition between health and disease. *Eur Resp* 3: 1206–1216.
75. Turner-Stokes L, Turner-Warwick M (1982) Intrathoracic manifestations of SLE. *Clin Rheum Dis* 8: 229–242.
76. Groen H, Aslander M, Bootsma H, Van der Mark ThW, Kallenberg CGM, Postma DS (1993) Bronchoalveolar lavage cell analysis and lung function impairment in patients with systemic lupus erythematosus. *Clin Exp Immun* 22: 323–325.
77. Wall CP, Gaesler EA, Carrington CB, Hayers JA (1981) Comparison of transbronchial and open biopsies in chronic infiltrative lung diseases. *Am Rev Respir Dis* 123: 280–285.
78. Koh WH, Boey ML (1993) Open lung biopsy in systemic lupus erythematosus with pulmonary disease. *Ann Acad Med Singapore* 22: 323–325.
79. Bell ME, Flye MW, Webber BL, Wesley RA (1981) Prospective evaluation of aspiration needle, cutting needle, transbronchial and open lung biopsy. *Ann Thorac Surg* 32: 146–153.
80. Bensard DD, McIntyre RC, Waring BJ, Simon JS (1993) Comparison of video thoracoscopic lung biopsy to open lung biopsy in the diagnosis of interstitial lung disease. *Chest* 103: 765–770.
81. Fanti S, De Fabritiis A, Aloisi D, Dondi M, Marengo M, Compagnone G, Fallani F, Cavalli A, Monnetti N (1994) Early pulmonary involvement in systemic sclerosis assessed by technitium-99m-DTPA clearance rate. *J Nucl Med* 35: 1933–1936.
82. Anaya JM, Diethelm L, Ortiz LA, Gutierrez M, Citera G, Welsh RA, Espinoza LR (1995) Pulmonary involvement in rheumatoid arthritis. *Semin Arthritis Rheum* 24: 242–254.

83. Eiser AR, Shanies HM (1994) Treatment of lupus interstitial lung disease with intravenous cyclophosphamide. *Arthritis Rheum* 37: 428–431.
84. Euler HH, Shroeder JO, Harten P, Zeuner RA, Gutschmidt HJ (1994) Treatment-free remission in severe systemic lupus erythematosus following synchronization of plasmapheresis with subsequent pulse cyclophosphamide. *Arthritis Rheum* 37: 1784–1794.
85. Raghu G, Depaso WJ, Cain K, Hammar SP, Wetzel CE, Dreis DF (1991) Azathoprine combined with prednisone in the treatment of idiopathic pulmonary fibrosis: A prospective double-blind, randomized, placebo-controlled clinical trial. *Am Rev Respir Dis* 144: 291–296.
86. St. Clair EW, Rice JR, Snyderman R (1985) Pneumonitis complicating low-dose methotrexate therapy in rheumatoid arthritis. *Arch Intern Med* 145: 2035–2038.
87. Arsura EL, Greenberg AS (1988) Adverse impact of interstitial pulmonary fibrosis on prognosis in polymyositis and dermatomyositis. *Semin Arthritis Rheum* 18: 29–37.
88. De Clerck LS, Dequeker J, Franox L, Demedts M (1987) D-penicillamine therapy and interstitial lung disease in scleroderma: A long-term follow-up study. *Arthritis Rheum* 30: 643–650.
89. Steen VD, Owens GR, Redmond C, Rodman GP, Medsger TA (1985) The effect of D-penicillamine on pulmonary findings in systemic sclerosis. *Arthritis Rheum* 28: 882–888.
90. Steen VD, Lanz JK, Conte C, Owens GR, Medsger TA (1994) Therapy for severe interstitial lung disease in systemic sclerosis. *Arthrit Rheum* 37: 1290–1296.
91. Freundlich B, Jimenez SA, Steen VD, Medsger TA, Szkolnicki M, Jaffe HS (1992) Treatment of systemic sclerosis with recombinant interferon-gamma A phase I/II clinical trial. *Arthritis Rheum* 35: 1134–1142.
92. Alpert MA, Pressly TA, Mukerji V, Lambert CR, Mukerji B (1992) Short- and long-term hemodynamic effects of captopril in patients with pulmonary hypertension and selected connective tissue disease. *Chest* 102: 1407–1412.
93. Arroliga AC, Podell DN, Matthay RA (1992) Pulmonary manifestations of scleroderma. *J Thorac Imag* 7: 30–45.
94. Martinez-Lavin M, Vaughan JH, Tan EM (1979) Autoantibodies and the spectrum of Sjögren's syndrome. *Ann Intern Med* 91: 185–190.
95. Duffy KN, Duffy CM, Gladman DD (1991) Infection and disease activity in systemic lupus erythematosus: A review of hospitalized patients. *J Rheum* 18: 1180–1184.
96. Gaensler EA, Carrington CB (1980) Open biopsy for chronic diffuse infiltrative lung disease: Clinical reontgenographic and physiologic correlations in 502 patients. *Ann Thor Surg* 30: 411–426.
97. Cupps TR, Fauci AS (1982) Corticosteroid-mediated immunoregulation in man. *Immunol Rev* 65: 133–155.
98. Spiro SG, Isenberg DA (1993) The respiratory system in rheumatic disease. In: Maddison PJ, Isenberg DA, Woo P, Glass DN (eds). *Oxford textbook of rheumatology, Oxford*: Oxford University Press, 125–138.
99. Kahl LE (1994) Herpes zoster infections in systemic lupus erythematosus: Risk factors and outcome. *J Rheum* 21: 84–86.
100. Turner-Warwick M (1981) Adverse reactions affecting the lung: Possible association with D-penicillamine. *J Rheum* (Suppl.) 7: 166–168.
101. Beyeler C, Jordi B, Gerber NJ, Hof V (1996) Pulmonary function in rheumatoid arthritis treated with low-dose methotrexate: A longitudinal study. *British J Rheum* 35: 446–452.
102. Hilliquin P, Renoux M, Perrot S, Puechal X, Menkes CJ (1996) Occurrence of pulmonary complications during methotrexate therapy in rheumatoid arthritis. *British J Rheum* 35: 441–445.
103. Schwarz MI, King TE (eds) (1993) *Interstitial lung disease*, 2nd ed. Philadelphia: Mosby Year Book.
104. Hargraves MR, Mowat AG, Benson MK (1992) Acute pneumonitis associated with low-dose methotrexate treatment for rheumatoid arthritis: Report of five cases and review of published reports. *Thorax* 47: 628–633.
105. Golden MR, Katz RS, Balk RA, Golden HE (1995) The relationship of pre-existing lung disease to the development of methotrexate pneumonitis in patients with rheumatoid arthritis. *J Rheumatol* 22: 1043–1047.

Autoimmune Aspects of Lung Disease
ed. by D. A. Isenberg and S. G. Spiro
© 1998 Birkhäuser Verlag Basel/Switzerland

CHAPTER 3
Pulmonary Manifestations of Systemic Vasculitides

Jan Willem Cohen Tervaert[1], Tjip S. van der Werf[2], Coen A. Stegeman[3], Wim Timens[4] and Cees G. M. Kallenberg[1]

[1] *Department of Clinical Immunology, University Hospital, Groningen, The Netherlands*
[2] *Department of Pulmonology, University Hospital, Groningen, The Netherlands*
[3] *Department of Nephrology, University Hospital, Groningen, The Netherlands*
[4] *Department of Pathology, University Hospital, Groningen, The Netherlands*

1. Introduction

The term "vasculitis" denotes a pathological process characterized by inflammation and necrosis of blood vessel walls. The vasculitic process can affect blood vessels of any type, size or location, and therefore can cause dysfunction in virtually any organ system, including the lungs. Pulmonary manifestations such as nodular shadows and/or infiltrative changes on the chest radiograph are often present in an early phase of the disease process, and in patients with arthralgias and/or constitutional symptoms, the presence of these pulmonary abnormalities should alert the clinician to the possibility of vasculitis. Vasculitis frequently affects the lung, and sometimes the lung is the only organ involved. Recent studies have shown that cytokines and adhesion molecules that mediate normal leukocyte function are involved in the pathogenesis of vasculitis [1, 2]. Pathological expression of adhesion molecules and production of cytokines may result from different initiating events. Indeed, several types of pathophysiological events that may lead to vessel wall damage are recognized currently. These include pathogenic immune complex deposition or *in situ* formation, a "Shwartzman-like" phenomenon in which intravascular activation and aggregation of neutrophils may be operative, antibody-dependent cell-mediated cytotoxicity, and cell-mediated immune responses [1, 3]. For therapeutic purposes, it would be useful to categorize different forms of vasculitis based on specific mechanisms of vessel damage. Classification of vasculitides is unfortunately, however, only partly based on our understanding of pathogenetic mechanisms. Although classification of vasculitides is still not perfect, enormous progress has been made in recent years. Firstly, a universally accepted classification scheme has emerged [4], and classification criteria for major vasculitic syndromes have been published [5], whereas at a consensus conference definitions for the most common forms of vasculitis have been adopted [4].

Vasculitides may be associated with a number of clinical syndromes (secondary forms of vasculitis; see Table 1), whereas classification of patients suffering from primary vasculitides is based on the predominant type and calibre of the blood vessel involved [4–8] (Table 2).

Diagnosing vasculitis as early as possible is crucial, because the disease may progress with time, and final outcome is determined by the extent of organ involvement. The demonstration of autoantibodies to myeloid lysosomal enzymes [9], i.e. antineutrophil cytoplasmic antibodies (ANCAs), in patients with vasculitis has facilitated the diagnostic assessment [10]. In addition, it has facilitated classification of those patients [11].

Table 1. Secondary forms of vasculitis

Infection-related vasculitis, e.g. hepatitis B, tuberculosis, HIV, endocarditis
Vasculitis secondary to collagen vascular diseases, e.g. rheumatoid arthritis, systemic lupus erythematosus
Vasculitis secondary to mixed essential cryoglobulinemia
Vasculitis secondary to sarcoidosis
Vasculitis in malignancies, e.g. lymphomatoid granulomatosis, hairy cell leukaemia
Vasculitis due to drug reactions, e.g. hydralazine, propylthiouracil (PTU), D-penicillamine
Vasculitis in substance abuse
Miscellaneous secondary forms of vasculitis, e.g. transplant vasculitis
Pseudovasculitis syndromes, e.g. atrial myxoma

Table 2. Classification of vasculitis

Idiopathic Vasculitides

Affecting large-, medium- and small-sized blood vessels
- Takayasu's arteritis
- Giant cell arteritis/temporal arteritis

Affecting predominantly medium-sized blood vessels
- Polyarteritis nodosa

Affecting predominantly medium- and small-sized blood vessels
- Churg-Strauss syndrome *
- Wegener's granulomatosis *
- Microscopic polyangiitis *

Affecting predominantly small-sized blood vessels
- ANCA-associated lung hemorrhage and nephritis *
- Henoch Schönlein purpura
- Cutaneous leukocytoclastic angiitis

Miscellaneous conditions
- Behçet's disease
- Kawasaki's disease

Secondary forms of vasculitis

---

* = ANCA-associated form of vasculitis; ANCA = anti-neutrophil cytoplasmic antibody.

This review will focus on clinical and therapeutic features of pulmonary vasculitis. Special attention will be paid to the role of ANCAs in classification, diagnosis and treatment of vasculitis affecting the lungs.

2. Clinical Characteristics of the Different Vasculitides

2.1. *Takayasu's Arteritis*

Takayasu's arteritis is a chronic, recurrent, inflammatory vascular disease that affects the aorta, proximal parts of its major branches and the pulmonary arteries [12].

The disease occurs predominantly but not exclusively in young women and is most common in Eastern countries such as Japan and China. Increasing reports from Europe, Africa, the Middle East and North America have established Takayasu's arteritis as a worldwide entity [13]. Takayasu's arteritis usually begins with non-specific symptoms of an inflammatory disease. These symptoms may merge with those resulting from arterial stenosis or occlusion, which dominate the later stages of the disease. Salient clinical features include absence or decrease of arterial pulses, claudication of arms or legs, intermittent or fluctuating visual loss, renovascular hypertension and congestive heart failure. Many patients also have neurological manifestations such as postural dizziness, vertigo, headache, syncope, seizures, diplopia and amaurosis fugax [10]. Aortic insufficiency and aortic aneurysms can be found as well.

Pulmonary symptoms are rare and include shortness of breath, cough, haemoptysis and pleuritic pain. Patients may be initially misdiagnosed as suffering from (chronic) pulmonary thromboembolic disease [14]. In addition, one case of Takayasu's arteritis presenting as idiopathic adult respiratory distress syndrome has been reported [15]. Chest radiographs may show pleural effusions, a prominent main pulmonary artery, a widened mediastinum or an infiltrate. Despite the fact that several studies have confirmed pulmonary artery involvement in more than 50% of Takayasu's patients [16, 17], this is seldom clinically recognized due to the absence of pulmonary symptoms. As a consequence of pulmonary arteritis, however, some patients develop symptomatic pulmonary hypertension and/or right-sided heart failure. On ventilation-perfusion scans, the pulmonary arteritis may cause defects which are indistinguishable from pulmonary embolism. Angiographically, however, the picture of arteritis is distinct from a pulmonary embolus [18].

The diagnosis of Takayasu's arteritis usually relies on the demonstration of aortic and arterial stenosis, obstruction, irregularities, narrowings and/or aneurysms by aortography and pulmonary arteriography [12]. Localized vascular lesions of the pulmonary artery and/or its subsegmental branches may occlude the blood vessels, producing segmental pulmonary infarcts [16]. Since angiograms demonstrate luminal changes, but not mural changes, computed tomographic angiography has been recently recommended to evaluate the activity and the extent of the disease [19]. As the diagnosis is often made based on radiographic findings, it is important that other causes of inflammatory arteritis such as infective arteritis and/or arteritis secondary to ankylosing spondylitis are excluded. The primary gross pathological lesion in Takayasu's arteritis is stenosis of the arterial ostium at its site of origin from the aorta. Histologically, in the early "prepulseless" phase and during recurrences of the disease, the vascular lesion is characterized by a granulomatous arteritis, whereas during the late "pulseless" phase there is transmural sclerosis with scanty or no inflammation. The pathological findings of the pulmonary arteries are similar to those of the systemic arteries. In addition, peculiar stenosis-recanalization lesions ("a vessel-in-vessel" lesion) of the pulmonary elastic arteries may be found [20].

Initial therapy is immunosuppression with corticosteroids, and this therapy is usually effective in controlling the disease at first. However, when the dose of corticosteroids is reduced, additional cytotoxic drugs such as methotrexate (MTX), azathioprine or cyclophosphamide are used in as many as 40% of patients, because the disease cannot be controlled with corticosteroids alone [13]. Once vascular fibrosis has occurred, various angioplastic and surgical interventions are sometimes warranted to prevent ischaemic damage.

2.2. Giant Cell Arteritis

Giant cell arteritis (GCA) is a systemic granulomatous arteritis with a pre-dilection for cranial vessels, especially the temporal arteries. The disease is rare under age 50, and the average age at onset is 70; it is almost exclusively reported in whites. Usually, patients present with non-specific symptoms such as malaise, weight loss and fever. Half of the patients suffer from morn-ing stiffness in combination with muscular aching and stiffness of the neck, shoulder and pelvic girdle regions ("polymyalgia rheumatica") [21, 22]. The most common and often most prominent complaint is headache, which is most severe in the temporal areas. Apart from tenderness to palpation of inflamed temporal arteries, there is also a more diffuse tenderness of the scalp, causing discomfort during combing the hair or wearing a cap. Jaw claudication, difficulty in swallowing and tongue pain are also well-recognized symptoms. Ophthalmological involvement is the most dreaded presentation of GCA. Partial or complete loss of vision occurs in 10–20% of cases, only infrequently preceded by amaurosis fugax [10]. In addition, diffuse cerebral dysfunction manifested by altered mental status is a not uncommon finding in patients with GCA [10]. Pulmonary involvement has been described in GCA [23–25]. A persistent dry cough is the most com-mon symptom [24], together with dyspnoea, haemoptysis, pleural effusions, pulmonary infiltrates and/or interstitial lung disease. In many of these reported cases, a coexisting other form of vasculitis such as Wegener's granulomatosis and/or the Churg-Strauss syndrome was probably present [26, 27]. In addition, rare cases of pulmonary infarction due to giant cell arteritis of the pulmonary artery and other pulmonary vessels have been described [28–30].

The diagnosis of GCA is based upon recognition of typical clinical symytoms and signs in combination with an elevated Erythrocyte Sedi-mentation Rate (ESR) and/or C-reactive protein. Histological examination of a temporal artery biopsy typically shows a granulomatous panarteritis. Prednisolone is the mainstay of therapy. In general, it is started at 40 to 60 mg/day (single dose). The majority of the patients respond quickly. After 4 weeks the prednisolone is reduced by 10 mg/day every 2 weeks until a dose of 30 mg/day is achieved. Subsequently, the dose can be de-creased by 5 mg/day every 2 weeks until a dose of 15 mg/day is reached. Then the dose can be reduced by 2.5 mg/day per 4 weeks down to a dose of 5 mg/day. Finally, the dose is decreased by 1 mg/day every month until prednisolone can be stopped. In some patients, the drug can be discon-tinued within 6 months. Many patients, however, have exacerbations of the disease that are often preceded by increases in C-reactive protein levels in the absence of infection. In most patients, flares can be treated with in-crements of prednisolone. In only a small percentage of patients additional treatment with azathioprine and/or MTX is needed.

2.3. Polyarteritis Nodosa

Polyarteritis nodosa (PAN) is a necrotizing vasculitis in which predominantly medium- and small-sized muscular arteries are affected. PAN is a diagnosis of exclusion, and therefore the diagnosis can only be made when the disease cannot fit into another recognized vasculitic syndrome [10, 31]. According to the Chapel Hill consensus conference definitions [4], PAN is a disease in which the vasculitic process is confined to arteries. So, PAN cannot be diagnosed if arterioles, capillaries and/or veins are also involved. A substantial proportion of patients with PAN have a hepatitis B virus (HBV) and/or human immunodeficiency virus (HIV) infection [32, 33].

At present, two different forms of PAN are recognized [11, 34]: (1) systemic PAN, i.e. with vasculitic involvement of visceral organs (kidneys, heart or gastrointestinal tract), and (2) limited PAN, i.e. vasculitis restricted to the skin, nerves and/or musculoskeletal system, also known as cutaneous PAN [35] and/or nonsystemic vasculitic neuropathy [36].

The disease is seen at any age; its mean age at onset is 45−55 years. Most patients initially present with non-specific symptoms such as weight loss, fever, arthralgias and (often severe) muscle weakness. Constitutional symptoms may be absent in a proportion of patients with limited PAN [36]. There is no consensus about the frequency of involvement of various organs, and widely ranging frequencies have been reported [31]. Organ systems frequently involved include peripheral nervous system, kidneys (vascular nephropathy but no glomerulonephritis), gastrointestinal tract, skin, central nervous system and heart.

In the past, pulmonary involvement was reported frequently. Almost all of these patients should now be classified under different diagnostic groups, especially one of the ANCA-associated forms of vasculitis [11]. So pulmonary involvement in PAN has to be regarded as controversial. In addition, in any patient with PAN and pulmonary lesions, the question must be raised whether the lesions are part of the vasculitic disease process or a complication, such as an infection.

PAN is an ANCA-negative form of vasculitis; that is, antibodies directed to either proteinase 3 or myeloperoxidase are only occasionally found in this disease [11, 33]. The diagnosis of PAN relies on clinical, histopathological and/or angiographic findings, and can only be made after exclusion of other recognized vasculitic syndromes. Diagnostic biopsies which show necrotizing arteritis are most frequently obtained from skeletal muscle, nerve, kidney, skin and/or subcutaneous tissue. Occasionally, necrotizing arteritis is found in biopsies of other organs such as testis, liver or rectum. In systemic PAN, visceral angiograms may demonstrate the presence of microaneurysms and/or stenoses in medium-sized vessels. Microaneurysms are, however, not pathognomonic and may also occur in ANCA-associated forms of vasculitis.

Initial treatment of PAN is with high-dose corticosteroid therapy. In patients with visceral organ involvement and/or with severe peripheral nerve disease, a cytotoxic agent has to be added. Cyclophosphamide, either pulse therapy or continuous oral therapy, is recommended. In less severe forms azathioprine or MTX can be used. Relapses of PAN are rare. In HBV- and/or HIV-related PAN, the mainstay of the treatment is the combination of antiviral agents and plasma exchange. Corticosteroids are only given for a short period, i.e. 2−4 weeks, to control the most severe life-threatening manifestations of PAN. In HBV-related PAN, interferon-α and/or vidarabine have been successfully used [33].

2.4. ANCA-Associated Vasculitides

During the last few years, ANCAs have been found in different forms of vasculitis [37]. The detection of these antibodies has dramatically changed the diagnostic approach of patients with clinically suspected vasculitis [10].

Two major types of ANCAs have been recognized (Figure 1). The first type is called c-ANCA ("classic" or "cytoplasmic" ANCA) and is associated strongly with Wegener's granulomatosis (WG) [38, 39]. These antibodies produce a characteristic granular cytoplasmic staining pattern on ethanol-fixed granulocytes when detected by a standard indirect immunofluorescence technique [40]. The antigen recognized by c-ANCA is proteinase 3 (PR3), a 29-kDa glycoprotein from azurophilic granules that has serine protease, antimicrobial and myeloblastic activity. The second type is called p-ANCA ("perinuclear" ANCA) and is found in many different inflammatory disorders [41]. These antibodies produce a perinuclear pattern on ethanol fixed granulocytes, but a cytoplasmic staining pattern when granulocytes are fixed with crosslinking fixatives [42]. The antigens recognized by p-ANCA are different myeloid proteins, i.e. myeloperoxidase (MPO), elastase, cathepsin G, lactoferrin, lysozyme, β-glucuronidase, α-enolase, bactericidal permeability-increasing protein, human lysosomal-associated membrane protein 2 and other uncharacterized proteins [43]. Antibodies to PR3, MPO and/or elastase are specifically associated with idiopathic necrotizing vasculitis [44, 45]. Antibodies to other myeloid proteins are found in a wide variety of different inflammatory disorders, such as autoimmune liver diseases and inflammatory bowel disease, and are not specific for a particular disease [43].

Antibodies to PR3 and to MPO are found predominantly in patients with either the Churg-Strauss syndrome or WG or microscopic polyangiitis, or in patients with isolated renal vasculitis and/or isolated alveolar capillaritis (Table 3). Anti-PR3 and/or anti-MPO are, however, also occasionally detected in patients with other diseases such as drug-induced vasculitis, systemic lupus erythematosus (SLE) and/or patients with antibodies to glomerular and alveolar basement membranes anti-(GBM) disease [37, 43].

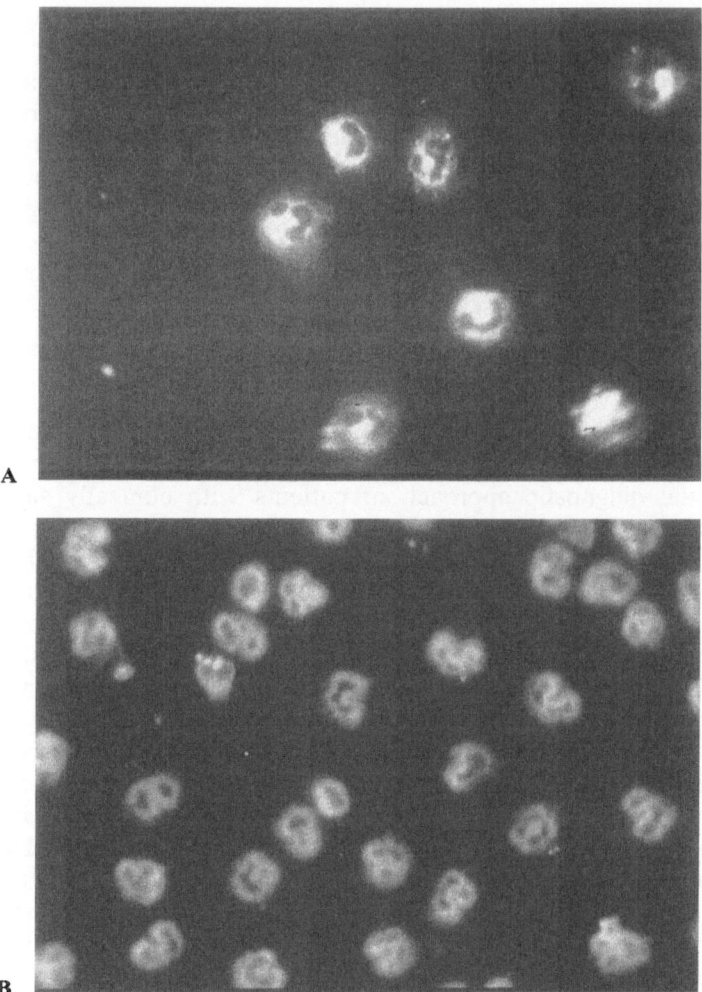

Figure 1. Staining of ethanol-fixed neutrophils by indirect immunofluorescence using a serum sample from a patient with active WG that produces a cytoplasmic pattern of fluorescence [c-ANCA (A)] and a serum sample from a patient with microscopic polyangiitis that produces a perinuclear pattern [p-ANCA (B)].

2.4.1. Churg-Strauss syndrome: Churg-Strauss syndrome (CSS) is a distinctive clinical condition characterized by asthma, allergic rhinitis, eosinophilia and systemic vasculitis.

The disease has been observed at any age; its peak incidence is in the third and fourth decades. Lanham and co-workers [46, 47] identified different phases of the disease: a prodromal phase characterized by allergic and eosinophilic infiltrative disease; a vasculitic phase which follows the prodromal phase after 5–10 years (range 0–58 years); and a postvasculitic

Table 3. Characteristics of ANCA-associated vasculitides

Disease	Clinical	Anti-PR3 antibody	Anti-MPO antibody
Churg-Strauss syndrome	Asthma, eosinophilia, neuropathy	+	++++
Wegener's granulomatosis	Nose bleeds, nephritis, lung infiltrates	++++	++
Microscopic polyangiitis	Nephritis, purpura, haemoptysis	+++	+++
ANCA-associated pulmonary-renal syndrome	Nephritis, haemoptysis, dyspnoea	++	+++

PR3 = proteinase 3; MPO = myeloperoxidase; ++++ = >70% of patients; +++ = 30–70% of patients; ++ = 10–30% of patients; + = 3–10% of patients; – = <1% of patients.

phase which is dominated by allergic disease, hypertension and incomplete recovery from major organ damage.

Patients initially present with rhinorrhoea, nasal polyposis, recurrent sinusitis and asthma. In addition, most patients have eosinophilia and a history of allergy. The vasculitic phase is often heralded by malaise, weight loss, fever, disabling muscle weakness and arthralgias [11, 47, 48]. Other features of the vasculitic phase are purpura or nodular lesions, abdominal pain, pericarditis and glomerulonephritis (Table 4). Involvement of the peripheral nervous system dominates the clinical picture of the vasculitic phase in most patients. Mononeuritis multiplex or a symmetrical polyneu-

Table 4. Clinical features of ANCA-associated vasculitides

	WG	CSS	MPA
	Organ involvement (%)		
Constitutional symptoms	70–80%	70–80%	70–80%
Arthralgias/myalgias	60–80%	60–80%	60–80%
Lung involvement	70–90%	90–100%	30–60%
– Alveolar haemorrhage	10 30%	rare	30–60%
ENT disease	90–100%	70–80%	rare
Glomerulonephritis	70–90%	25–50%	90–100%
Cutaneous manifestations	40–50%	50–60%	50–60%
Gastrointestinal disease	rare	30–60%	30–60%
Eye involvement	30–60%	20–30%	20–30%
Neuropathy	20–40%	70–80%	15–30%

ANCA = anti-neutrophil cytoplasmic antibody; WG – Wegener's granulomatosis; CSS Churg-Strauss syndrome; MPA = microscopic polyangiitis; ENT = ear, nose and throat.

ropathy can be found in 65–80% of patients [10], which can be extremely painful and severe. In addition, other manifestations such as cranial nerve palsies, vasculitis of the central nervous system, myocarditis and endocarditis have been documented in a substantial number of cases.

Pulmonary disease is a hallmark of CSS. In the prodromal phase, reversible airways obstruction is usually present. The onset of asthma usually occurs after childhood and follows episodes of recurrent rhinitis and sinusitis. Asthma predates the vasculitic phase by months to years, and it frequently worsens before the onset of vasculitis. Asthma, however, may also abruptly disappear as vasculitic symptoms become manifest. Pulmonary infiltrates are found frequently and typically are transient and patchy [47]. Patients may also present with chronic eosinophilic pneumonia [44, 49], miliary lesions and/or fixed, nodular lesions. Cavitation of the lesion is rare and suggests an infectious complication [50]. Other pulmonary manifestations may include alveolar haemorrhage, diffuse interstitial disease, hilar adenopathy and pleuritic chest pain with pleural effusions (Figure 2). Pleural fluid analysis may reveal an exudate with many eosinophils and a low glucose level [51]. Bronchoalveolar lavage in patients with pulmonary infiltrates show an increased percentage of alveolar eosinophils [52].

Patients with active vasculitic disease have an elevated ESR, an elevated C-reactive protein level, leukocytosis and peripheral eosinophilia. In addition, in about 65–80% of patients with CSS, ANCAs with specificity for MPO are found [43]. In addition, a substantial number of patients have ANCA with specificity for bactericidal permeability increasing protein [53].

The diagnosis of CSS is based on the presence of asthma, peripheral eosinophilia, clinical signs of systemic vasulitis, histopathological findings and/or angiographic abnormalities. Biopsy of skin lesions, peripheral nerves and/or muscles may reveal necrotizing vasculitis often with many eosinophils in the infiltrate, but only occasionally with granulomas. Kidney biopsies may show focal necrotizing and/or crescentic glomerulonephritis. The classic triad of necrotizing vasculitis, tissue infiltration by eosinophils and extravascular granulomas is found rarely in biopsy specimens [47]. Histological examination of the lungs typically reveals changes of asthma such as plugging of bronchi by mucus, thickening of the basement membrane and eosinophilic inflammation of the bronchiolar walls. Damage to the bronchi may cause bronchiectasis. In addition, infiltration of the alveolar septa with eosinophils and a considerable admixture of

Figure 2. (A) Chest radiograph of a 50-year-old woman with Churg Strauss Syndrome (CSS) showing pleural effusion and diffuse interstitial and alveolar shadowing predominantly in the lower lung fields. (B) Chest radiograph of the same patient as in (A) showing resolution and normalisation of chest radiograph after 6 weeks of immunosuppressive therapy.

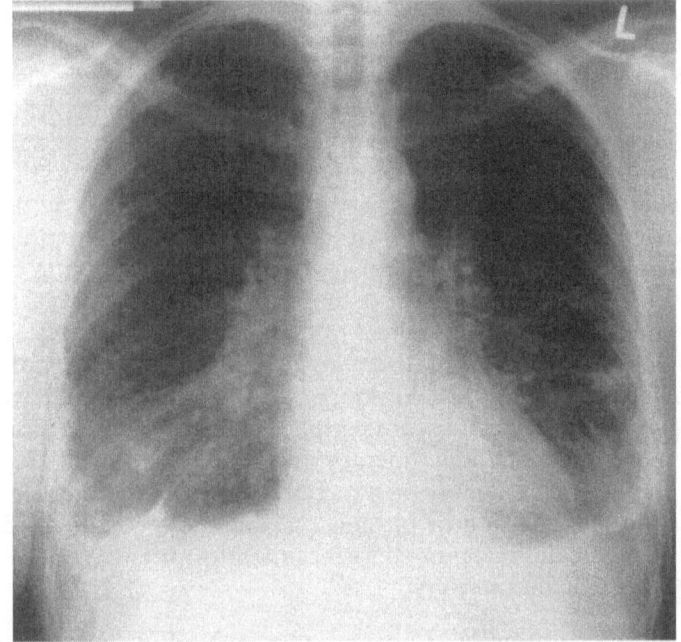

A

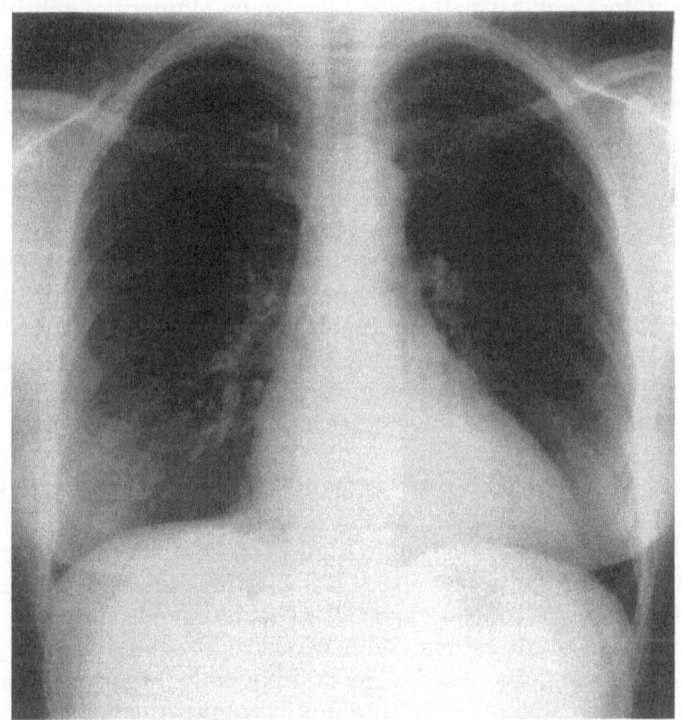

B

multinucleated giant cells can be found. Finally, granulomas, vasculitis and/or necrotizing capillaritis may be present [47].

Corticosteroids are the mainstay of treatment, and the response to treatment is often dramatic. Chumbley et al. followed 30 patients with CSS; 25 patients were treated with corticosteroids only. Survival at 1 year was 90%, survival at 5 years 62%. The authors concluded that corticosteroids without cytotoxic agents are sufficient in this form of vasculitis [54]. In 10–20% of the cases, however, the disease progresses despite adequate steroid therapy, and in 20–40% relapses occur during tapering of corticosteroids. Since irreversible organ damage may develop quickly, the use of immunosuppressive drugs has been recommended in patients with renal involvement, gastrointestinal tract involvement and/or central nervous system involvement [55]. In addition, based on our experience we suggest immunosuppressives when severe peripheral nerve disease occurs. Cyclophosphamide, either as pulse therapy or continuous oral therapy, is the drug of choice. In extremely severe cases, e.g. life-threatening alveolar haemorrhage, the addition of plasma exchange is recommended. During tapering of medication, asthma becomes manifest in many cases and may be treated with inhaled steroids.

2.4.2. *Wegener's granulomatosis:* Wegener's granulomatosis (WG) is characterized by chronic necrotizing inflammatory lesions of the upper and/or lower respiratory tracts usually accompanied by glomerulonephritis and/or systemic vasculitis. The course of the disease may be rapidly progressive or indolent, and relatively mild disease may go unrecognized for months to years. The disease has been observed at any age; its peak incidence is in the fourth and fifth decades. The disease affects both sexes equally and is more commonly seen in white patients [56].

Initial symptoms of the disease may vary from patient to patient [57, 58], but most present with upper airway illness such as serosanguinous nasal discharge, nasal obstruction and recurrent sinusitis [56–59]. Other frequently observed presenting symptoms and signs are otitis media, haemoptysis, episcleritis, arthralgias, palpable purpura, cutaneous ulcers, microscopic haematuria and asymptomatic pulmonary infiltrates. Finally, at the time of diagnosis roughly two out of three patients have nose, sinus, lung, kidney and joint involvement, whereas half have ear, eye and skin involvement (Table 4).

Pulmonary involvement in WG may be due to vasculitis or to granulomatous inflammatory lesions. At the time of diagnosis, 50–70% of the patients have abnormal chest radiographs [60–62]. Computerized tomography (CT) of the chest may reveal lesions which are undetected on conventional radiographs [63, 64], and CT is a recommended procedure for the initial evaluation of all patients with WG. Usually the pulmonary abnormalities are asymptomatic. The most frequently reported symptom is cough, which can also result from either laryngitis/tracheitis or postnasal

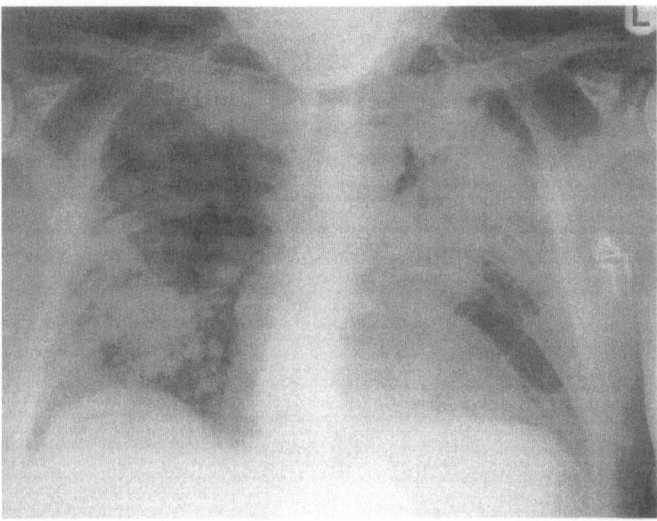

Figure 3. Chest radiograph of a 78-year-old man with diffuse bilateral alveolar haemorrhage due to WG.

drip due to ethmoiditis or generalized sinusitis. In the study of Cordier et al. 78% of the patients presented with cough, which was unproductive in nearly 90% of cases [65]. Hoffman et al. found cough to be a presenting symptom in 19% of the patients [58]. Dyspnoea, chest pain, inspiratory stridor and/or haemoptysis are reported to be present in less than 20% of patients at presentation. Dyspnoea is generally mild, but may be more severe due to alveolar haemorrhage [66], which may cause respiratory failure for which mechanical ventilation is needed occasionally (Figure 3). Chest radiographs may show nodular shadows, infiltrative changes, pleural effusions, and/or atelectasis or different combinations of these radiographic abnormalities [56, 62, 65] (Figures 4 and 5). Hilar and/or mediastinal lymphadenopathy is extremely rare [67–69]. Spontaneous pneumothorax with bronchopleural fistula has been reported [70]. With fiberoptic bronchoscopy, endobronchial inflammatory lesions and/or ulceration are found occasionally. More frequently bronchial stenosis due to involvement of the surrounding parenchyma is seen [65]. Bronchoalveolar lavage reveals a marked increased percentage of neutrophils and often eosinophils [71]. Neutrophilic alveolitis may be present in patients with active WG who have completely normal chest radiographs and CT scans [71]. Pulmonary function tests may reveal obstructive and/or restrictive defects [72], and a reduced diffusing capacity [72]. Pleural fluid analysis reveals an exudate with a predominance of neutrophils [65].

Sixty to 70% of patients with WG and lung disease have nodular shadows on the chest radiograph. Nodules consist of rounded lesions with well-defined margins. In our patients with active disease about one-third of

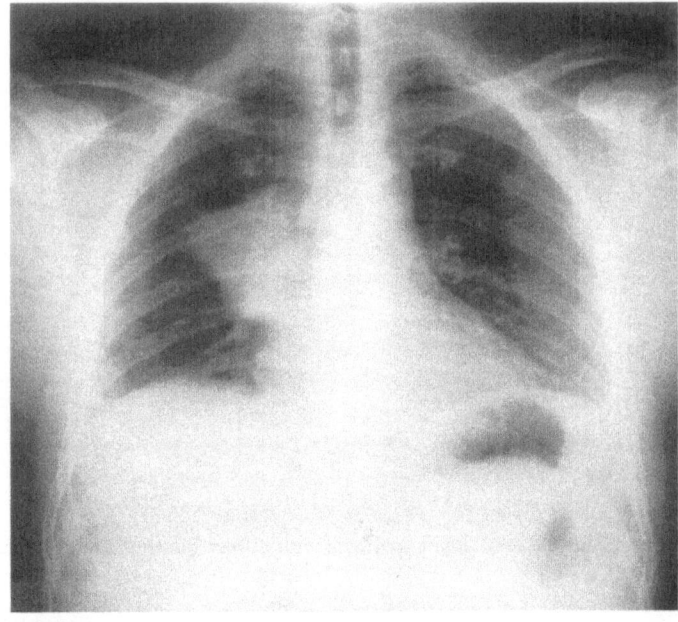

A

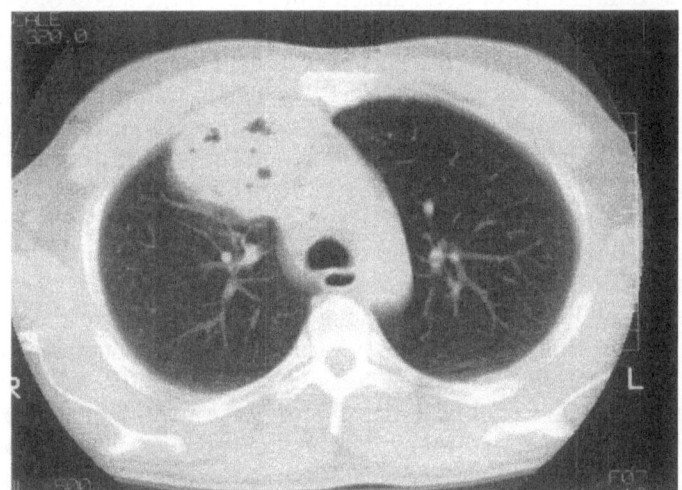

B

Figure 4. (A) Chest radiograph of a 68-year-old man with WG showing a large infiltrative lesion in the medial segment of the middle lobe at initial presentation. (B) CT scan of the same patient as in (A) showing dense consolidation and scant aeration, suggesting early cavitation. (C) CT scan of the same patient as in (A) and (B) 6 months later, showing progression in the right upper lobe with multiple (cavitating) nodular lesions and extensive cavitation of the lesion in the middle lobe.

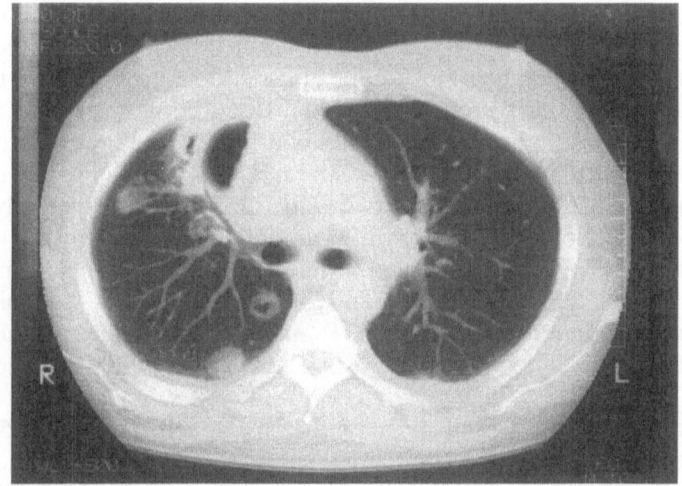

C

Figure 4. (continued)

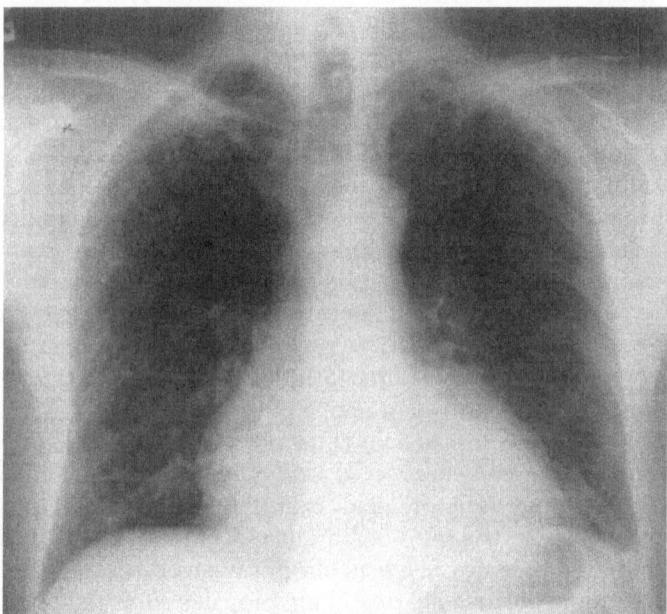

Figure 5. Chest radiograph of a 64-year-old man with WG showing diffuse pulmonary interstitial shadowing, pleural involvement (left upper field) and pericardial effusion.

patients with nodules had single nodules, whereas the remainder had multiple nodules. The size of the nodules varies between 0.5 cm and 10 cm, but most (>65%) are small (<2 cm). No predilection for either lung has been observed in our patient group [62]. In addition, corrected for lung volume, nodules are distributed evenly over upper and lower fields. Most nodules are peripheral in distribution and subpleural [73]. Cavitation occurs in about half of the cases during the disease, especially in the largest nodules. Sometimes cavitation can only be detected by CT scan and not on chest radiograph. Cavitated nodules usually have thick to medium-sized walls and are only infrequently filled with fluid. Secondary infection with *Staphylococcus aureus, Pseudomonas aeruginosa*, anaerobic organisms and/or other microorganisms may occur. Finally, lesions may calcify.

Infiltrates consisting of ill-defined alveolar opacities occur in 50–60% of patients with WG and lung involvement [62]. About 60% of the infiltrates are diffuse, the remainder being more localized. The right lung is more often affected than the left, and perihilar localization is common.

Lobar or segmental atelectasis is found in less than 5% of cases. In addition, 5–20% of patients have pleural effusions that may be attributed to WG [56]. Finally, bronchovascular bundling is often found and is distributed mainly around lobar, segmental and subsegmental bronchi. Occasionally, involvement of the pulmonary artery can be seen on CT [73].

During follow-up most infiltrates and small nodules (<2 cm) disappear within 3–4 months of treatment. Large nodules, however, disappear more slowly and sometimes result in scarring. A substantial number of patients develop pulmonary infections during follow-up, which may be due to a variety of microorganisms and are the cause of death in a significant proportion of cases. In addition, progressive respiratory insufficiency due to diffuse interstitial lung disease may develop during treatment. The aetiology of this abnormality is often unclear. Possible causes are opportunistic infections such as cytomegalovirus infection and/or *Pneumocystis carinii* infection, cyclophosphamide-induced interstitial lung disease, pulmonary embolism, pulmonary fibrosis or active pulmonary WG.

The diagnosis of WG is based upon the presence of typical clinical symptoms and signs, the demonstration of antibodies to PR3 or MPO and histopathological findings. Histological examination of nasal and/or sinus biopsies frequently shows granulomatous inflammation occasionally with vasculitis, kidney biopsies show pauci-immune necrotizing and/or crescentic glomerulonephritis, and open lung biopsies show pathological findings considered to be diagnostic for WG in more than 90% of cases [58]. The most characteristic pathological finding of WG is "pathergic" necrosis and granulomatous inflammation in the absence of infectious or foreign body granulomas, angio-invasive lymphomas and/or rheumatoid nodules [74]. Necrosis may involve large areas of tissue destruction with irregular borders (geographic necrosis). Adjacent to the necrotic areas, neutrophils, eosinophils, lymphocytes, plasma cells, mononuclear histocytes, frequently with an epitheloid appearance, and scattered multinucleated histocytes are found (Figure 6). In addition to extravascular lesions, vasculitis is observed frequently (Figure 7). The vasculitic process may show granulomatous features or may be indistinguishable from other forms of necrotizing angiitis. In addition, focal necrotizing capillaritis ("microvasculitis") may be found. Finally, cicatrical vasculitis is found as the only abnormality in some cases.

Bronchiolitis obliterans organizing pneumonia (BOOP) occurs in a substantial number of patients [75] (see also Chapter 5). Other histological findings include necrotizing chondritis, bronchiectasis, bronchocentric granulomatous inflammation, infiltrates predominantly composed of lymphocytes, sometimes with multiple germinal centers, and interstitial fibrosis. Histological findings of pleural lesions include fibrinous pleuritis and necrotizing granulomatous lesions. Immunohistochemical studies of pulmonary tissue revealed that the lymphocytes within the infiltrates are predominantly T lymphocytes [76]. No immune complexes are found in pulmonary lesions on electron microscopy [77].

Treatment consists of the combination of high-dose steroids and cyclophosphamide. Typically, prednisolone 40−60 mg/day in combination with oral cyclophosphamide 2−2.25 mg/kg body weight per day are used [78]. Predisolone is tapered in 6 to 8 months, and cyclophosphamide over a period of 1 to 2 years. Alternative therapeutic options include pulse cyclophosphamide, MTX, azathioprine or cyclosporine A [78]. In patients with life-threatening disease, pulse methylprednisolone and/or plasma exchange may be added to the standard regimen. Finally, in a few patients with disease localized to the nose or lungs, treatment with sulfamethoxazole/trimethoprim is sufficient to include a prolonged remission [79].

It is possible to induce remissions in most patients, although serious treatment-related morbidity, e.g. opportunistic infections, is frequently observed. However, many patients relapse, either during tapering of the immunosuppressive treatment or after treatment has been stopped. Early detection of relapses may prevent morbidity and treatment-related complications. Careful follow-up is mandatory, with patients instructed to contact a physician in case symptoms of the disease recur. In addition, laboratory abnormalities such as an elevated C-reactive protein level strongly suggest disease activity if infections are not detected. Previously, we found that relapses in WG are preceded by recurrence or increase of ANCAs [38]. In a prospective study of 16 months duration, increases in the ANCA titre preceded all 17 observed relapses. Increases in the ANCA titre were not only a sensitive predictor of disease activity but were also highly specific in this regard [38]. Most ANCA titre rises occur between 3 and 6 months before the relapse is diagnosed and before a rise in C-reactive protein level occurs [80]. These data were confirmed, but disputed by others (reviewed

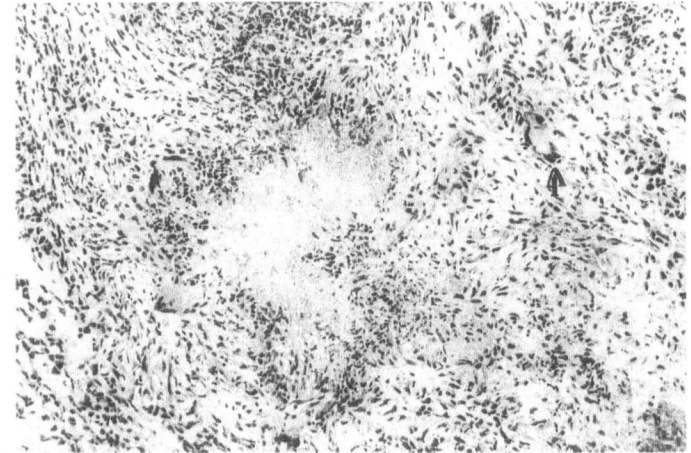

Figure 6. Photomicrograph of a lobectomy (right upper lobe) specimen from a patient with WG. A typical example of granulomatous inflammation is shown with "pathergic" necrosis surrounded by a granulomatous reaction with multi-nucleated giant cells (arrow), other inflammatory cells, and extensive fibrosis (hematoxylin and eosin stain; original magnification ×160).

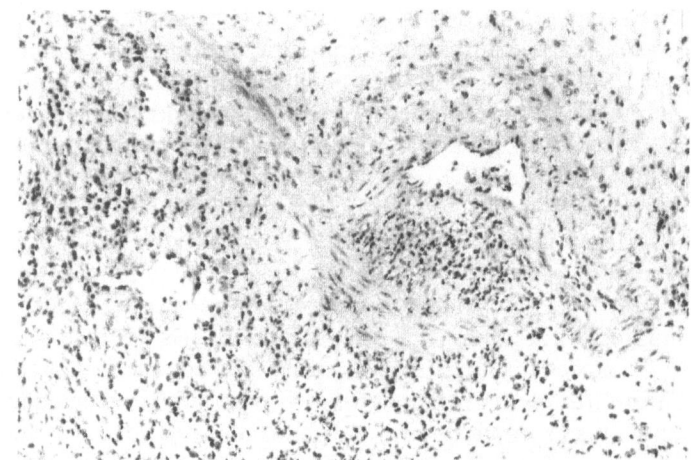

Figure 7. Photomicrograph of a lobectomy (right upper lobe) specimen from a patient with WG showing a medium-sized artery with an active eosinophilic inflammatory infiltate in media and intima. At the left, two alveolar remnants are observed (hematoxylin and eosin stain; original magnification ×160).

in [43]). Based on the aforementioned data, a prospective study was undertaken by our group in which patients were randomized for treatment or no treatment once an increase in the ANCA titre had occurred [81]. During an observation period of 24 months, none of nine patients assigned to immunosuppressive treatment relapsed, as compared with 9 of 11 patients who were not treated at the time their ANCA titres had risen. Interestingly, the total amount of immunosuppressive medication used was lower in the former group than in the latter. Thus, serial quantitation of ANCA levels is useful for following and predicting disease activity in WG. In patients with microscopic polyangiitis (MPA) and CSS serial quantitation of MPO antibody levels may also be useful [43]. At present, however, no prospective studies have been reported in patients with MPO antibodies.

Another risk factor for relapse is the chronic nasal carriage of *S. aureus*. In a prospective study of 3.5 years, we found that *S. aureus* carriers relapse nearly eight times more frequently than non-carriers [82]. In another study of the relation between chronic nasal carriage and disease reactivation, we started a prospective placebo-controlled randomized study with sulfamethoxazole/trimethoprim 800/160 mg b.i.d. for a period of 2 years. Eighty-one patients with WG in complete remission entered the study. During treatment, patients with WG had a 60% decreased risk for a relapse [83]. Furthermore, patients treated with sulfamethoxazole/trimethoprim had significantly fewer respiratory and other infections. Based on these findings, we recommend sulfamethoxazole/trimethoprim therapy during the first years after diagnosis. Furthermore, sequential ANCA determination is useful for monitoring, as an increase in titre alerts the physician that a relapse may occur within the next 3–6 months.

2.4.3. Microscopic polyangiitis: Microscopic polyangiitis (MPA) is characterized by necrotizing and/or crescentic glomerulonephritis (NCGN) ("renal vasculitis") and a multisystem vasculitis involving medium- and/or small-sized vessels but without granulomas. MPA shares many features with WG [84]. Clinically, the most important difference is the lack of ear, nose and throat (ENT) involvement and/or other respiratory tract manifestations – apart from alveolar haemorrhage – in MPA. Only recently has consensus been reached about the definition of this disease [4]. In the past, many patients said to have MPA in one center may have been considered to have WG or CSS in another [85].

Patients with MPA present with malaise, fever, arthralgias and purpura in combination with impaired renal function, proteinuria and microscopic haematuria [84, 86–90] (Table 4). Renal involvement is the major feature of MPA, and most patients have rapidly progressive glomerulonephritis. Often patients present with renal failure for which renal replacement therapy is needed. In addition, 30–60% of patients have haemoptysis with or without alveolar haemorrhage (see later). Chest radiographs show localized or diffuse alveolar shadowing. In contrast to PAN, but similar to other ANCA-associated forms of vasculitis, relapses are common during follow-up.

The diagnosis of MPA is based on clinical findings, the presence of either PR3 or MPO antibodies, and the histopathological finding of necrotizing vasculitis. The diagnosis can only be made after exclusion of other recognized vasculitic syndromes, most notably WG. Histological examination of the kidney shows pauci-immune necrotizing glomerulonephritis with crescent formation and (in a minority of the cases) vasculitis involving arterioles and/or small interlobular arteries. Skin biopsies show leukocytoclastic angiitis involving capillaries, arterioles and venules. If Immunoglobulin A (IgA) deposits are detected in the skin and/or kidney biopsy, a diagnosis of Henoch-Schönlein purpura must be considered. Open lung biopsies in patients with MPA complicated by alveolar haemorrhage show intra-alveolar red blood cells and capillaritis that is only occassionally accompanied by necrotizing vasculitis involving arteries, arterioles and/or venules. In addition, chronic haemorrhage evident by hemosiderin deposition within alveolar macrophages and/or in the interstitium is often found. Therapy of MPA is similar to that of WG and consists of the combination of high-dose steroids and cyclophosphamide. In patients with fulminant disease such as dialysis-dependent renal failure, severe lung haemorrhage or other life-threatening complications, pulse methylprednisolone (1 gm/day for the first 3 days) and/or plasma exchange (6–10 exchanges during the first 2–3 weeks) are added. Currently, multicentre trials are in progress to define the optimal treatment [78].

As in WG, aggressive immunosuppressive therapy is effective in inducing remission in about 80 to 90% of the patients. Recovery of renal function, i.e. being dialysis-independent, occurs in more than half of the patients that are initially dialysis-dependent. Patient survival is 60–80% at 1 year and 60–70% at 5 years [91]. Early deaths, i.e. within the first 2 months, are primarily from active vasculitis, whereas deaths occurring after 2 months of follow-up are primarily due to pulmonary infections, sepsis or vascular disease. In the Chapel Hill experience, the relative risk of death was 8.6 times greater in patients who presented with pulmonary haemorrhage compared with patients without haemorrhage, and 3.8 times greater in patients with c-ANCA compared with patients with ANCA with specificity for MPO [92].

2.4.4. ANCA-associated lung haemorrhage and nephritis: The syndrome of lung haemorrhage and glomerulonephritis is usually called Goodpasture's syndrome. The syndrome has been reported to occur in ANCA-associated vasculitides, including WG, CSS and MPA, and in patients with antibodies to glomerular and alveolar basement membranes (i.e. Goodpasture's *disease*). In addition, this syndrome has also been reported in other diseases, such as drug-induced vasculitis, SLE, Henoch-Schönlein purpura, Behçet's disease and mixed cryoglobulinemia [93].

The majority of patients with this syndrome have ANCA-associated vasculitis. Niles et al. [94] found ANCA in 55 of 88 patients with pulmonary-renal syndrome. Eight of these 55 patients had biopsy-proven WG, 7 had clinical features suggestive of WG, 2 had MPA and 3 had hydralazine-induced vasculitis. Furthermore, 7 other patients with ANCA-associated pulmonary-renal syndrome had linear IgG staining along the GBM in the kidney biopsy, and in 5 of these patients anti-GBM antibodies were detected as well. The remaining 28 patients had isolated pulmonary renal syndrome. Since these patients may have WG at autopsy, Niles et al. [94] suggested that a better clinical term for these patients might be simply "ANCA-associated lung haemorrhage and nephritis" rather than MPA, as was suggested at the consensus meeting at Chapel Hill [4]. In 1990, we reported 8 patients with an ANCA-associated pulmonary renal syndrome [95], in whom 2 had biopsy-proven WG. Since symptoms and signs suggestive of ENT disease were present in all remaining 6 patients, these patients were diagnosed as having "clinically suspected WG" [95]. Ter Maaten et al. [96] reported respiratory failure requiring mechanical ventilation in 9 of 62 patients with ANCA-associated vasculitis and pulmonary involvement. Two of these patients had staphylococcal infection, and the remaining 7 had pulmonary haemorrhage. Two of 7 patients had biopsy-proven WG, 1 additional patient had ENT involvement suggestive of WG, 3 had symptoms suggestive of MPA and the remaining 1 had isolated pulmonary renal syndrome [96]. In addition, Bosch et al. [97] reported 3 patients with isolated necrotizing alveolar capillaritis and anti-MPO. Finally, we reported 1 patient with anti-MPO who was not treated with immunosuppressive treatment and who had recurrent uncomplicated pulmonary haemoptysis and haematuria during an observation period of more than 3 years [44].

The diagnosis of ANCA-associated lung haemorrhage and nephritis is based on clinical findings, the presence of either PR3 or MPO antibodies, and histopathological findings. The diagnosis can only be made after exclusion of other recognized vasculitic syndromes, most notably WG and MPA. Clinical and radiological findings include haemoptysis, localized or diffuse infiltrates on the chest radiograph, anaemia and dyspnoea [93]. The quantity of alveolar bleeding is variable and may only be detected by bronchoscopy and/or bronchoalveolar lavage. Massive haemoptysis is extremely unusual even if lung haemorrhage is life-threatening. The chest radiograph is abnormal in almost all cases, with an alveolar or a mixed alveolar-interstitial pattern. Alveolar haemorrhage should be suspected if the uptake of carbon monoxide (CO) by the lung is increased. The diffusing capacity for CO expressed as the carbon monoxide transfer coefficient (KCO) is increased due to the large pool of extravascular erythrocytes that will bind inhaled CO. Monitoring the activity of the disease process can be done using a single-breath technique of measuring CO uptake. Increases of KCO of 30% or more over baseline are a reliable indicator of active lung hemorrhage [93]. Other markers are sequential hemoglobin levels and serum levels of lactate dehydrogenase (LDH). Patients with ANCAs specific for PR3 are more prone to develop respiratory failure for which mechanical ventilation is needed than patients with ANCAs specific for MPO antibodies [98]. ANCAs in patients with pulmonary-renal syndrome are frequently of both the IgM and IgG isotype [99]. Occasionally IgM ANCAs without IgG ANCAs are found [100].

Histological findings of the kidney and/or lung are similar to the findings in MPA (see above). Vasculitis of arteries, arterioles and/or venules, however, is not found. Treatment is similar to the treatment of MPA and has been described above.

2.5. Henoch-Schönlein Purpura

Henoch-Schönlein purpura (HSP) is a multisystem disease predominantly affecting the skin, joints, gastrointestinal tract and kidneys. HSP, generally, is an illness of childhood, although it can occur in adults of any age. The median age of onset is 4 years.

Patients initially present with palpable purpura. Characteristically, the lesions chiefly involve the buttocks and the legs, and are associated with mild oedema of the lower extremities. As the lesions fade, new crops develop after a few days interval, up to 3 months from onset [101]. The rash is often preceded by an upper respiratory infection. Colicky abdominal pain, vomiting, bloody diarrhoea, melaena, arthralgias and/or arthritis involving the knees or ankles may be associated with or follow the skin lesions. Renal involvement occurs in over one-half of patients. Involvement of other organs is extremely rare [102].

Pulmonary involvement is rare, but does occur [103]. Occasionally, pleuritic chest pain with pleural effusion has been found. Most frequently, however, acute pulmonary haemorrhage has been reported [60, 104–106]. Many reported patients, however, would currently be classified as microscopic polyangiitis, since IgA deposits in skin and/or kidney were not detected. Nearly all children with acute HSP have an impaired diffusion capacity as measured by the lung transfer for CO [107]. The low diffusion capacity was found to be related to disease activity, and return to normal occurred only after complete clinical recovery. Clinical examination, arterial oxygen tensions, and lung volumes were all normal in these children, and the impaired diffusion capacity was the only abnormal pulmonary function test.

HSP is an ANCA-negative disease. The diagnosis of HSP is based on clinical findings in combination with the occurrence of IgA in skin and/or kidney biopsies. Skin biopsies show leukocytoclastic angiitis involving capillaries, arterioles and venules. IgA and C3 deposits are found both in lesions and normal skin [108, 109]. Kidney biopsies show either minimal glomerular abnormalities or mesangial proliferation with or without crescents. Immunofluorescence studies show mesangial dense deposits of IgA often in combination with C3 and/or IgG. In two fatal cases of pulmonary haemorrhage, IgA deposits were found in the alveolar septal vessels [104, 105]. HSP is usually a self-limiting disease. In the case of pulmonary haemorrhage, however, aggressive immunosuppressive treatment as in ANCA-associated pulmonary renal syndrome has to be started [93] (see above). The efficacy of this therapy is not well known, but it is likely that aggressive therapy contributes to improved outcome. For instance, in the report by Olsen et al. [106], three of four children demonstrated a dramatic improvement during immunosuppressive treatment.

2.6. Cutaneous Leukocytoclastic Angiitis

Cutaneous leukocytoclastic angiitis (LCA) or cutaneous necrotizing vasculitis is a form of vasculitis that predominantly involves the skin. Idiopathic cutaneous LCA is a diagnosis of exclusion. At least three clinically distinctive types of idiopathic cutaneous LCA exist [110]:

1. idiopathic palpable purpura, the most common form of idiopathic cutaneous LCA; lesions are most often located on the lower extremities and tend to be chronic and/or recurrent,
2. urticarial (or hypocomplementemic) vasculitis; patients have urticaria-like lesions that tend to persist longer (more than 24 h) than typical urticaria and are associated with a burning sensation of the skin,
3. erythema elevatum diutinum; patients have persistent red to purple papules usually localized to the extensor surfaces of the extremities especially over the joints.

Symptoms such as low-grade fever, malaise and/or arthralgias are present in only a small proportion of cases. Even during long-term follow-up there is no progression to systemic disease. By definition, pulmonary involvement is not seen in this form of vasculitis.

The diagnosis of idiopathic cutaneous LCA is based on clinical and histopathological findings. The diagnosis can only be made after exclusion of other idiopathic or secondary vasculitic disorders. Histological examination of the skin shows leukocytoclastic angiitis involving capillaries, arterioles and venules. No IgA deposits are detected by immunofluorescence microscopy. Therapy is often not necessary. For patients with severe or recurrent episodes of skin vasculitis, treatment with dapsone, colchicine or prednisolone may be considered. Only occasionally are steroids indicated. Forty to sixty milligrams per day of prednisolone is very effective and will promptly control most episodes of skin vasculitis. A rapid taper over approximately 1 to 2 months should be attemped after disease activity has been controlled. In patients with a chronic course, dapsone 50–150 mg/day is often helpful. An alternative therapy is the use of 0.6–1.2 mg/day of colchicine. Its success rate is variable, and its usefulness is often limited by diarrhoea.

2.7. Miscellaneous Vasculitic Syndromes

2.7.1. Behçet's disease: This disease is a multisystem vasculitis in which virtually any organ system may be involved. The combination of ulcers of the mouth and genitalia with relapsing uveitis comprises Behçet's classic triad. In addition, venous thrombosis, thrombophlebitis and skin lesions such as erythema nodosum are frequently encountered. Involvement of the central nervous system (CNS) occurs in a substantial number of patients. Neuropsychiatric manifestations usually develop years after the onset of the disease, but may also be the presenting symptom. The neurological manifestations have a tendency to relapse and remit; in fact, this is one of the most characteristic features of the disease [10]. Furthermore, arthritis and involvement of the heart, kidneys and the gastrointestinal tract have been reported. Finally, pulmonary involvement has been reported [111]. Pulmonary symptoms include dyspnoea, cough, haemoptysis and pleuritic chest pain. Chest radiographs and/or CT scans may show infiltrates, pleural effusions and/or mediastinal widening, which may be caused by thrombosis of the superior vena cava [112].

Haemoptysis and dyspnoea may be caused by alveolar haemorrhage [111]. In addition, haemoptysis may be due to pulmonary arteritis, which frequently results in arterial aneurysm formation [113, 114]. This complication is associated with a bad prognosis, and rupture of pulmonary aneurysms is a leading cause of death in Behçet's disease. Other complications of pulmonary artery vasculitis include pulmonary vascular thromboses, infarcts, massive haemoptysis due to bronchial erosion by pulmonary artery aneurysms and formation of an arteriobronchial fistula [113–115]. The association of haemoptysis, dyspnoea and pleuritic chest pain in these patients is suggestive of pulmonary infarction secondary to thromboembolism. Differentiation between pulmonary thromboembolism and pulmonary arteritis complicated by thrombosis in these patients is difficult, and only occasionally is the correct diagnosis suggested by the angiographic finding of pulmonary artery aneurysms. Finally, it is felt that the Hughes-Stovin syndrome, which is characterized by major vessel venous thrombosis and pulmonary arterial aneurysms, is a variant of Behçet's disease [116].

Pulmonary manifestations of Behçet's need aggressive immunosuppressive treatment with corticosteroids and cyclophosphamide, similar to the treatment described for WG. If haemoptysis continues and a bleeding site can be established, arterial embolisation or surgery has to be considered [113].

2.7.2. Kawasaki's disease: or mucocutaneous lymph node syndrome is a disease characterized by high fever, conjunctivitis, strawberry tongue, diffuse reddening of oral and pharyngeal mucosa, swelling of cervical lymph nodes, polymorphous exanthema and erythema with desquamation of the skin of the hands and/or fingertips. Most cases occur in young children usually under 4 years of age. The disease is complicated by a systemic necrotizing vasculitis predominantly symptomatic in the coronary arteries. Other organs may be affected as well, and pulmonary manifestations have been found during the acute phase [117]. Cough is present in about 30% of the patients. In addition, about 15% have an abnormal chest radiograph. Abnormal findings include an interstitial pattern, peribronchial cuffing, pleural effusion and atelectasis [117]. On autopsy, interstitial pneumonia, bronchopneumonia, pleuritis and pulmonary arteritis have been documented [118, 119]. Treatment of Kawasaki's disease consists of a combination of aspirin and intravenous gamma globulin. The overall outlook for children with Kawasaki disease is good. Acute mortality due to myocardial infarction is rare. There may, however, be a late morbidity and occasionally mortality due to coronary arterial stenotic lesions in later life.

2.8. Secondary Forms of Vasculitis

Vasculitis may be the primary pathological process or secondary to other conditions (Table 1).

2.8.1. Drug-induced vasculitis: This can result in a pulmonary renal syndrome (see also Chapter 11). Drugs that are especially involved include hydralazine, D-penicillamine and propylthiouracil. Recently, it has been demonstrated that in these cases ANCAs with specificity for MPO and elastase are nearly always found [43].

2.8.2. Lymphomatoid granulomatosis: This is a disease characterized by infiltration of small- and medium-sized blood vessels by lymphocytes, predominantly T-cells [120]. It is one of the so-called angiocentric immunoproliferative lesions, i.e. a malignant lymphoproliferative disorder, and not strictly a form of vasculitis, since vessels are not inflamed but infiltrated. Patients present with weakness, fatigue, fever and weight loss. The lungs, skin and nervous system are involved frequently. The chest radiograph typically shows multiple nodular densities, which may cavitate. Other findings include hilar adenopathy, reticular infiltrates and pleural effusions. Therapy is similar as for other lymphomas with either radiotherapy and/or chemotherapy.

2.8.3. Sarcoidosis: This may involve virtually any organ, and the lungs are involved frequently (see also Chapter 4). Arteries and veins are affected in typical pulmonary sarcoid granulomas. Elastic stains often reveal destruction of the elastica. Vessels may be occluded, but overt vascular necrosis is extremely rare. So sarcoidosis may be considered a form of pulmonary vasculitis [121]. Liebow described a variant of sarcoidosis, i.e. nodular necrotizing sarcoidosis, in which the pulmonary sarcoid lesions have features similar to those in patients WG [122]. In these cases the lesions are nodular, may be solitary or multiple, and unilateral or bilateral and can cavitate. In addition, hilar lymphadenopathy is often present. By histological examination, typical sarcoid-type granulomas, central necrosis and granulomatous vasculitis are found [121]. In contrast to WG, clinical outcome with corticosteroid therapy alone is excellent in most cases.

2.8.4. Autoimmune rheumatic diseases: Autoimmune rheumatic diseases such as SLE, rheumatoid arthritis, scleroderma, mixed connective tissue disease and Sjögren's syndrome are often accompanied by pulmonary involvement (see also Chapter 2). Documented vasculitis, however, is relatively uncommon in these diseases. In SLE, acute necrotizing vasculitis involving small vessels, including capillaries, has been implicated in pulmonary haemorrhage [123]. Pulmonary hypertension in SLE may be due to vasculitis [124]. In addition, a more or less non-inflammatory vascular disease may affect the pulmonary arteries, also resulting in pulmonary hypertension. It has been hypothesized that this form of vascular disease is also related to vasculitis, although the exact pathogenesis is not known [125]. In rheumatoid arthritis, pulmonary vasculitis usually presents with pulmonary hypertension. In addition, vasculitic lesions have been shown in the pathology of rheumatoid nodules and, occasionally, rheumatoid interstitial lung disease [28].

2.8.5. Mixed cryoglobulinaemia: This is a form of vasculitis which is often seen as an idiopathic form of vasculitis [4]. It has been known for years that cryoglobulinemia can be a primary disorder or a disorder associated with haematological malignancies, infections and/or autoimmune rheumatic diseases such as Sjögren's syndrome. Recently it became evident that the primary or "essential" form of mixed cryoglobulinaemia is related to hepatitis C infection in most cases [126, 127]. Patients with cryoglobulinaemia often complain of weakness. Classic clinical findings include purpura, arthralgias and glomerulonephritis, and alveolar haemorrhage due to pulmonary vasculitis has been described [93]. A small decrease in diffusing capacity has been reported as well [128].

2.8.6. Infection-related vasculitis: Polyarteritis-type necrotizing vasculitis may occur during hepatitis B and HIV infection. In addition, necrotizing granulomatous vasculitis, which is indistinguishable from that seen in WG has been reported in patients with mycobacterial and fungal infections [60].

3. Summary

The vasculitides frequently involve the lung. Pulmonary manifestations of ANCA-associated vasculitides such as Wegener's granulomatosis, the Churg-Strauss syndrome, and microscopic polyangiitis, are often a presenting symptom. Lesions may be due to granulomatous inflammation or vasculitis of arteries or arterioles. In addition, alveolar haemorrhage due to pulmonary capillaritis may be found. Alveolar haemorrhage may also rarely be found in Henoch-Schönlein purpura and secondary forms of small-vessel vasculitis. Other vasculitides, in particular, Takayasu arteritis, giant cell arteritis, and Behçet's disease may result in vasculitis of the pulmonary arteries.

Therapy consists of corticosteroids, which are often combined with cyclophosphamide or other immunosuppressive agents. In cases with severe forms of vasculitis plasma exchange may be attempted.

Acknowledgement

Dr. Cohen Tervaert is supported by a grant from the Royal Netherlands Academy of Arts and Sciences.

References

1. Sundy JS, Haynes BF (1995) Pathogenic mechanisms of vessel damage in vasculitis syndromes. *Rheum Dis Clin N Am* 21: 861–881.
2. Cohen Tervaert JW, Kallenberg CGM (1997) Cell adhesion molecules in vasculitis. *Curr Opin Rheumatol* 9: 16–25.
3. Cohen Tervaert JW, Kallenberg CGM (1996) The role of autoimmunity to myeloid lysosomal enzymes in the pathogenesis of vasculitis. In: Hansson GK, Libby P (eds). *Immune functions of the vessel wall*. London: Harwood Academic Publishers, 99–120.
4. Jennette JC, Falk RJ, Andrassy K, Bacon PA, Churg J, Gross WL, Hagen EC, Hoffman GS, Hunder GG, Kallenberg CGM, et al. (1994) Nomenclature of systemic vasculitides: The proposal of an international consensus conference. *Arthritis Rheum* 37: 187–192.
5. Hunder GG, Arend WP, Bloch DA, Calabrese LH, Fauci AS, Fries JF, Leavitt RY, Lie JT, Lightfoot RW, Masi AT, et al. (1990) The American College of Rheumatology 1990 criteria for the classification of vasculitis. *Arthritis Rheum* 33: 1065–1136.
6. Alarcón-Segovia D (1980) Classification of the necrotizing vasculitides in man. *Rheum Dis Clin N Am* 6: 223–231.
7. Lie JT (1992) Vasculitis, 1815 to 1991: classification and diagnostic specificity. *J Rheumatol* 19: 83–89.
8. Lie JT (1994) Nomenclature and classification of vasculitis: Plus ça change, plus c'est la meme chose. *Arthritis Rheum* 37: 181–186.

9. Kallenberg CGM, Mulder AHL, Cohen Tervart JW (1992) Antineutrophil cytoplasmic antibodies: A still-growing class of autoantibodies in inflammatory disorders. *Am J Med* 93: 675–682.
10. Cohen Tervaert JW, Kallenberg CGM (1993) Neurologic manifestations of systemic vasculitides. *Rheum Dis Clin N Am* 19: 913–940.
11. Cohen Tervaert JW, Limburg PC, Elema JD, Huitema MG, Horst G, The TH, Kallenberg CGM (1991) Detection of autoantibodies against myeloid lysosomal enzymes: A useful adjunct to classification of patients with biopsy-proven necrotizing arteritis. *Am J Med* 91: 59–66.
12. Lie JT (1991) Takayasu's arteritis. In: Churg A, Churg J (eds). *Systemic vasculitides*. New York: Igaku-Shoin, 159–179.
13. Kerr GS (1995) Takayasu's arteritis. *Rheum Dis Clin N Am* 21: 1041–1058.
14. Hayashi K, Nagasaki M, Matsunaga N, Hombo Z, Imamura T (1986) Initial pulmonary artery involvement in Takayasu arteritis. *Radiology* 159: 401–403.
15. Kreidstein SH, Lytwyn A, Keystone EC (1993) Takayasu arteritis with acute interstitial pneumonia and coronary vasculitis: Expanding the spectrum. Report of a case. *Arthritis Rheum* 36: 1175–1178.
16. Lupi-Herrera E, Sanchéz Torres G, Horwitz S, Gutierrez E (1975) Pulmonary artery involvement in Takayasu's arteritis. *Chest* 67: 69–74.
17. Yamato M, Lecky JW, Hiramatsu K, Kohda E (1986) Takayasu arteritis: Radiographic and angiographic findings in 59 patients. *Radiology* 161: 329–334.
18. Kawai C, Ishikawa K, Ishii Y, Kato M, Nakao K (1978) Pulmonary pulseless disease: Pulmonary involvement in so-called Takayasu's disease. *Chest* 73: 651–657.
19. Park JH, Chung JW, Im JG, Kim SK, Park YB, Han MC (1995) Takayasu arteritis: Evaluation of mural changes in the aorta and pulmonary artery with CT angiography. *Radiology* 196: 89–93.
20. Matsubara O, Yoshimura N, Tamura A, Kasuga T, Yamada I, Numano F, Mark EJ (1992) Pathological features of the pulmonary artery in Takayasu arteritis: *Heart Vessels* (Suppl.) 7: 18–25.
21. Fauchald P, Rygvold O, Oystese B (1972) Temporal arteritis and polymyalgia rheumatica: clinical and biopsy findings. *Ann Intern Med* 77: 845–852.
22. Huston KA, Hunder GG, Lie JT, Kennedy RH, Elveback LR (1978) Temporal arteritis: A 25-year epidemiologic, clinical and pathologic study. *Ann Intern Med* 88: 162–167.
23. Sonnenblick M, Nesher G, Rosin A (1989) Nonclassical organ involvement in temporal arteritis. *Sem Arthritis Rheum* 19: 183–190.
24. Larson TS, Hall S, Hepper NGG, Hunder GG (1984) Respiratory tract symptoms as a clue to giant cell arteritis. *Ann Intern Med* 101: 594–597.
25. Gur H, Ehrenfeld M, Izsak E (1996) Pleural effusion as a presenting manifestation of giant cell arteritis. *Clin Rheumatol* 15: 200–203.
26. Nishino H, DeRemee RA, Rubino FA, Parisi JE (1993) Wegener's granulomatosis associated with vasculitis of the temporal artery: Report of five cases. *Mayo Clin Proc* 68: 115–121.
27. Amato MBP, Barbas CSV, Delmonte VC, Carvalho CRR (1989) Concurrent Churg-Strauss syndrome and temporal arteritis in a young patient with pulmonary nodules. *Am Rev Respir Dis* 139: 1539–1542.
28. Staudt LS, Silver RM (1992) The lung and vasculitis. In: LeRoy EC (ed). *Systemic vasculitis: The biologic basis*. New York: Marcel Dekker, 273–301.
29. Chassagne P, Gligorov J, Dominique S (1995) Pulmonary artery obstruction and giant cell arteritis. *Ann Intern Med* 122: 732.
30. De Heide LJM, Pieterman H, Henneman G (1995) Pulmonary infarction caused by giant-cell arteritis of the pulmonary artery. *Neth J Med* 46: 36–40.
31. Rosen S, Falk RJ, Jennette JC (1991) Polyarteritis nodosa, including microscopic form and renal vasculitis. In: Churg A, Churg J (eds). *Systemic vasculitides*. New York: Igaku-Shoin, 57–77.
32. Somer T, Finegold SM (1995) Vasculitides associated with infections, immunization and antimicrobial drugs. *Clin Infect Dis* 20: 1010–1036.
33. Guillevin L, Lhote F, Cohen P, Sauvaget F, Jarrousse B, Lortholary O, Noël L-H, Trépo C (1995) Polyarteritis nodosa related to hepatitis B: A prospective study with long-term observation of 41 patients. *Medicine* 74: 238–253.

34. Conn DL, McDuffie FC, Holley KE, Schroeter AL (1976) Immunologic mechanisms in systemic vasculitis. *Mayo Clin Proc* 51: 511–518.
35. Moreland LW, Ball GV (1990) Cutaneous polyarteritis nodosa. *Am J Med* 88: 426–430.
36. Dyck PJ, Benstead TJ, Conn DL, Stevens JC, Windebank AJ, Low PA (1987) Nonsystemic vasculitic neuropathy. *Brain* 110: 843–853.
37. Kallenberg CGM, Brouwer E, Weening JJ, Cohen Tervaert JW (1994) Anti-neutrophil cytoplasmic antibodies: Current diagnostic and pathophysiological potential. *Kidney Int* 46: 1–15.
38. Cohen Tervaert JW, van der Woude FJ, Fauci AS, Ambrus JL, Velosa J, Keane WF, Meyer S, van der Giessen M, The TH, van der Hem GK, Kallenberg CGM (1989) Association between active Wegener's granulomatosis and anticytoplasmic antibodies. *Arch Int Med* 149: 2461–2465.
39. Nölle B, Specks V, Lüdemann J, Rohrbach MS, DeRemee RA, Gross WL (1989) Anticyto-plasmic autoantibodies: Their immunodiagnostic value in Wegener's granulomatosis. *Ann Intern Med* 111: 28–40.
40. Wiik A, Rasmussen N, Wieslander J (1993) Methods to detect autoantibodies to neutro-philic granulocytes. In: *Manual of biological markers of disease A9*. Amsterdam: Kluwer Academic Publishers, 1–14.
41. Cohen Tervaert JW, Mulder AHL, Kallenberg CGM (1993) Perinuclear antineutrophil cytoplasmic antibodies (P-ANCA): Clinical significance and relation to antibodies against myeloid lysosomal enzymes. *Adv Exp Med Biol* 336: 253–256.
42. Falk RJ, Jennette JC (1988) Anti-neutrophil cytoplasmic autoantibodies with specificity for myeloperoxidase in patients with systemic vasculitis and idiopathic necrotizing and crescentic glomerulonephritis. *N Engl J Med* 318: 1651–1657.
43. Cohen Tervaert JW (1996) The value of serial ANCA testing during follow-up studies in patients with ANCA-associated vasculitides: A review. *J Nephrol* 9: 232–240.
44. Cohen Tervaert JW, Goldschmeding R, Elema JD, Limburg PC, van der Giessen M, Huitema MG, Koolen MI, Hené RJ, The TH, van der Hem GK, et al. (1990) Association of autoantibodies to myeloperoxidase with different forms of vasculitis. *Arthritis Rheum* 33: 1264–1272.
45. Cohen Tervaert JW, Mulder AHL, Stegeman CA, Huitema MG, The TH, Kallenberg CGM (1993) The occurrence of autoantibodies to human leukocyte elastase in Wegener's granulomatosis and other inflammatory disorders. *Ann Rheum Dis* 52: 115–120.
46. Lanham JG, Elkon KB, Pusey CD, Hughes GR (1984) Systemic vasculitis with asthma and eosinophilia: A clinical approach to the Churg-Strauss syndrome. *Medicine* 63: 65–81.
47. Lanham JG, Churg J (1991) Churg-Strauss syndrome. In: Churg A, Churg J (ed). *Systemic vasculitides*. New York: Igaku-Shoin, 101–120.
48. Masi AT, Hunder GG, Lie JT, Michel BA, Bloch DA, Arend WP (1990) The American College of Rheumatology 1990 criteria for the classification of Churg-Strauss syndrome (allergic granulomatosis and angiitis). *Arthritis Rheum* 33: 1094–1100.
49. Hueto-Perez-de-Heredia JJ, Dominguez-del-Vall FJ, Garcia E, Gomez ML, Gallego J (1994) Chronic eosinophilic pneumonia as a presenting feature of Churg-Strauss syndrome. *Eur Respir J* 7: 1006–1008.
50. Amundsen DE (1992) Cavitary pulmonary cryptococcosis complicating Churg-Strauss vasculitis. *South Med J* 85: 700–702.
51. Erzerum SC, Underwood GA, Hamilos DL, Waldron JA (1989) Pleural effusion in Churg-Strauss syndrome. *Chest* 95: 1357–1359.
52. Wallaert B, Gosset P, Prin L, Bart F, Marquette CH, Tonnel AB (1993) Bronchoalveolar lavage in allergic granulomatosis and angiitis. *Eur J Respir J* 6: 413–417.
53. Siegert CEH, Cohen Tervaert JW, Heemskerk E, Kallenberg CGM, van Es LA, Daha MR (1996) Occurrence of antibodies to bactericidal permeability-increasing protein in sera with perinuclear anti-neutrophil cytoplasmic antibody (P-ANCA) reactivity. *Sarcoidosis Vasc Diffuse Lung Dis* 13: A279.
54. Chumbley LC, Harrison EG, DeRemee RA (1977) Allergic granulomatosis and angiitis (Churg-Strauss syndrome): Report and analysis of 30 cases. *Mayo Clinic Proc* 52: 477–484.
55. Lhote F, Guillevin L (1995) Polyarteritis nodosa, microscopic polyangiitis and Churg-Strauss syndrome: Clinical aspects and treatment. *Rheum Dis Clin N Am* 21: 911–947.

56. Duna GF, Galperin C, Hoffman GS (1995) Wegener's granulomatosis. *Rheum Dis Clin N Am* 21: 949–986.
57. Cohen Tervaert JW, van der Woude FJ, Kallenberg CGM (1987) Analysis of the symptoms preceding the diagnosis of Wegener's disease. *Ned Tijdschr Geneesk* 131: 1391–1394.
58. Hoffman GS, Kerr GS, Leavitt RY, Hallahan CW, Lebovics RS, Travis WD (1992) Wegener granulomatosis: An analysis of 158 patients. *Ann Intern Med* 116: 488–498.
59. Specks U, DeRemee RA (1990) Granulomatous vasculitis: Wegener's granulomatosis and Churg-Strauss syndrome. *Rheum Dis Clin N America* 16: 377–397.
60. Leavitt RY, Fauci AS (1986) Pulmonary vasculitis. *Am Rev Respir Dis* 134: 149–166.
61. Lieberman K, Churg A (1991) Wegener's granulomatosis. In: Churg A, Churg J (eds). *Systemic vasculitides*. New York: Igaku-Shoin, 79–99.
62. Van der Werf TS, Vrieze A, Cohen Tervaert JW, Stegeman CA (1997) Chest radiographic pattern in Wegener's granulomatosis. *Am J Respir Crit Care Med* 153: A984
63. Kuhlman JE, Hruban RH, Fishman EK (1991) Wegener granulomatosis: CT features of parenchymal lung disease. *J Comput Assist Tomogr* 15: 948–952.
64. King TE Jr (1996) A lung biopsy is necessary in the management of ANCA positive patients with chest roentgenographic abnormalities. *Sarcoidosis Vasc Diffuse Lung Dis* 13: 232–234.
65. Cordier JF, Valeyre D, Guillevin L, Loire R, Brechot JM (1990) Pulmonary Wegener's granulomatosis: A clinical and imaging study of 77 cases. *Chest* 97: 906–912.
66. Haworth SJ, Savage COS, Carr D, Hughes JMB, Rees AJ (1985) Pulmonary haemorrhage complicating Wegener's granulomatosis and microscopic polyarteritis. *Br Med J* 290: 1775–1778.
67. Boudes P (1990) Mediastinal tumour as the presenting manifestation of Wegener's granulomatosis. *J Intern Med* 227: 215–217.
68. Gutiérrez-Ravé VM, Ayerza MA (1991) Hilar and mediastinal lymphadenopathy in the limited form of Wegener's granulomatosis. *Thorax* 46: 219–220.
69. Van der Werf TS, Stegeman CA, Meuzelaar KJ, Timens W (1994) Late recurrence of Wegener's granulomatosis presenting as solitary upper lobe mass. *Eur Respir J* 7: 1365–1368.
70. Jaspan T, Davison AM, Walker WC (1982) Spontaneous pneumothorax in Wegener's granulomatosis. *Thorax* 37: 774–775.
71. Hoffman GS, Sechler JMG, Gallin JI, Shelhamer JH, Suffredini A, Ognibene FP, Baltaro RJ, Fleisher TA, Leavitt RY, Travis WD, et al. (1991) Bronchoalveolar lavage analysis in Wegener's granulomatosis: A method to study disease pathogenesis. *Am Rev Respir Dis* 143: 401–407.
72. Rosenberg DM, Weinberger SE, Fulmer JD, Flye MW, Fauci AS, Crystal RG (1980) Functional correlates of lung involvement in Wegener's granulomatosis: Use of pulmonary function tests in staging and follow-up. *Am J Med* 69: 387–394.
73. Papiris SA, Manoussakis MN, Drosos AA, Kontogiannis D, Constantopoulos SH, Moutsopoulos HM (1992) Imaging of thoracic Wegener's granulomatosis: The computed tomographic appearance. *Am J Med* 93: 529–536.
74. Fienberg R, Mark EJ, Goodman M, McKluskey RT, Niles JL (1993) Correlation of antineutrophil cytoplasmic antibodies with the extrarenal histopathology of Wegener's (pathergic) granulomatosis and related forms of vasculitis. *Hum Pathol* 24: 160–168.
75. Gaudin PB, Askin FB, Falk RJ, Jennette JC (1995) The pathologic spectrum of pulmonary lesions in patients with antineutrophil cytoplasmic autoantibodies specific for anti-proteinase 3 and anti-myeloperoxidase. *Am J Clin Pathol* 104: 7–16.
76. Gephardt GN, Ahmad M, Tubbs R (1983) Pulmonary vasculitis (Wegener's granulomatosis). *Am J Med* 74: 700–704.
77. Brown RW, Clarkson DR, Coalson JJ (1991) Ultrastructural observations in Wegener's granulomatosis. *Arch Pathol Lab Med* 115: 426.
78. Rasmussen N, Jayne DRW, Abramowicz D, Andrassy K, Bacon PA, Cohen Tervaert JW, Dadonlené J, Feighery C, van Es LA, Ferrario F, et al. (1995) European therapeutic trials in ANCA-associated systemic vasculitis: Disease scoring, consensus regimens and proposed clinical trials. *Clin Exp Immunol* (S1) 101: 29–34.

79. Kallenberg CGM, Stegeman CA, Cohen Tervaert JW (1996) Staphylococcus aureus, Trimethoprim-Sulfamethoxazole and Wegener's granulomatosis. *Sarcoidosis Vasc Diffuse Lung Dis* 13: 253–255.
80. Stegeman CA, Cohen Tervaert JW, Huitema MG, Kallenberg CGM (1993) Serum markers of T-cell activation in relapses of Wegener's granulomatosis. *Clin Exp Immunol* 91: 415–420.
81. Cohen Tervaert JW, Huitema MG, Hene RJ, Sluiter WJ, The Th, van der Hem GK, Kallenberg CGM (1990) Prevention of relapses of Wegener's Granulomatosis by treatment based on antineutrophil cytoplasmic antibody titre. *Lancet* 336: 709–711.
82. Stegeman CA, Cohen Tervaert JW, Manson WL, Sluiter WJ, de Jong PE, Kallenberg CGM (1994) Chronic nasal carriage of *Staphylococcal aureus* in Wegener's granulomatosis identifies a subgroup of patients more to relapses. *Ann Int Med* 120: 12–17.
83. Stegeman CA, Cohen Tervaert JW, De Jong PE, Kallenberg CGM, on behalf of the Dutch Co-trimoxazole Study Group (1996) Trimethoprim-sulfamethoxazole (co-trimoxazole) for the prevention of relapses of Wegener's granulomatosis. *N Engl J Med* 335: 16–20.
84. Savage COS, Winearls CG, Evans DJ, Rees AJ, Lockwood CM (1985) Microscopic polyarteritis: Presentation, pathology and prognosis. *Q J Med* 56: 467–483.
85. Hoffman GS (1996) ANCAs: Are they important? *J Nephrol* 9: 216–218.
86. Serra A, Cameron JS, Turner DR, Hartley B, Ogg CS, Neild GH et al. (1984) Vasculitis affecting the kidney: Presentation, histopathology and long-term outcome. *Q J Med* 53: 181–207.
87. D'Agati V, Chander P, Nash M, Mancilla-Jiminez R (1986) Idiopathic microscopic polyarteritis nodosa: Ultrastructural observations on the renal vascular and glomerular lesions. *Am J Kidney Dis* 7: 95–110.
88. Adu D, Howie AJ, Scott DGI, Bacon PA, McGonigle RJ, Michael J (1987) Polyarteritis and the kidney. *Q J Med* 62: 221–237.
89. Rodgers H, Guthrie JA, Brownjohn AM, Turney JH (1989) Microscopic polyarteritis: Clinical features and treatment. *Postgrad Med J* 65: 515–518.
90. Andrews M, Edmunds M, Campbell A, Walls J, Feehally J (1990) Systemic vasculitis in the 1980s: Is there an increasing incidence of Wegener's granulomatosis and microscopic polyarteritis? *J Royal Coll Physicians London* 24: 284–288.
91. Gaskin G, Pusey CD (1992) Systemic vasculitis. In: Cameron JS, Davison AM, Grunfeld J, Kerr DNS, Ritz E (eds). *Oxford textbook of clinical nephrology*. Oxford: Oxford University Press, 612–636.
92. Hogan SL, Nachman PH, Wilkman AS, Jennette JC, Falk RJ and the glomerular disease collaborative network (1996) Prognostic markers in patients with antineutrophil cytoplasmic autoantibody-associated microscopic polyangiitis and glomerulonephritis. *J Am Soc Nephrol* 7: 23–32.
93. Leatherman JW (1987) Immune alveolar hemorrhage. *Chest* 91: 891–897.
94. Niles JL, Böttinger EP, Saurina GR, Kelly KJ, Pan G, Collins B, McCluskey RT (1996) The syndrome of lung hemorrhage and nephritis is usually an ANCA-associated condition. *Arch Intern Med* 156: 440–445.
95. Cohen Tervaert JW, Goldschmeding R, Elema JD, van der Giessen M, Huitema MG, van der Hem GK, The TH, von dem Borne AEGKr, Kallenberg CGM (1990) Autoantibodies against myeloid lysosomal enzymes in crescentic glomerulonephritis. *Kidney Int* 37: 799–806.
96. Ter Maaten JC, Franssen CFM, Gans ROB, Strack van Schijndel RJM, Hoorntje SJ (1996) Respiratory failure in ANCA-associated vasculitis. *Chest* 110: 357–362.
97. Bosch X, Font J, Mirapeix E, Revert L, Ingelmo M, Urbano-Márquez (1992) Antimycloperoxidase autoantibody-associated necrotizing alveolar capillaritis. *Am Rev Respir Dis* 146: 1326–1329.
98. Goldschmeding R, Cohen Tervaert JW, Gans ROB, Dolman KM, van den Ende ME, Kuizinga MC, Kallenberg CGM, von dem Borne AEGKr (1990) Different immunological specificities and disease assocations of c-ANCA and p-ANCA. *Neth J Med* 36: 114–116.
99. Esnault VLM, Soleimani B, Keogan MT, Brownlee AA, Jayne DRW, Lockwood CM (1992) Association of IgM with IgG ANCA in patients presenting with pulmonary hemorrhage. *Kidney Int* 41: 1304–1310.

100. Jayne DRW, Jones SJ, Severn A, Shaunak S, Murphy J, Lockwood CM (1989) Severe pulmonary hemorrhage and systemic vasculitis in association with circulating anti-neutrophil cytoplasm antibodies of IgM class only. *Clin Nephrol* 32: 101–106.
101. White RHR (1991) Henoch-Schönlein purpura. In: Churg A, Churg J (eds). *Systemic vasculitides.* New York: Igaku-Shoin, 203–217.
102. Ilan Y, Naparstek Y (1991) Schönlein Henoch syndrome in adults and children. *Sem Arthritis Rheum* 21: 103–109.
103. Cream JJ, Gumpel JM, Peachey RDG (1970) Schönlein-Henoch purpura in the adult: A study of 77 adults with anaphylactoid or Schönlein-Henoch purpura. *Q J Med* 39: 461–484.
104. Kathuria S, Chejfec G (1982) Fatal pulmonary Henoch-Schönlein syndrome. *Chest* 82: 654–656.
105. Yokose T, Aida J, Ito Y, Ogura M, Nakagawa S, Nagai T (1993) A case of pulmonary hemorrhage in Henoch-Schönlein purpura accompanied by polyarteritis nodosa in an elderly man. *Respiration* 60: 307–310.
106. Olson JC, Kelly KJ, Pan CG, Wortmann DW (1992) Pulmonary disease with hemorrhage in Henoch-Schönlein purpura. *Pediatrics* 89: 1177–1181.
107. Chaussain M, de Boissieu D, Kalifa G, Epelbaum S, Niaudet P, Badoual J, Gendrel D (1992) Impairment of lung diffusion capacity in Schönlein-Henoch purpura. *J Pediatr* 121: 12–16.
108. Baart de la Faille-Kuyper EH, Kater L, Kooiker CL, Corhout Mees EJ (1973) IgA-deposits in cutaneous blood-vessel walls and mesangium in Henoch-Schönlein syndrome. *Lancet* 1: 892–893.
109. Baart de la Faille-Kuyper EH, Kater L, Kuyten RH, Kooiker CL, Wagenaar SS, van der Zouwen P, Dorhout Mees EJ (1976) Occurrence of vascular IgA-deposits in clinically normal skin of patients with renal disease. *Kidney Int* 9: 424–429.
110. Swelick RA, Lawley TJ (1991) Small-vessel vasculitis and cutaneous vasculitis. In: Churg A, Churg J (eds). *Systemic vasculitides.* New York: Igaku-Shoin, 193–201.
111. Cadman EC, Lundberg WB, Mitchell MS (1976) Pulmonary manifestations in Behçet syndrome: Case report and review of the literature. *Arch Intern Med* 136: 944–947.
112. Ahn JM, Im JG, Ryoo JW, Kim SJ, Do YS, Choi YW, Oh YW, Yeon KM, Han MC (1994) Thoracic manifestations of Behçet syndrome: Radiographic and CT findings in nine patients. *Radiology* 194: 199–203.
113. Efthimiou J, Johnston C, Spiro SG, Turner-Warwick W (1986) Pulmonary disease in Behçet's syndrome. *Q J Med* 227: 259–280.
114. Numan F, Islak C, Berkmen T, Tüzün H, Cokyüksel O (1994) Behçet disease: Pulmonary arterial involvement in 15 cases. *Radiology* 192: 465–468.
115. Oezer ZG, Palali Z, Cengiz M, Oezdemir IA (1991) Die vaskularen Läsionen des Morbus Behçet. *Vasa* 20: 181–185.
116. Durieux P, Bletry O, Huchon G, Wechsler B, Chretien J, Godeau P (1981) Multiple pulmonary arterial aneurysms in Behçet's disease and Hughes-Stovin syndrome. *Am J Med* 71: 736–741.
117. Umezawa T, Saji T, Matsuo N, Odagiri K (1989) Chest X-ray findings in the acute phase of Kawasaki disease. *Pediatr Radiol* 20: 48–51.
118. Amano S, Hazama F, Kubagawa H, Tasaka K, Haebara H, Hamashima Y (1980) General pathology of Kawasaki disease: On the morphological alterations corresponding to the clinical manifestations. *Acta Pathol Jpn* 30: 681–694.
119. Amano S, Hazama F, Hamashima Y (1979) Pathology of Kawasaki disease. II. Distribution and incidence of the vascular lesions. *Jpn Circ J* 43: 741–748.
120. Churg A (1991) Vasculitis and mimics of vasculitis involving the lung. In: Churg A, Churg J (eds). *Systemic vasculitides.* New York: Igaku-Shoin, 121–132.
121. Churg A (1991) Vasculitis in sarcoidosis. In: Churg A, Churg J (eds). *Systemic vasculitides.* New York: Igaku-Shoin, 299–304.
122. Liebow AA (1973) Pulmonary angiitis and granulomatosis. *Am Rev Respir Dis* 108: 1–18.
123. Myers JL, Katzenstein ALA (1986) Microangiitis in Lupus-induced pulmonary hemorrhage. *Am J Clin Pathol* 85: 552–556.
124. Simonson JS, Schiller NB, Petri M, Hellman DB (1989) Pulmonary hypertension in systemic lupus erythematosus. *J Rheum* 16: 918–925.

125. Bacon PB, Carruthers DM (1995) Vasculitis associated with connective tissue disorders. *Rheum Dis Clin N Am* 21: 1077–1096.
126. Misiani R, Bellavita P, Fenili D, Borelli G, Marchesi D, Massazza M, Vendramin G, Comotti B, Tanzi E, Scudeller G, et al. (1992) Hepatitis C virus infection in patients with essential mixed cryoglobulinemia. *Ann Intern Med* 117: 573–577.
127. Zignego AL, Ferri C, Giannini C, Monti M, La Cavita L, Careccia G, Longombardo G, Lombardini F, Bomardieri S, Gentilini P (1996) Hepatitis C virus genotype analysis in patients with type II mixed cryoglobulinemia. *Ann Intern Med* 124: 31–34.
128. Viegi G, Fornai E, Ferri C, Di Munno O, Begliomini E, Vitali C, Melocchi F, Bombardieri S, Paoletti P (1989) Lung function in essential mixed cryoglobulinemia: A short-term follow-up. *Clin Rheumatol* 8: 331–338.

Autoimmune Aspects of Lung Disease
ed. by D.A. Isenberg and S.G. Spiro
© 1998 Birkhäuser Verlag Basel/Switzerland

CHAPTER 4
The Lung in Granulomatous Diseases

Monica A. Spiteri[1] and Graham A.W. Rook[2]

[1] *Department of Respiratory Medicine, North Staffordshire Hospital Trust/Keele University,
Stoke-on-Trent, Staffordshire, UK*
[2] *Department of Bacteriology, UCL Medical School, London, UK*

1. Introduction

Sarcoidosis is a disease of unknown aetiology, for which autoimmunity is
one of several candidate aetiologies. A condition which may or may not be
related to sarcoidosis is necrotising sarcoid granulomatosis (NSG), and this

is also considered in this chapter. Other conditions that are primarily vasculitides are considered in Chapter 3 in spite of their associated granulomata. Much of what we know about the immunology of the lung, and of granulomatous inflammation in this organ, is derived from a study of granuloma-inducing infections [1]. The distinction between immunological mechanisms involved in chronic infection and autoimmune disease (and immunity to cancer) is not absolute. Many of the autoimmune diseases considered in this volume may eventually turn out to be triggered by cryptic infections [2], and chronic infections can be accompanied by autoimmune manifestations that are remarkably similar to those seen in systemic lupus erythematosus (SLE) or rheumatoid arthritis (RA), though we do not know what role they play in pathogenesis [2, 3]. Thus a study of granulomata known to be caused by infection (human and murine tuberculosis, and schistosomal egg granulomata in the lungs of mice) can increase our understanding of the factors that determine which patients with sarcoidosis develop severe lung fibrosis, or why necrosis is a major feature of NSG but not of sarcoidosis. In these infectious models we can now implicate patterns of cytokine release and disturbances of the immunoregulatory role of the hypothalamo-pituitary-adrenal axis, and of local glucocorticoid and anti-glucocorticoid metabolism in target organs.

2. Peculiarities of the Lung as an Immunological Organ

The lung is unusual because immune responses within this tissue can be primed both by the mucosal route and by parenteral immunisation. Both mucosal and systemic immunisation can prevent lung infection [4], and both peripheral lymph node and Peyer's patch cells will bind to bronchus-associated lymphoid tissue [5], indicating the presence of "addressin" receptors for cells of both origins. (This is a generic term for cell membrane receptors that determine adhesion to endothelial cells, and hence the recirculation patterns and organ-specific homing of lymphocytes.) This relationship may explain the facts that the gut can be subtly abnormal in sarcoidosis [6], and alveolar lavage cell populations can be abnormal in Crohn's disease [7]. Whenever, therefore, we see lung abnormalities, we must think about other mucosal sites.

The lung is a very rich source of lymphocytes. There is a large interstitial pool [8], but an even larger number of T-cells is found in the vascular compartment of the lungs [9–11], where they are held by a physiological process. Their role is unclear. They may be important in infection [12], but their involvement in autoimmunity is unknown. They appear to be functionally different from the circulating peripheral blood lymphocyte pool, suggesting selective trapping or a transient influence of local factors [13].

3. Tuberculosis and Autoimmunity

3.1. Mycobacterioses, Autoimmunity and Arthritis

Tuberculosis (and leprosy) are accompanied by autoantibody production [3]. The spectrum of autoantibodies in these conditions is similar to that seen in SLE [3]. Another occasional manifestation of autoimmunity in the mycobacterioses is a sterile arthritis [14, 15]. This rare condition (called Ponçet's disease when it occurs in tuberculosis) is one reason for the development of the concept of "slow bacterial infections". Tuberculosis, leprosy, *Mycobacterium avium* infection, and immunotherapy with the Bacille Calmette-Guérin (BCG) can all be accompanied by syndromes resembling diseases conventionally labelled as "autoimmune", such as RA or SLE or sarcoidosis [2]. Because several non-mycobacterial infections (Whipple's disease, Lyme disease and syphilis) can also do this, the aetiology of these "autoimmune" diseases must be questioned [2]. When present in small numbers such organisms can be very difficult to detect, and mycobacteria can persist in normal tissues for prolonged periods without causing disease. Attempts to prove an infectious aetiology for sarcoidosis by culture, passage into animals or polymerase chain reaction have yielded conflicting results [16–18]. Thus the matter is not settled, and it remains possible that several autoimmune diseases are really ongoing cryptic infections, or alternatively, that they are triggered by transient infections, but become independent of the continuing presence of that infection.

3.2. Stress (Heat Shock) Proteins and Autoimmunity

Probably all chronic infections are accompanied by some manifestations of autoimmunity. This is partly because the T-lymphocyte repertoire generated in the thymus does not exclude self-reactive cells, though it may weed out some cells bearing receptors with a particularly high avidity for major histocompatibility complex (MHC) plus self peptides (Figure 1). Cells recognising self with lower avidity are positively selected, and so provide the immune system with a repertoire that is relevant to the biological relative of our surroundings. Random mutation, followed by selection of T-cells with no ability to recognise self, would generate many cells unlikely to recognise anything useful, whereas a T-cell that recognises a self peptide with low avidity stands a good chance of recognising the bacterial homologue of this peptide rather well. However, even this concept, which would have sounded wild a few years ago, understates the current revolution in our thinking about the T-cell repertoire. Part of the repertoire, far from recognising self badly, recognises a restricted set of autoantigens efficiently and deliberately. There appears to be a set of conserved self antigens, notably including certain stress proteins, "against which there exists in healthy individuals a kind of benign autoimmunity" [19].

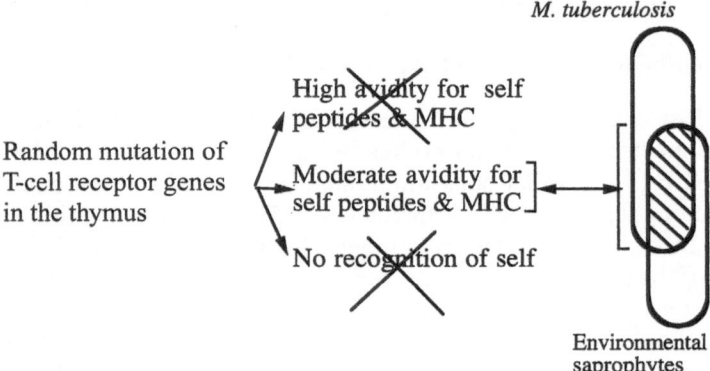

Figure 1. The thymus does not eliminate all T-cells that recognise self peptides presented by the MHC during repertoire development. The cells that are eliminated are those that recognise self with very high avidity and those that are unresponsive. Thus the T-cell-mediated response to bacteria is inevitably biased towards conserved proteins that are similar in humans and bacteria. The heat shock proteins (hsps) fall into this category and are particularly immunodominant targets for recognition of infection. Responses to the hsps also appear to play complex regulatory roles (see main text). When the response to hsps is dysregulated, autoimmunity can result. (We do not yet know what such dysregulation means at a molecular level.)

The fact that stress proteins (such as hsp60) are found within this subset of autoantigens adds a further level of interest. Stress proteins may be upregulated in the host's cells when these are infected, or undergo malignant transformation, or are exposed to cytokines or inflammation. Thus recognition of stress proteins or of peptides derived from them may alert the immune response to the existence of a problem. In fact, T-cells from animals immunised with mycobacterial hsp can kill stressed autologous macrophages in the absence of the bacterial homologue [20], and a similar phenomenon has been observed with T-cells from human joints [21]. Autoimmunity to hsp60 may then play a role as an amplifier of inflammation, as a restrainer of inflammation, or when something goes wrong, as a cause of specific autoimmune disease [19]. Similarly, stress protein homologues, perhaps associated with tumour-derived peptides, may play a role as targets for the recognition of malignant cells [22]. The next intellectual challenge will be understand the regulation of these various functions of benign autoimmunity. When is it a "restrainer", as may be desirable in autoimmune disease, and when does it attack, as may be desirable in cancer and infection?

3.3. Mycobacterial hsp65 and Models of Autoimmunity

In rodent models, the regulation of responses evoked by the mycobacterial hsp65 is easily deranged, and in several models of autoimmune disease (arthritis and diabetes) this hsp is a critical immunogen. This was first documented in the rat model of adjuvant arthritis evoked by an injection of killed mycobacteria emulsified in oil (complete Freund's adjuvant) [23, 24], but this protein, or mammalian proteins cross-reactive with it, has also been proven to play a role in several other models [19, 25–27], and has been more tentatively implicated in human RA, particularly the juvenile form [28].

3.4. Agalactosyl IgG in Tuberculosis and Autoimmune Disease

There is a change in the glycosylation of immunoglobulin G (IgG) heavy chain tuberculosis [29], with loss of terminal galactose from the N-linked oligosaccharides situated on the CH2 domain. The presence of this glycosylation change constitutes a further parallel between tuberculosis and autoimmune disorders because it is also seen in RA [30] and Crohn's disease [31]. This glycoform of IgG has been shown to be directly pathogenic in transfer experiments in mice [32]. It is therefore probable that complexes of antigen and agalactosyl IgG contribute to immunopathology. There is also circumstantial evidence that when autoantigens are complexed with agalactosyl antibodies the T-cell component of autoimmunity is activated [33], and this is also the simplest interpretation of the rodent data [32]. Agalactosyl IgG is raised in a subset of patients with sarcoidosis, as outined below in Section 4.7.2.

4. Sarcoidosis

Sarcoidosis commonly affects young adults, and frequently presents with bilateral hilar lymphadenopathy with or without pulmonary infiltration, ocular and/or cutaneous lesions. The diagnosis is established when well-recognized clinical and radiograpic findings are supported by histological evidence of discrete non-caseating epithelioid cell granulomata in one or more organs. In addition, a positive Kveim-Siltzbach skin test and cutaneous anergy to tuberculoprotein are often present. Immunological features suggest aberrant cell-mediated reactions at the site of inflammation, in the presence of hypergammaglobulinaemia [34]. The disease is frequently self-limiting with spontaneous resolution. However, in a few patients there is a progressive downhill course culminating in irreversible fibrosis and severe impairment of organ function.

4.1. Possible Aetiological Factors in Sarcoidosis

Despite extensive research there is no identifiable aetiological agent to account for the granulomata that characterise sarcoidosis. There is some epidemiological evidence for an environmental factor [35]. Infectious agents are one possibility. Early studies suggested viral involvement, and as outlined above, a mycobacterial aetiology for this and other diseases of obscure or "autoimmune" aetiology has frequently been suggested, but attempts to prove it in relation to sarcoidosis have yielded conflicting results [16–18].

Exhaustive skin testing with metals and other inorganic substances in sarcoid patients and controls has not revealed any peculiar hypersensitivity to chemicals. Beryllium [36] and zirconium [37] produce granulomata in the sensitized individual. Although such granulomata are found at the injection site 1 month after inoculation, and are histologically similar to those produced in the Kveim response in patients with sarcoidosis, each skin test is specific for its own disorder, and there is no overlap.

Other possible environmental factors that have been suggested include inhalation of pine pollen, peanut dust, clay soil, talc and secondary oxalosis. The role of these factors in the pathogenesis of sarcoidosis remains speculative.

4.2. The Role of Genetic Factors in Sarcoidosis

The occurrence of sarcoidosis in members of the same family has suggested that genetic factors might be involved [38], but no firm relationship has been demonstrated. Sarcoidosis has been reported to be more common in monozygotic than heterozygotic twins [39]. Various features of sarcoidosis may be associated with specific antigens of MHC loci. Human lymphocyte antigen HLA-B8 has been associated with erythema nodosum [40] and arthritis [41], while HLA-B27 is found in a high percentage of patients with uveitis [42]. Persson et al. reported a statistically significant increase of HLA-B7 in 47 patients with negative reactivity to tuberculin [43]. In contrast, the frequency of this allele was zero in the group with positive response to tuberculin. The most interesting HLA association in sarcoidosis has been that of B8, DR3 in patients with acute sarcoidosis and arthritis [44]. Kremer suggested that B8, DR3 phenotype identifies a group of patients who are more likely to develop acute sarcoid arthritis and hilar adenopathy, progressing to chronic disease [45]. It is interesting that the B8, DR3 haplotype is overexpressed by patients with several "classical" autoimmune diseases, including SLE and myositis [46]. Others have shown an association of HLA-B8 with early resolution of the disease [47], while patients expressing HLA-B13 are more prone to persistent disease [48]. Despite such findings there is no definitive evidence for the "linkage" of the HLA-associated alleles with disease susceptibility gene(s) in sarcoidosis.

4.3. Pulmonary Manifestations of Sarcoidosis

The lung is the organ most commonly involved. At least 90% of patients with sarcoidosis exhibit abnormalities on their chest X-rays. Twenty to twenty-five percent of these patients have permanent loss of lung function, and of these 5–10% die from complications of the disease [49]. Patients are commonly asymptomatic, or there may be insidious onset of respiratory symptoms with dry cough, progressive dyspnoea, exercise intolerance and chest pain [50]. Lung function typically shows a decrease in diffusion capacity, with or without a fall in lung volume [49]. The type and quantity of the physiological abnormality relate to the location and the extent of the pathology [51, 52].

The inflammatory process seems to extend through the lymphatics to the hilar and mediastinal nodes. Over 85% of patients with pulmonary sarcoidosis have radiographically apparent mediastinal and hilar lymph node enlargement. Spread may then occur throughout the lung as well as to other favoured organs such as the liver [53].

The clinical course of pulmonary sarcoidosis may be related, at least in part, to the radiological appearance of the disease. Patients have been divided into clinical groups according to the appearance of the chest film, ranging from the commoner, usually asymptomatic, bilateral hilar lymphadenopathy without parenchymal involvement [54] to diffuse dense progressive and irreversible parenchymal fibrosis with respiratory failure [55]. Using this radiological staging, Siltzbach noted a clear relationship between the prognosis of sarcoidosis and the initial radiological appearance as well as associated extrathoracic features [56].

4.4. Staging of Disease Activity in Sarcoidosis

In particular groups of affected patients, while the disease is often graded as intense by certain indices, the majority of the patients recover spontaneously within a short time and without treatment. Another aspect to be considered is the multisystem involvement of sarcoidosis. In practice, patients who have intense granulomatous inflammation within one organ do not necessarily have serious systemic involvement. The old concept of a single or multiple extrathoracic organ involvement as an indicator of poor prognosis remains unconfirmed [57]. Recent guidelines on the management of sarcoidosis suggest that routine tests to stage disease activity can be limited to clinical indices that include worsening respiratory symptoms, deterioration of lung function and/or chest radiography [58]. Sometimes the following may also be useful: biochemical markers such as serum angiotensin converting enzyme (ACE), gallium-67 (^{67}Ga) scanning, high-resolution computed tomography and bronchoalveolar lavage (BAL) cell populations, and CD4/CD8 ratio [58].

4.5. Assessing Pulmonary Sarcoidosis by BAL

The lung in sarcoidosis appears to be the site of a compartmentalised inflammatory response not reflected in the peripheral blood [59]. The types and numbers of cells retrieved by BAL are similar to those found in lung biopsies from the same patients [60]. They parallel the severity of the acute illness, resolving as the disease abates or responds to treatment [61].

The correlation between a high initial lymphocyte count in BAL and disease prognosis is controversial. A number of investigations have suggested that BAL may be superior to any clinical, radiological and physiological parameters in assessing the present status of the alveolitis and subsequent events in any individual patient, but this has not been confirmed. Others have observed that a BAL lymphocytosis present on two successive investigations tends to correlate well with a deterioration of lung function [62]. Ward et al. [63] found that an acute onset of sarcoidosis with high lymphocytosis in BAL offered a better prognosis than disease of more insidious onset with low lavage lymphocyte counts. Foley et al. concluded that the presence of a high BAL lymphocytosis could indicate a favourable prognosis for the outcome of lung function in pulmonary sarcoidosis even in those patients with chronic disease [64]. This suggests that the absence of a lymphocytosis in lavage does not necessarily indicate burnt-out disease. In patients with more extensive long-standing radiographic shadows, BAL neutrophils may be as important as lymphocytes in the assessment of disease activity, perhaps serving as an indicator for therapy [65].

Inconsistent correlations are found in the literature relating the proportion of lavage T-cells recovered by BAL to the amount of ^{67}GA uptake by lung parenchyma [66]. This may be because BAL fluid analysis mirrors the alveolitis, while gallium uptake reflects granuloma load. BAL is now believed to yield more information, at least in the initial stages of the disease [66].

Delineation of specific lavage lymphocyte and macrophage subpopulations may be more informative. A close relationship between the CD4/CD8 ratio and more progressive disease has been reported [67], and a correlation between phenotypically distinct macrophage subsets and radiographic staging has also been identified [68].

4.6. The Pathogenesis of Sarcoidosis

The histology of early sarcoidosis is characterised by a mononuclear cell infiltrate of macrophages and T lymphocytes. This lymphocytic response distinguishes sarcoidosis from other interstitial lung diseases such as fibrosing alveolitis, where polymorphonuclear cells usually predominate in early disease [69, 70].

4.6.1. The lymphocytes in sarcoid BAL: The lymphocytes associated with granulomata are larger than usual and have features of activated cells such as expression of class II MHC, receptors for interleukin-2 (IL-2 or TAc antigen) and spontaneous secretion of IL-2 [71]. Some of these lymphocytes are in the proliferative phase of their cell cycle (S/G2) [71, 72].

The accumulation of lymphocytes around the granulomata and in BAL is more prominent within fresh active lesions, and tends to diminish as the granulomata mature. These lymphocytes are mainly CD4+, so the CD4+/CD8+ T-lymphocyte ratio in active sarcoid lavage is 4–10 times greater than in normal BAL [73]. As the lesions become less active, CD4+ cells decrease, and CD8+ T-cells predominate [70].

Raised levels of IL-2 have been found in active sarcoid BAL, and T lymphocytes recovered from active sarcoid BAL spontaneously release IL-2 [71], monocyte chemotactic factor (MCF) and monocyte migration inhibition factor (MIF) [74]. Pulmonary T-cells release approximately 25 times more MCF on a per cell basis than blood T-cells from the same patients. Consequent recruitment of monocytes to the pulmonary interstitium may be an initial step in the assembly of granulomata. Interferon γ (IFNγ), a potent activator of macrophages, is also released by lung T lymphocytes from patients with active sarcoidosis and may contribute to the activation and differentiation of recruited monocytes into activated macrophages, giant cells and epithelioid cells [75]. Alveolar macrophages are also said to express IL-2 receptors, so the IL-2 release by T-cells may be a further activation signal [76].

In sarcoid BAL, the vast majority of T lymphocytes express the $\alpha\beta$ T-cell receptor (TCR), with significant expression of markers of recent activation [77]. In contrast, although $\gamma\delta$ T-cells are increased in the peripheral blood of active long-term sarcoidosis, they are scarcely seen in BAL and in biopsy specimens, suggesting that these cells may not be directly related to granuloma formation [78].

In summary, studies of the T-cells in sarcoidosis have proved disappointing in terms of aetiology. The findings suggest an essentially "normal" immune response driven by a persistent, exogenous and/or self-specific antigen. The problem is to identify that antigen.

4.6.2. The alveolar macrophages in sarcoid BAL: BAL samples, as well as lung biopsies, have revealed an increase in the total number of macrophages present in active sarcoid. These alveolar macrophages (AM) have enhanced expression of HLA-DR [79] and may serve as antigen-presenting cells that initiate the alveolitis seen in pulmonary sarcoidosis by presenting the as yet unidentified antigen(s) to locally resident and recruited T lymphocytes [80].

Sarcoid AM show other characteristics of activated cells, including increased expression of Fc receptors and increased phagocytosis, spontaneous secretion of IL-1, IL-6, granulocyte-macrophage colony-stimulating factor (GMCSF) [81], and increased potential for endotoxin-induced secretion of tumour necrosis factor α (TNFα) [82]. However, the mRNA for TNFα may not be expressed *in vivo* in the AM of active sarcoidosis [83]. This is interesting in view of the important role of TNFα in de development and maintenance of granulomata [84], and probably of tissue damage in tuberculosis (see below) and could contribute to the self-limiting nature of many cases of sarcoidosis, and to the lack of caseating necrosis in this disease.

Sarcoid AM also show increased conversion of circulating 25(OH) cholecalciferol into the active 1,25-dihydroxy derivative. This occurs because macrophage 1α-hydroxylase is activated by IFNγ. A similar phenomenon occurs to a lesser extent in tuberculosis [85]. This is a powerful effect that probably explains the hypercalcaemia seen in some patients with sarcoidosis, and has complex immunological consequences [86].

Release of IL-1β, IL-6 and GMCSF by sarcoid peripheral blood mononuclear cells correlates with neutrophil influx into the BAL compartment [81], but there appears to be no correlation between local or systemic cytokine release and the severity of the disease as assessed by radiographic staging and detailed lung function testing.

Recent studies have shown that the presence of sarcoid inflammation in the lung induces the energence of an AM subset that suppresses T-cell proliferation [87]. There is circumstantial evidence that this suppressive activity may occur *in vivo*, because reduced levels of CD7 (expressed on a subset of activated T-cells) and of HLA-DR expression on CD4$^+$ T-cells were seen at the same time as the percentage of the "suppressor"-type AM was increasing in sarcoid BAL [68]. These macrophages appear in direct proportion to the degree of local lymphocytosis, and show increased expression of an antigen that identifies epithelioid cells in tissue, and an enhanced fibronectin content.

In the relatively small number of patients who progress to fibrosis, reduced numbers of lymphocytes and increased neutrophils are found in the BAL. In addition, there are increased levels of fibronectin, AM-derived growth factors and enhanced expression of membrane fibronectin receptors on macrophages. The role of suppressor AM in these patients remains unknown.

4.7. Systemic Immune Events in Sarcoidosis

Although lung T-cells appear to be activated in sarcoidosis, the opposite is true in the peripheral blood, where there is an absolute decrease in the number of circulating T-cells. Functionally, the response of peripheral lymphocytes to mitogen and recal antigen is partially impaired, and B-cell function (*in vitro*) is consequently depressed.

4.7.1. Delayed hypersensitivity responses in sarcoidosis: Many patients with active sarcoidosis have a partial to complete skin-test anergy to tuberculin purified protein derivative (PPD), and this extends to other antigens such as *Trichophyton*, mumps virus, streptokinase/streptodornase and *Candida*, as well as to dinitrochlorobenzene. The anergy appears to parallel disease severity, and its incidence in sarcoid patients varies from 30 to 70% depending on the number of antigens used [49]. This observation is almost certainly not disease-specific, since anergy accompanies the presence of lung granulomata in experimental animals whether these are induced by BCG, antigen-conjugated sepharose beads, talcum powder, polymerised dextran or latex [88, 89].

While patients with sarcoidosis do not respond to these skin-test antigens, they are uniquely capable of mounting a cutaneous response to a Kveim preparation (prepared from sarcoid granulomata). Although Kveim test lesions exhibit histopathological similarities to sarcoid granulomata, there are marked differences between the Kveim reaction and the classic delayed-type hypersensitivity skin reaction. The most obvious difference is in the kinetics of the two reactions. The delayed-type hypersensitivity reaction begins at 8 h, peaks at 24–48 h and resolves by 96–120 h. By contrast, the Kveim reaction takes 4–6 weeks to develop. Furthermore, no specific antigen in the Kveim preparation has bene identified as the inducing agent in this response.

4.7.2. Humoral events in sarcoidosis: There appears to be a hyper-reactivity of the humoral immune system in sarcoidosis [90]. This is expressed by an increased response to exogenous antigens and the development of autoantibodies [91]. Immunoglobulin formation in patients with sarcoidosis is probably a by-product of the presence of large numbers of activated T-cells at the site of granuloma formation. A polyclonal hypergammaglobulinaemia is also found in active sarcoid BAL. Lung CD4$^+$ T-cells, but not blood T lymphocytes, from patients with active sarcoidosis are capable of polyclonally activating normal B-cells without added antigen or mitogen. In contrast, lung T lymphocytes from normal subjects or patients with idiopathic pulmonary fibrosis do not have this property [90].

As described earlier in relation to tuberculosis, there is a change in the glycosylation of IgG heavy chains in some patients with sarcoidosis, leading to formation of agalactosyl IgG [92]. Interestingly, however, the switch to the agalactosyl glycoform of IgG is characteristic of the patients who present with florid disease, and who have a relatively good prognosis [92].

The prevalence of immune complexes ranges from 23 to 70% of sarcoid patients. Complexes appear to persist in active disease but disappear with resolution. A high prevalence of immune complexes is noted in sarcoid patients who present with erythema nodosum and arthritis. It is possible that agalactosyl IgG (characteristic of RA) takes part in this complex formation, but the matter has not been investigated. It is unclear what role the complexes play in the evolution of the disease, and serious clinical effects of immune complexes, such as renal damage seen in other diseases (e.g. SLE) do not occur in sarcoidosis.

4.8. The Histopathology and Electron Microscopy of Sarcoidosis

Macroscopic descriptions of the very early stage of sarcoidosis are not available, because cases coming to autopsy are extremely rare. However, an accumulation of mononuclear cells in the lung precedes granuloma formation, and in patients with early disease there are greater numbers of inflammatory cells and fewer granulomata and a less prominent alveolitis. The definition of sarcoidosis is based on the formation of granulomata, even though these appear after the lymphocytic alveolitis [93]. The recommended definition is a disease characterised by the formation in all or several affected organs or tissues of discrete non-caseating epithelioid-cell tubercles [94]. Fibrinoid necrosis may be present at the centres of the granulomata, proceeding either to resolution or conversion into hyaline fibrous tissue. These granulomata may involve the walls of bronchi and bronchioles, and follow the lines of the pulmonary lymphatics in the interstitium as well as lymph nodes, especially those in peribronchial, hilar and mediastinal locations. A vascular component of sarcoid may be seen with extensive disease, such as non-caseating granulomata in the intima, media and adventitia of the vessels. There is no fibrinoid necrosis of the vessel walls, but rarely pulmonary hypertension may occur secondary to this occlusion. Also rarely, pulmonary veins may be affected, stimulating veno-occlusive disease, without pulmonary arterial involvement.

In addition to severe end-stage fibrosis involving both parenchyma and the pleura, there may be emphysema. A rare complication is systemic amyloidosis [93, 95].

The heart may be involved in sarcoidosis, and this can cause sudden death. The common sites of involvement are the free wall of the left ventricle [94], the basal aspect of the ventricular septum, the free wall of the right ventricle, the sino-atrial node, atrio-ventricular node and Purkinje system. Uncommon locations of cardiovascular involvement are the atrial walls, pericardium, valves, aorta, the main pulmonary arteries and veins and superior vena cava.

The ultrastructure of a typical well-developed granuloma shows two characteristic zones [96, 97]. The central zone is composed of closely opposed epithelial cells, a few giant cells, lymphocytes, histiocytes and intermediate cells. The intermediate cells resemble both histiocytes and epithelioid cells. Cytoplasmic organelles are profuse, with many mitochondria, much rough endoplasmic reticulum and some membrane-lined vesicles. There is a well-developed Golgi apparatus but only a few lysosomes. The peripheral zone contains loosely arranged cellular elements, including fibroblasts, myofibroblasts, occasional epithelioid cells, collagen, fibrils and a mixture of chronic inflammatory cells including lymphocytes, plasma cells and eosinophils.

5. Necrotising Sarcoid Granulomatosis

This is a rare condition, originally described by Liebow in 1973 [98]. There have been three subsequent large series describing a total of 86 cases [99–101]. The aetiology is unknown, and there is doubt whether it should even be classified along with sarcoid. Churg argued that NSG was in fact a form of sarcoid, based on the frequency of hilar lymphadenopathy, the occasional occular abnormalities, especially uveitis, and liver damage [100].

Saldana believes the disease is unrelated to classic sarcoid for several reasons [99]. NSG patients may have normal ACE levels, negative Kveim tests [101] and no hilar lymphadenopathy. In contrast, they may have extensive necrosis, and extensive granulomatous vasculitis, as well as systemic vasculitis.

5.1. Clinical Features of NSG

This disease is rare in children and adolescents and is most common in the fifth decade of life. It affects females more than males, with a ratio M:F = 1:4 [100]. There are chest symptoms, including chest pain, dyspnoea and non-productive cough, but with extensive disease there may be fever, malaise and weight loss [102]. The lesions tend to involve the lower lobes, and the incidence of cavitation ranges from 0 [100] to 23% [101]. There are multiple nodular infiltrates which can measure up to 5 cm in diameter. Bilateral hilar lymphadenopathy is rare, being present in less than 10% of cases [98, 99, 101].

Only a small percentage of patients have extrapulmonary signs and symptoms [100]. There may be diabetes insipidus due to hypothalamic deficiency, uveitis, iritis [101] and leg weakness due to spinal cord involvement. Some may be asymptomatic and are diagnosed on routine chest radiography [100].

The prognosis of NSG is good, and patients with bilateral infiltrates respond well to corticosteroids [103]. Relapse may occur in up to 25% of patients [98, 101].

5.2. The Pathology of NSG

Typically these are solid masses or irregular infiltrates measuring up to 8 cm in diameter. They are yellow-white, firm and less necrotic than in Wegener's granulomatosis. Histological examination reveals sarcoid-like granulomata with variable necrosis and vasculitis. Between the granulomata there are large numbers of chronic inflammatory cells with lymphocytes and plasma cells as well as desquamated alveolar cells and macrophages. As in typical sarcoid the granulomata are sited in the bronchovascular bundles and interlobular septa. Bronchial and bronchiolar involvement is common. The granulomata tent to confluency. Necrosis may affect small central areas of the granulomata. Rare cases have been described, where the necrosis was suppurative, resembling Wegener's or bronchocentric granulomatosis. Vascular involvement is prominent and affects both arteries and veins. The granulomata may extend through arterial walls, causing thrombosis and obliteration. Similar lesions are seen in veins. More rarely a giant cell arteritis is noted in larger pulmonary arteries up to elastic-type vessels.

6. Granulomatous Lesions Leading to Fibrosis and Necrosis – Lessons from Tuberculosis

6.1. Cytokine Profiles, Granulomata and Necrosis

We have little understanding of the factors that lead to irreversible fibrosis in a subset of patients with sarcoidosis or to necrosis in NSG. However, studies of various experimentally induced granulomata, and of tuberculosis, provide evidence that cytokine profiles profoundly influence both the size of granulomata and the likelihood of permanent tissue damage. For

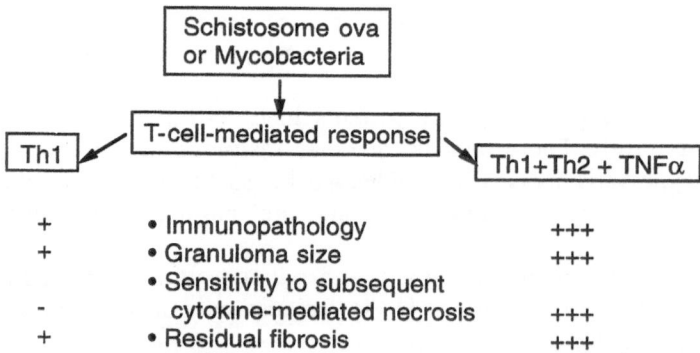

Figure 2. Schistosome ova and mycobacteria evoke granulomata in the lungs of mice. These are much larger, and leave more permanent residual fibrosis if the T-cell response is providing a mixed Th1 + Th2 cytokine profile. TNFα is also needed for granuloma formation. Removal of any one of the three components (Th2, Th1 or TNFα) reduces granuloma size. But TNFα has a dual role, and in sites of mixed Th1 + Th2 inflammation, injection of further TNFα can induce frank necrosis, whereas in inflammatory sites mediated only by Th1 cells, TNFα is not toxic, and promotes granuloma formation and macrophage activation. It is not yet clear to what extent these findings in mice apply to T-cell-mediated inflamation in humans.

instance, the granulomata evoked by the eggs of *Schistosoma mansoni* in the lungs of mice involve Th1 cytokines, Th2 cytokines [104] and TNFα [105]. All three factors are needed. Neutralisation of Th1 or Th2 cytokines, or neutralisation of TNFα with appropriate antibodies, will diminish the size of the lesions (Figure 2). The same is true in murine pulmonary tuberculosis, where a massive inflammatory response correlates with the presence of an inappropriate Th2 cytokine component superimposed on the usual Th1 response [106]. The absence of any recorded Th2 component in sarcoidosis may therefore be significant, and it will be interesting to study cytokine profiles of cells from NSG.

6.2. Cytokine Profiles and Necrosis within T-Cell-Mediated Inflammatory Sites

A similar point can be made in relation to cytokine-mediated necrosis. Granulomata evoked by mycobacteria [107] or by *Schistosoma* [108] will undergo acute necrosis when high systemic levels of cytokines such as TNFα are induced by injecting endotoxin intravenously. A similar phenomenon occurs in delayed hypersensitivity sites and has allowed the toxicity of TNFα to be related to the cytokine profile. If mice are immunised with mycobacterial antigens, and then challenged in the footpad with soluble mycobacterial antigen, a delayed hypersensitivity reaction occurs, that peaks 24 h later. If TNFα is then injected into the same site, local tissue damage is induced if the animal has a mixed Th1 + Th2 (or perhaps Th0) pattern of response to the mycobacterial antigen (i.e. similar production of both IFNγ and IL-4) but not if the response was "pure" Th1 (i.e. IFNγ production, but no IL-4) [109]. The same is true in mice with pulmonary tuberculosis (Figure 2). TNFα injected into a tuberculin test site causes no local toxicity early in the infection when the Th1 response dominates, but does cause local damage later in the disease when there is an equal balance of Th1 and Th2 cytokine production [106]. Thus it may be that a mixed cytokine profile (Th1 + Th2 or Th0) causes a type of inflammation that is inherently more likely to undergo irreversible damage. There is clear evidence of TNFα release and of a Th2 component in the immune response of severe tuberculosis [110, 111], but not in sarcoidosis, where, although the alveolar macrophages are primed for excessive TNFα release *in vitro* [82], this cytokine may not be expressed in the lesions *in vivo* [83].

6.3. Cytokines, Granulomata and Fibrosis

As discussed above, both Th1 and Th2 cytokines and TNFα are implicated in the formation of schistosome egg-induced granulomata [104, 105]. These normally progress to irreversible fibrosis. However, if mice are preimmunised with egg antigens mixed with IL-12 (a potent inducer of a

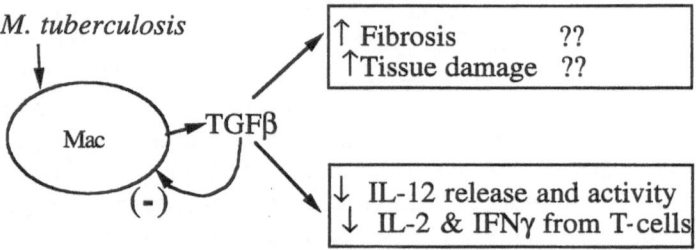

Figure 3. Possible mechanisms for the role of TGFβ in the tissue damage and immune dysfunction in tuberculosis based on known *in vitro* properties of TGFβ. However, it is clear that TGFβ is expressed in sarcoidosis at levels that are at least as high as in tuberculous tissue, so a direct role in necrosis is unlikely. Moreover, in a murine model, expression of TGFβ is a very late event that occurs long after the crucial Th1- to -Th2 switch has taken place (see Figure 2).

Th1 cytokine pattern) before infection, the eggs are unable to evoke a Th2 component, and the resulting granulomata are not only smaller but also generate less permanent fibrosis [112].

According to another (and not mutually incompatible) view, overproduction of TGFβ (Figure 3) may also play a role in tissue damage in tuberculosis [113]. Sustained excessive production of this cytokine is associated with fibrosis, and mice injected intraperitoneally with TGFβ for 10 days develop cachexia and generalised fibrosis [114]. In normal lung, expression of TGFβ is negligible [115], though some claim to find expression in the bronchial epithelium [116]. However, there is increased expression of TGFβ in monocytes of tuberculosis patients, and in the Langerhans and epithelioid cells in the granulomata [117]. On the other hand, TGFβ is strongly expressed in sarcoidosis [115, 118] and colocalises in the granulomas with procollagen type 1, fibronectin, decorin (a TGFβ-binding proteoglycan) and integrin receptors for fibronectin ($\alpha5\beta1$) and collagen ($\alpha2\beta1$). Since TGFβ is a feature of sarcoidosis, it is unlikely to be involved in the tissue necrosis of tuberculosis, but it may play a role in fibrosis. PDGFβ is also produced by alveolar macrophages activated by IFNγ, and this may also add to fibrotic lung damage [119].

7. Endocrine Control of Immune Mechanisms and Fibrosis

The endocrine system has potent effects on the regulation of necrosis, fibrosis and Th1/Th2 balance. If naive T-cells are driven by mitogens or via the T-cell receptor in the presence of glucocorticoids, they develop into lymphocytes expressing a Th2 cytokine profile [120, 121], though glucocorticoids will reduce cytokine production by most memory T-cells (including Th2). Similarly, glucocorticoids reduce TNFα production while enhancing expression of TGFβ in T-cells [122]. Glucocorticoids also downregulate numerous molecular processes involved in fibrosis (see Chapter 1, this volume). For all these reasons glucocorticoids are commonly used in the treatment of the lung conditions discussed here, but success is variable. Recent studies in tuberculosis have drawn attention to the lung as an important organ for the regulation of glucocorticoid activity, and revealed subtle changes in the hypothalamo-pituitary-adrenal axis that may have important consequences for T-lymphocyte and macrophage function [123].

7.1. Regulation of Glucocorticoid Activity within the Lung

Tuberculosis patients show several metabolic changes that may result in increased glucocorticoid effects within the lung, contributing to changes in Th1/Th2 balance and macrophage function [123]. They lack the normal evening trough in plasma cortisol levels so glucocorticoid receptors in their T-cells are occupied 24 h/day [124]. They also have low ratios of dehydro-epiandrosterone (DHEA) to cortisol. DHEA opposes glucocorticoid effects *in vivo* [125], so this relative DHEA deficiency further enhances cortisol activity. Moreover, some of the DHEA that tuberculosis patients do make becomes 16α-hydroxylated [123], and these 16α-hydroxylated DHEA derivatives are inactive as anti-glucocorticoids *in vivo*. Finally, analysis of cortisol metabolites in the urine reveals that there is a gross failure of conversion of cortisol into inactive cortisone (or accelerated conversion of cortisone back to active cortisol) [123].

These changes will all tend to enhance cortisol-mediated effects. However, the last of these phenomena (high cortisol/cortisone ratio) may depend directly upon regulatory events taking place within the lung itself that become abnormal during inflammatory lung diseases. In normal lung cortisol is rapidly converted to inactive cortisone [126, 127]. The enzyme responsible is known as 11β-hydroxysteroid dehydrogenase type 1 (11βHSD-1), though it is in fact an NADPH-dependent reversible oxi-doreductase. This is of great potential interest, because in the liver 11βHSD-1 functions as a reductase (i.e. in the opposite direction), converting inactive cortisone back into cortisol. Thus 11βHSD-1 is reversible. Moreover, it behaves unidirectionally or bidirectionally in different cell types into which it has been cloned, but efforts to understand its regulation have failed [128]. It is, however, known to be subject to regulation by T-lymphocyte-derived cytokines, at least in granulosa cell preparations [129].

It remains to be discovered whether lung 11βHSD-1 switches from dehydrogenase to reductase when exposed to inflammatory cytokines, but it would explain some of the changes seen in tuberculosis [123]. Meanwhile, we are unaware of studies of the HPA axis and urinary steroid metabolites in NSG or sarcoidosis, but these would clearly be fruitful areas of investigation, and would perhaps cast light on the variable glucocorticoid sensitivity of the latter.

References

1. Zumla A, James DG (1996) Granulomatous infections. *Clin Inf Dis* 23: 146–158.
2. Rook GAW, Lydyard PM, Stanford JL (1993) A reappraisal of the evidence that rheumatoid arthritis and several other idiopathic diseases, are slow bacterial infections. *Ann Rheum Dis* 52(Suppl): S30–S38.
3. Shoenfeld Y, Isenberg DA (1988) Mycobacteria and autoimmunity. *Immunol Today* 9: 178–182.
4. Cripps AW, Dunkley ML, Clancy RL (1994) Mucosal and systemic immunisations with killed *Pseudomonas aeruginosa* protect against acute respiratory infection in rats. *Infect Immun* 62: 1427–1436.
5. van der Brugge-Gamelkoorn GJ, Kraal G (1985) The specificity of the high endothelial venule in bronchus-associated lymphoid tissue (BALT). *J Immunol*134: 3746–3750.
6. McCormick PA, Feighery C, Dolan C, O'Farelly C, Kelliher P, Graeme-Cook F, Finch A, Ward K, Fitzgerald MX, O'Donoghue DP, et al. (1988) Altered gastrointestinal immune response in sarcoidosis. *Gut* 29: 1628–1631.
7. Douglas JG, McDonald CF, Leslie MJ, Gillon J, Crompton GK, McHardy GJR (1989) Respiratory impairment in inflammatory bowel disease: Does it vary with disease activity? *Resp Med* 83: 389–394.
8. Holt PG, Robinson BWS, Reid M, Kees UR, Warton A, Dawson VH, Rose A, Schon-Hegrad M, Papadimitriou JM (1986) Extraction of immune and inflammatory cells from human lung parenchyma: Evaluation of an enzymatic digestion procedure. *Clin Exp Immunol* 66: 188–200.
9. Pabst R (1990) Compartmentalization and kinetics of lymphoid cells in the lung. *Reg Immunol* 3: 62–71.
10. Pabst R (1994) In: Busse WW, Holgate ST (ed) (1994) *Astma and rhinitis*. Oxford: Blackwell Scientific, 415–425.
11. Pabst R, Binns RM, Licence T, Peter M (1987) Evidence of a selective major vascular marginal pool of lymphocytes in the lung. *Am Rev Resp Dis* 136: 1213–1218.
12. Pabst R, Binns RM (1989) Heterogeneity of lymphocyte homing physiology: Several mechanisms operate in the control of migration to lymphoid and non-lymphoid organs *in vivo*. *Immunol Rev* 108: 83–109.
13. Holt PG, Kees UR, Shon-Hegrad MA, Rose A, Ford J, Bilyk N, Bowman R, Robinson BWS (1988) Limiting dilution analysis of T-cells extracted from solid human lung tissue. Comparison of precursor frequencies for proliferative responses and lymphokine production between lung and blood T-cells from individual donors. *Immunology* 64: 649–654.
14. Moreland LW, Koopman WJ (1991) Infection as a cause of arthritis. *Curr Opin Rheumatol* 3: 639–649.
15. Isaacs AJ, Sturrock RD (1974) Poncet's disease – fact or fiction? A reappraisal of tuberculous rheumatism. *Tubercle* 55: 135–142.
16. Graham DY, Markesich DC, Kalter DC, Yoshimura HH (1988) Isolation of cell-wall-defective acid-fast bacteria from skin lesions of patients with sarcoidosis. In: Grassi C, Rizzato G, Pozzi E (eds). *Sarcoidosis and other granulomatous disorders*. Amsterdam: Elsevier Science Publishers, 161–163.
17. Bocart D, Lecossier D, de Lassence A, Valeyre D, Battesti J-P, Hance A (1992) A search for mycobacterial DNA in granulomatous tissues from patients with sarcoidosis using the polymerase chain reaction. *Am Rev Resp Dis* 145: 1142–1148.
18. Saboor S, Johnson NM, McFadden J (1992) Use of the polymerase chain reaction to detect mycobacterial DNA in tuberculosis and sarcoidosis. *Lancet* 339: 1012–1015.
19. Cohen IR (1996) Heat shock protein 60 and the regulation of autoimmunity. In: van Eden W, Young DB (eds). *Stress proteins in medicine*. New York: Marcel Dekker, 93–102.
20. Koga T, Wand-Wurttenberger A, DeBruyn J, Munk ME, Schoel B, Kaufmann SH (1989) T cells against a bacterial heat shock protein recognise stressed macrophages. *Science* 245: 1112–1115.
21. Hermann E, Lohse AW, van der Zee R, van Eden W, Mayet WJ, Probst P, Poralla T, Meyer zum Buschenfelde KH, Fleischer B (1991) Synovial fluid-derived Yersinia-reactive T-cells responding to human 65-kDa heat-shock protein and heat-stressed antigen-presenting cells. *Eur J Immunol* 21: 2139–2143.

22. Suto R, Srivastava PK A (1995) A mechanism for the specific immunogenicity of heat shock proteinchaperoned peptides. *Science* 269:1585–1588.
23. van Eden W, Thole JER, van der Zee R, Noordzij A, van Embden JDA, Hensen EJ, Cohen IR (1988) Cloning of the mycobacterial epitope recognised by T lymphocytes in adjuvant arthritis. *Nature* 331: 171–173.
24. Anderton SM, van Eden W (1996) T-lymphocyte recognition of hsp60 in experimental arthritis. In: van Eden W, Young DB (ed). *Stress proteins in medicine*. New York: Marcel Dekker, 73–91.
25. Thompson SJ, Rook GAW, Brealey R, van-der-Zee R, Elson CJ (1990) Autoimmune reactions to heat shock proteins in pristane-induced arthritis. *Eur J Immunol* 20: 2479–2484.
26. Elias D, Markovits D, Reshef T, van der Zee R, Cohen IR (1990) Induction of autoimmune diabetes in the non-obese diabetic (NOD/Lt) mouse by a 65kDa heat shock protein. *Proc Natl Acad Sci USA* 87: 1576–1580.
27. Billingham MEJ, Carney S, Butler R, Colston MJ (1990) A mycobacterial 65kDa heat shock protein induces antigen-specific suppression of adjuvant arthritis, but is not itself arthritogenic. *J Exp Med* 171: 339–344.
28. De-Graeff-Meeder ER, van der Zee R, Rijkers GT, Schurman HJ, Kuis W, Bijlsma JW, Zegers BJ, van Eden W (1991) Recognition of human 60 kD heat shock protein by mononuclear cells from patients with juvenile chronic arthritis. *Lancet* 337: 1368–1372.
29. Pilkington C, Wang Y, Rook GAW (1996) The disease distribution and pathogenetic significance of a raised percentage of agalactosyl IgG. In: Isenberg DA, Rademacher TW, Roitt I (eds). *Abnormalities of IgG glycosylation and immunological disorders*. Chichester: John Wiley & Sons 200–219.
30. Parekh RB, Isenberg D, Rook GAW, Roitt I, Dwek R, Rademacher T (1989) A comparative analysis of disease associated changes in galactosylation of serum IgG. *J Autoimmun* 2: 101–114.
31. Dube R, Rook GA, Steele J, Brealey R, Dwek R, Rademacher T, Lennard-Jones J (1990) Agalactosyl IgG in inflammatory bowel disease: Correlation with C-reactive protein. *Gut* 31: 431–434.
32. Rademacher TW, Jones RHV, Williams PJ (1995) Significance and molecular basis for IgG glycosylation changes in rheumatoid arthritis. *Adv Exp Med Biol* 376: 193–204.
33. Pilkington C, Taylor PV, Silverman E, Isenberg DA, Costello AMdL, Rook GAW (1996) Agalactosyl IgG and maternofetal transmission of autoimmune neonatal lupus. *Rheumatol Int.* 16: 89–94.
34. James DG, Turiaf J, Hosoda Y, Williams WJ, Israel HL, Douglas AC, et al. (1976) Description of Sarcoidosis: Report of the subcommittee on classification and definition. *Ann NY Acad Sci* 278: 742.
35. Hills SE, Parkes SA, Baker SB (1987) Epidemiology of sarcoidosis in the Isle of Man. 2. Evidence for space-time clustering. *Thorax* 42: 427–430.
36. Williams WJ, Williams R (1983) The value of beryllium lymphocyte transformation tests in chronic beryllium disease and in potentially exposed workers. *Thorax* 38: 41–44.
37. Shelley WB, Hurley HJ (1958) The allergic origin of zirconium deodorant granuloma. *Br J Dermatol* 70: 75–77.
38. Prendiville J, Robinson A, Young M (1982) Familial sarcoidosis. *Int J Med Sci* 151: 258–260.
39. Sharma OP, Neville E, Walker AN, James DG (1976) Familial sarcoidosis: A possible genetic influence. *Ann NY Acad Sci* 278: 335–346.
40. Guyatt GH, Bensen WG, Stolman IP, Fagnilli L, Singal DP (1982) HLA-B8 and erythema nodosum. *Can Med Assoc J* 127: 1005–1006.
41. James DG, Neville E (1977) Pathology of sarcoidosis. *Pathobiol Ann* 7: 31–36.
42. Scharf Y, Zonis S (1980) Histocompatibility antigens (HLA) and uveitis. *Surv Ophthalmol* 24: 220–228.
43. Persson IB, Ryder LP, Nielsen SL, Svejgaard A (1975) The HLA-B histocompatibility antigen in sarcoidosis in relation to tuberculin sensitivity. *Tissue Antigens* 6: 50–53.
44. Hedfors E, Lindstrom F (1983) HLA-B8/DR3 in sarcoidosis: Correlation to acute onset disease with arthritis. *Tissue Antigens* 22: 200–203.
45. Kremer JM (1986) Histologic findings in siblings with acute sarcoid arthritis: Association with the B8, DR3 phenotype. *J Rheumatol* 13: 593–597.

46. Shoenfeld Y, Isenberg DA (1989) *The Mosaic of autoimmunity*. Amsterdam: Elsevier, 183–186.
47. Smith MJ, Turton CW, Mitchell DN, Turner-Warwick M, Morris LM, Lawler SD (1981) Association of HLA-B8 with spontaneous resolution in sarcoidosis. *Thorax* 36: 296–298.
48. Neville E, James DG, Brewerton DA (1980) HLA antigens and features of sarcoidosis. In: Jones Williams W, Davies BH (eds). *Sarcoidosis*. Cardiff: Alpha and Omega Press, p 201
49. Mitchell DN, Scadding JG (1974) Sarcoidosis. *Am Rev Resp Dis* 110: 774–802.
50. Israel HL (1970) Prognosis of sarcoidosis. *Ann Intern Med* 73: 1038–1039.
51. Westcott JL, Noehren TH (1973) Bronchial stenosis in chronic sarcoidosis. *Chest* 63: 893–897.
52. Dines DE, Stubbs SE, McDougall JC (1978) Obstructive disease of the airways associated with stage 1 sarcoidosis. *Mayo Clin Proc* 53: 788–791.
53. Katz S (1983) Clinical presentation and natural history of sarcoidosis. In: Fanburg BL (ed). *Sarcoidosis and other granulomatous diseases of the lung*, vol. 20. Marcel Dekker, 3–36.
54. Kirks DR, McCormick VD, Greenspan RH (1973) Pulmonary sarcoidosis: Roentgenologic analysis of 150 patients. *Am J Radiol* 117: 777–786.
55. Freundlich IM, Libschitz I, Glassman LM, Israel HL (1970) Sarcoidosis, typical and atypical thoracic manifestations and complications. *Clin Radiol* 21: 373–383.
56. Siltzbach LE (1967) Sarcoidosis: Clinical features and management. *Med Clin North Am* 51: 483–502.
57. Chretien J, Venet A, Israel-Biet D, Clavel F, Sandron D (1986) Summary statement on disease activity assessment. *Ann NY Acad Sci* 465: 479–481.
58. Panel of the World Association of Sarcoidosis and Other Granulomatous Diseases (1994) Consensus conference. *Eur Resp J* 7: 624–627.
59. Hudspith BN, Flint KC, James GD, Brostoff J, Johnson NM (1987) Lack of immune deficiency in sarcoidosis: Compartmentalisation of the immune response. *Thorax* 42: 250–255.
60. Campbell D, Poulter LW, duBois RM (1985) Immunocompetent cells in bronchoalveolar lavage reflect the cell populations in transbronchial biopsies in pulmonary sarcoidosis. *Am Rev Resp Dis* 132: 1300–1306.
61. Spiteri MA, Poulter LW (1988) Autologous mixed lymphocyte reactions probe macrophage function in sarcoidosis. In: Grassi C, Rizzato G, Pozzi E (eds). Sarcoidosis and other granulomatous disorders. Amsterdam: Elsevier Science Publishers, 173–176.
62. Bjermer L, Rosenhall L, Angstrom T, Hallgren R (1988) Predictive value of bronchoalveolar lavage cell analysis in sarcoidosis. *Thorax* 43: 284–288.
63. Ward K, O'Connor C, Odlum C, Fitzgerald MX (1989) Prognostic value of bronchoalveolar lavage in sarcoidosis: The critical influence of disease presentation. *Thorax* 44: 732–738.
64. Foley NM, Coral AP, Tung K, Hudspith BN, James DG, Johnson NM (1989) Bronchoalveolar lavage cell counts as a predictor of short-term outcome in pulmonary sarcoidosis. *Thorax* 44: 732–738.
65. Lin YH, Haslam PL, Turner-Warwick M (1985) Chronic pulmonary sarcoidosis: Relationships between lung lavage cell counts, chest radiograph and results of standard lung function tests. *Thorax* 40: 501–507.
66. Line BR, Hunninghake GW, Keogh BA, Jones AE, Johnston GS, Crystal RG (1982) Gallium-67 scanning to stage the alveolitis of sarcoidosis: Correlation with clinical studies, pulmonary function tests and bronchoalveolar lavage. *Am Rev Resp Dis* 123: 440–446.
67. Costabel U, Bross KJ, Guzman J, Nilles A, Ruhle KH, Matthys H (1986) Predictive value of bronchoalveolar lavage T cell subsets for the course of pulmonary tuberculosis. *Ann NY Acad Sci* 465: 418–426.
68. Ainslie G, duBois RM, Poulter LW (1989) Relationship between immunocytological features of bronchoalveolar lavage and clinical indices in sarcoidosis. *Thorax* 44: 501–509.
69. Hunninghake GW, Gadek JE, Kawanami O, Ferrans VJ, Crystal RG (1979) Inflammatory and immune processes in the human lung in health and disease: Evaluation by bronchoalveolar lavage. *Am J Pathol* 97: 149–206.

70. Paradis IL, Dauber JH, Rabin BS (1986) Lymphocyte phenotypes in bronchoalveolar lavage and lung tissue in sarcoidosis and idiopathic pulmonary fibrosis. *Am Rev Resp Dis* 133: 858–860.
71. Pinkston P, Bitterman PB, Crystal RG (1983) Spontaneous release of interleukin-2 by lung T lymphocytes in active pulmonary sarcoidosis. *N Engl J Med* 308: 793–800.
72. Mornex JF, Cordier G, Pages J, Lefebure R, Revillard JP, Vergnon JM, et al. (1985) Pulmonary sarcoidosis: Flow cytometry measurement of lung T-cell activation. *J Lab Clin Med* 105: 70–76.
73. Hunninghake GW, Crystal RG (1981) Pulmonary sarcoidosis a disorder mediated by excess helper T lymphocyte activity at sites of disease activity. *N Engl J Med* 305:429–434.
74. Hunninghake GW, Gadek JE, Young RC, Kawanami O, Ferrans VJ, Crystal RG (1980) Maintenance of granuloma formation in pulmonary sarcoidosis by T lymphocytes within the lung. *N Engl J Med* 302: 594–598.
75. Robinson BWS, McLemore TL, Crystal RG (1985) Gamma interferon is spontaneously released by alveolar macrophages and lung T lymphocytes in patients with pulmonary sarcoidosis. *J Clin Invest* 75: 1488–1495.
76. Hancock WW, Kobzik L, Colby AJ, O'Hara CJ, Cooper AG, Gooleski JJ (1986) Detection of lymphokines and lymphokine receptors in pulmonary sarcoidosis: Immunohistologic evidence that inflammatory macrophages express IL-2 receptors. *Am J Pathol* 123: 1–8.
77. duBois RM, Kirby M, Balbi B, Saltini C, Crystal RG (1992) T-lymphocytes accumulating in the lung in sarcoidosis have evidence of recent stimulation of the T-cell antigen receptor. *Am Rev Resp Dis* 145: 1205–1211.
78. Nakata K, Sugie T, Nakano H, Sakai T, Aoki M (1994) Gamma-delta T-cells in sarcoidosis: Correlation with clinical features. *Am J Respir Crit Care Med* 149: 981–988.
79. Campbell DA, duBois RM, Butcher RG, Poulter LW (1986) The density of HLA-DR antigen expression on human alveolar macrophages isolated by bronchoalveolar lavage. *Clin Exp Immunol* 65: 165–171.
80. Venet A, Hance AJ, Saltini C, Robinson BW, Crystal RG (1985) Enhanced alveolar macrophage-mediated antigen-induced T lymphocyte proliferation in sarcoidosis. *J Clin Invest* 75: 293–301.
81. Prior C, Knight RA, Herold M, Ott G, Spiteri MA (1996) Pulmonary sarcoidosis: Patterns of cytoline release *in vitro. Eur Resp J* 9: 47–53.
82. Bachwich PR, Lynch JP, Larrick J, Spengler M, Kunkel SL (1986) Tumour necrosis factor production by human sarcoid alveolar macrophages. *Am J Pathol* 125: 421–425.
83. Kaneshima H, Nagai S, Shimoji T, Tsutsumi T, Mikuniya T, Satake N, Izumi T (1994) TNF alpha mRNA but not IL-1 beta is differentially expressed in lung macrophages of patients with active pulmonary sarcoidosis. *Sarcoidosis* 11: 19–25.
84. Lukacs NW, Chensue SW, Strieter RM, Warmington K, Kunkel SL (1994) Inflammatory granuloma formation is mediated by TNFα-inducible intercellular adhesion molecule-1. *J Immunol* 152: 5883–5889.
85. Rook GAW (1988) The role of vitamin D in tuberculosis. *Am Rev Resp Dis* 138: 768–770.
86. Lemire JM (1995) Immunomodulatory actions of 1,25-dihydroxyvitamin D3. *J Steroid Biochem Mol Biol* 53: 599–602.
87. Spiteri MA, Clarke SW, Poulter LW (1992) Alveolar macrophages that suppress T-cell responsiveness may be crucial to the pathogenic outcome of pulmonary sarcoidosis. *Eur Resp J* 5: 394–403.
88. Kobayashi K, Allred C, Yoshida T (1989) Suppression of interleukin 2 production by sera obtained from hypersensitivity granuloma-bearing mice with defective T-cell-mediated immune responses. *Immunobiology* 178: 329–339.
89. Radic I, Vucak I, Milosevic J, Marusic A, Vukicevic S, Marusic M (1988) Immunosuppression induced by talc granulomatosis in the rat. *Clin Exp Immunol* 73: 316–321.
90. Hunninghake GW, Crystal RG (1981) Mechanisms of hypergammaglobulinaemia in pulmonary sarcoidosis: Site of increased antibody production and role of T lymphocytes. *J Clin Invest* 67: 86–92.
91. Lobop I, Suratt PM (1979) Studies on the autoantibody to lymphocytes in sarcoidosis. *J Lab Clin Immunol* 1: 283–288.
92. O'Connor CM, Rook GAW, Fitzgerald MX (1992) Proceedings of the World Conference on Sarcoidosis and Other Granulomatous diseases: Serum agalactosyl IgG levels in sarcoidosis. In: James G, Izumi T (eds). *Sarcoidosis*, vol. 9 (Suppl 1), 453–454.

93. Bernaudin JF, LaCronique J, Soler P, Lange F, Kawanami O, Basset F (1981) Alveolitis and granulomas: Sequential onset and evolution in pulmonary sarcoidosis. *Bull Eur Physiopathol Respir* 17: 27–64.
94. Crystal RG, Roberts WC, Hunninghake GW, Gadek JE, Fulmer JD, Line BR (1981) Pulmonary sarcoidosis: A disease characterised and perpetuated by activated T lymphocytes. *Ann Intern Med* 94: 73–94.
95. Rosen Y, Athanassiades TJ, Moon S, Lyons HA (1978) Non-granulomatous interstitial pneumonitis in sarcoidosis: Relationship to the development of epithelioid granulomas. *Chest* 74: 122–125.
96. Carr I, Norris P (1977) The fine structure of human macrophage granules in sarcoidosis. *J Pathol* 122: 29–32.
97. Spector WG (1976) Epithelioid cells, giant cells and sarcoidosis. *Ann NY Acad Sci* 278: 3–6.
98. Liebow AA (1973) The J. Burns Amberson lecture: Pulmonary angiitis and granulomatosis. *Am Rev Resp Dis* 108: 1–18.
99. Saldana MJ (1978) Necrotising sarcoid granulomatosis: Clinicopathologic observations in 24 patients. *Lab Invest* 38: 364.
100. Churg A (1983) Pulmonary angiitis and granulomatosis revisited. *Hum Pathol* 14: 868–883.
101. Koss MN, Hocholzer L, Faigan S, Garancis TC, Ward PA (1980) Necrotising sarcoid-like granulomatosis: Clinical, pathologic and immunopathologic findings. *Hum Pathol* 11: 510–519.
102. Saldana MJ, Israel HL (1989) Necrotising sarcoid granulomatosis, benign lymphocytic angiitis and granulomatosis: Do they exist? *Semin Resp Med* 10: 182–188.
103. Spiteri MA, Gledhill A, Campbell D, Clarke SW (1987) Necrotising sarcoid granulomatosis. *Br J Dis Chest* 81: 70–75.
104. Wynn TA, Eltoum I, Cheever AW, Lewis FA, Gause WC, Sher A (1993) Analysis of cytokine mRNA expression during primary granuloma formation induced by eggs of *Schistosoma mansoni*. *J Immunol* 151: 1430–1440.
105. Joseph AL, Boros DL (1993) Tumour necrosis factor plays a role in *Schistosoma mansoni* egg-induced granulomatous inflammation. *J Immunol* 151: 5461–5471.
106. Rook GAW, Hernandez-Pando R (1996) The pathogenesis of tuberculosis. *Ann Rev Microbiol* 50: 259–284.
107. Shands JW, Senterfitt VC (1972) Endotoxin-induced hepatic damage in BCG-infected mice. *Am J Pathol* 67: 23–40.
108. Ferluga J, Doenhoff MJ, Allison AC (1979) Increased hepatotoxicity of bacterial lipopolysaccharide in mice infected with *Schistosoma mansoni*. *Parasite Immunol* 1: 289–294.
109. Hernandez-Pando R, Rook GAW (1994) The role of TNFα in T-cell-mediated inflammation depends on the Th1/Th2 cytokine balance. *Immunology* 82: 591–595.
110. Schauf V, Rom WN, Smith KA, Sampaio EP, Meyn PA, Tramontana JM, Cohn ZA, Kaplan G (1993) Cytokine gene activation and modified responsiveness to interleukin-2 in the blood of tuberculosis patients. *J Infect Dis* 168: 1056–1059.
111. Yong AJ, Grange JM, Tee RD, Beck JS, Bothamley GH, Kemeny DM et al. (1989) Total and anti-mycobacterial IgE levels in serum from patients with tuberculosis and leprosy. *Tubercle* 70: 273–279.
112. Wynn TA, Cheever AW, Jankovic D, Poindexter RW, Caspar P, Lewis FA, Sher A (1995) An IL-12-based vaccination method for preventing fibrosis induced by schistosome infection. *Nature* 376: 594–596.
113. Toossi Z (1996) Cytokine circuits in tuberculosis. *Infect Agents Dis* 5: 98–107.
114. Zugmaier G, Paik S, Wilding G et al. (1991) Transforming growth factor b1 induces cachexia and systemic fibrosis without an anti-tumour effect in nude mice. *Cancer Res* 51: 3590–3594.
115. Roman J, Jeon YJ, Gal A, Perez RL (1995) Distribution of extracellular matrices, matrix receptors, and transforming growth factor beta 1 in human and experimental lung granulomatous inflammation. *Am J Med Sci* 309: 124–133.
116. Magnan A, Frachon I, Rain B, Peuchmaur M, Monti G, Lenot B et al. (1994) Transforming growth factor beta in normal lung: Preferential location in bronchial epithelial cells. *Thorax* 49: 789–792.

117. Toossi Z, Gogate P, Shiratsuchi H, Young T, Ellner JJ (1995) Enhanced production of TGFβ by blood monocytes from patients with active tuberculosis and presence of TGFβ in tuberculous granulomatous lung lesions. *J Immunol* 154: 465–473.
118. Limper AH, Colby TV, Sanders MS, Asakura S, Roche PC, DeRemee RA (1994) Immuno-histochemical localisation of transforming growth factor-β in the non-necrotising granulomas of pulmonary sarcoidosis. *Am J Respir Crit Care Med* 149: 197–204.
119. Wangoo A, Taylor IK, Haynes AR, Shaw RJ (1993) Upregulation of alveolar macrophage platelet-derived growth factor-β mRNA by interferon gamma from *Mycobacterium tuberculosis* antigen (PPD)-stimulated lymphocytes. *Clin Exp Immunol* 94: 43–50.
120. Ramirez F, Fowell DJ, Puklavec M, Simmonds S, Mason D (1996) Glucocorticoids promote a Th2 cytokine response by CD4+ T-cells *in vitro*. J Immunol 156: 2405–2412.
121. Brinkmann V, Kristofic C (1995) Regulation by corticosteroids of Th1 and TH2 cytokine production in human CD4+ effector T-cells generated from CD45RO- and CD45RO+ subsets. *J Immunol* 155(7): 3322–3328.
122. Batuman OA, Ferrero AP, Diaz A, Jimenez SA (1991) Regulation of transforming growth factor-beta 1 gene expression by glucocorticoids in normal human T lymphocytes. *J Clin Invest* 88: 1574–1580.
123. Rook GAW, Honour J, Kon OM, Wilkinson RJ, Davidson R, Shaw RJ (1996) Urinary steroid metabolites in tuberculosis. A new clue to pathogenesis. *Q J Med* 89: 333–341.
124. Sarma GR, Chandra I, Ramachandran G, Krishnamurthy PV, Kumaraswami V, Prabhakar R (1990) Adrenocortical function in patients with pulmonary tuberculosis. *Tubercle* 71: 277–282.
125. Blauer KL, Poth M, Rogers WM, Bernton EW (1991) Dehydroepiandrosterone antagonises the suppressive effects of dexamethasone on lymphocyte proliferation. *Endocrinology* 129(6): 3174–3179.
126. Schleimer RP (1991) Potential regulation of inflammation in the lung by local metabolism of hydrocortisone. *Am J Respir Cell Mol Biol* 4: 166–173.
127. Hubbard WC, Bickel C, Schleimer RP (1994) Simultaneous quantitation of endogenous levels of cortisone and cortisol in human nasal and bronchoalveolar lavage fluids and plasma via gas chromatography-negative ion chemical ionization mass spectrometry. *Anal Biochem* 221: 109–117.
128. Jamieson PM, Chapman KE, Edwards CR, Seckl JR (1995) 11 Beta-hydroxysteroid dehydrogenase is an exclusive 11 beta-reductase in primary cultures of rat hepatocytes: Effect of physicochemical and hormonal manipulations. *Endocrinology* 136: 4754–4761.
129. Evangelatou M, Antoniw J, Cooke BA (1996) The effect of leukocytes on 11β-HSD activity in human granulosa cell cultues. *J Endocrinol* 148(Suppl): Abstract P55.

Autoimmune Aspects of Lung Disease
ed. by D. A. Isenberg and S. G. Spiro
© 1998 Birkhäuser Verlag Basel/Switzerland

CHAPTER 5
The Diagnosis and Treatment of Respiratory Infections in Autoimmune Disease, Excluding Tuberculosis

Graham H. Bothamley[1] and Penny Shaw[2]

[1] *Department of Respiratory Medicine, Homerton Hospital, London, UK*
[2] *Department of Imaging, University College London Hospitals, London, UK*

1. Introduction

Respiratory infections play an important role in the morbidity and mortality associated with autoimmune disease. A patient with autoimmune disease who presents with a fever, cough breathlessness or pleuritic pain may have a respiratory infection, but these symptoms can also occur if there is an exacerbation of the autoimmune process or adverse reaction to medication. A general approach to such a patient is outlined as an algorithm in Figure 1. A complete drug history is essential. Empirical treatment with antibiotics for common respiratory infections (e.g. a penicillin and a macrolide), while awaiting the results of blood cultures, sputum examination and serology, will cover the majority of such episodes. Patients with low numbers of circulating neutrophils or lymphocytes require special consideration. High-resolution computed tomography (CT) may reveal parenchymal lesions where the chest radiograph appears normal, such as ground-glass shadowing with *Pneumocystis carinii* pneumonia (PCP), nodules with *Aspergillus* or an early drug reaction, or may be diagnostic, e.g. the "halo sign" in *Aspergillus* infection. A more invasive approach is dictated by a lack of response to treatment, and again CT is valuable in planning the procedure and anatomical site to be sampled. The choice of bronchoscopy, thoracoscopy or open-lung biopsy is determined by the patient's condition: rapid worsening of the patient's clinical state or hypoxia recommend an open-lung biopsy. Transbronchial biopsies are frequently too small to provide adequate material to make a diagnosis, and there is a greater risk to the patient who is approaching respiratory failure from pneumothorax and haemorrhage.

This chapter will confirm the greater frequency of respiratory infections in patients with autoimmune disease and suggest some reasons for this finding, review the differential diagnosis of patients whose chest radiographs show diffuse alveolar infiltration, focal pulmonary shadowing, nodules or a pleural effusion, note the effect of treatment as a cause or a mimic of respiratory infections and examine the evidence for a role for respiratory infections in the pathogenesis of autoimmune disease.

2. Increased Risk of Respiratory Infection

2.1. Pneumonia

Pneumonia occurs frequently in patients with rheumatoid arthritis (RA) and systemic lupus erythematosus (SLE) and may be related to the disease process itself or its treatment. Walker [1] was one of the first to suggest that pulmonary infections were especially common in RA. Suzuki et al. [2] noted that infection was the cause of death in almost a quarter of a series of 81 patients with RA, 14 of whom had pneumonia. This frequency was

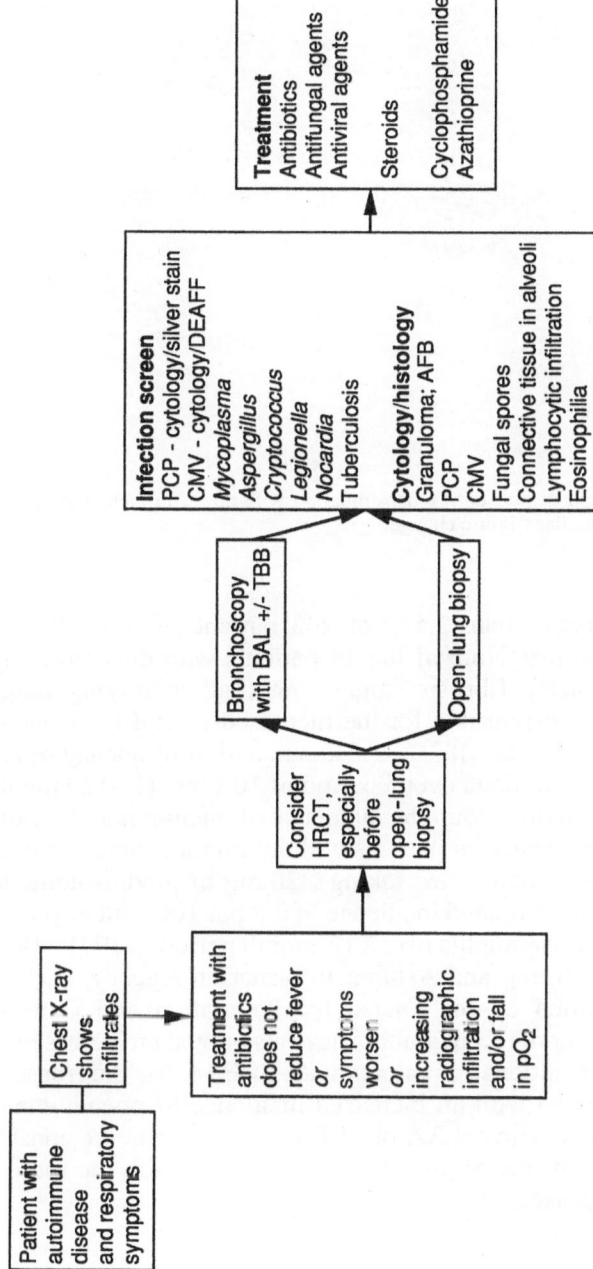

Figure 1. An algorithm for attaining the diagnosis of pulmonary infiltrates in patients with autoimmune disease.

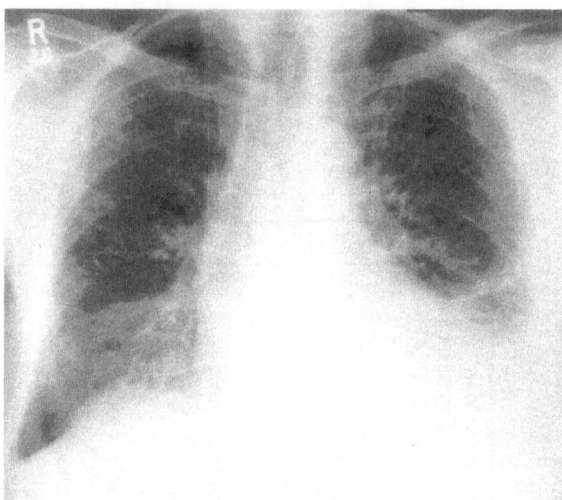

Figure 2. Radiograph demonstrating consulidation with an air bronchogram at the left base, with background nodular fibrotic change.

significantly greater than 2.5% of 243 patients without RA who were examined at autopsy. Nine of the 14 patients who died from pneumonia also had pulmonary fibrosis, suggesting that underlying lung damage might be in part responsible for the increased mortality of pneumonia in RA (Figure 2). Patients with SLE also had a high frequency of respiratory infections when examined over a period of 10 years (1–120 months, mean 35 months) [3]. In this group the incidence of pneumonia was calculated at 35 per 100 patient years for patients without immunosuppressive treatment and 179 per 100 patient years taking >20 mg of prednisolone daily. This compares with an estimated incidence of 0.5 per 100 patient years from GP consultations for pneumonia over a 12-month period in 1991–1992 in England and Wales (Lung and Asthma Information Agency, Factsheet 95/3, from data supplied by the Office for Population and Census Studies (OPCS)). Other more recent authors have also noted an increased frequency of respiratory infections in patients with SLE [4, 5]. Sjögren's syndrome was also associated with an increased incidence of pneumonia, although frequently with concurrent RA or SLE [6]. These data are consistent with an increased incidence of pneumonia in patients with the more common autoimmune diseases.

2.2. Bronchiectasis

There have been sporadic reports of bronchiectasis associated with RA (Figure 3), but the majority have implied merely a chance association

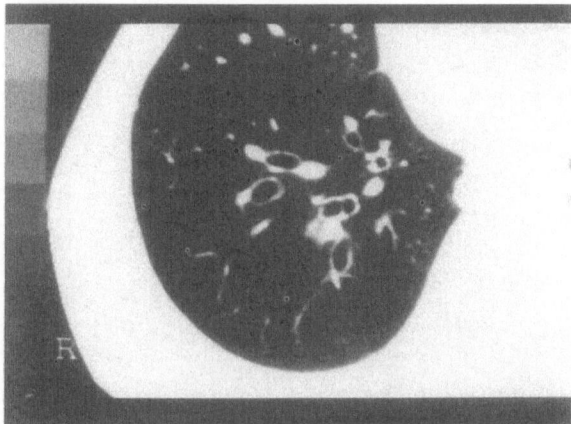

Figure 3. CT scan with typical changes of bronchiectasis in the right lower lobe (signet ring appearance) in a patient with rheumatoid arthritis.

[7, 8]. In these studies bronchiectasis has often preceded the development of arthritis. Shadick et al. [9] compared patients with RA who developed bronchiectasis before and after the diagnosis of RA. The majority of those who developed bronchiectasis after the diagnosis of RA had severe joint disease with extra-articular features and rheumatoid nodules and had an unfavourable prognosis. As expected, those patients with more severe disease had received more immunosuppressive therapy, and a role for drug treatment in the pathogenesis of bronchiectasis could not be excluded.

2.3. Possible Reasons for Increased Susceptibility to Respiratory Infections

Patients with autoimmune disease might be especially susceptible to respiratory infections for a number of reasons. The antibody response may be disturbed. Lower levels of naturally occurring antibodies to *Brucella* and *Escherichia coli* and possibly a poorer response to immunization with influenza and tetanus toxoid have been reported in SLE [10]. Hypogammaglobulinaemia might play a role. However, in patients with Sjögren's syndrome and immunoglobulin A (IgA) with IgG2 deficiency, only 2 of 34 patients had more infections than other patients with Sjögren's syndrome alone [11], while chronic respiratory infections were not associated with an increase in autoantibodies found in patients with IgA and/or IgG2 deficiency [12]. There is general agreement that delayed hypersensitivity is reduced in patients with SLE and RA [10, 13].

Non-specific immunity may also be affected. Levels of tumour necrosis factor are reduced in some patients with SLE [14]. Cytotoxicity due to monocytes is impaired in patients with RA [15]. Autoimmune neutropaenia

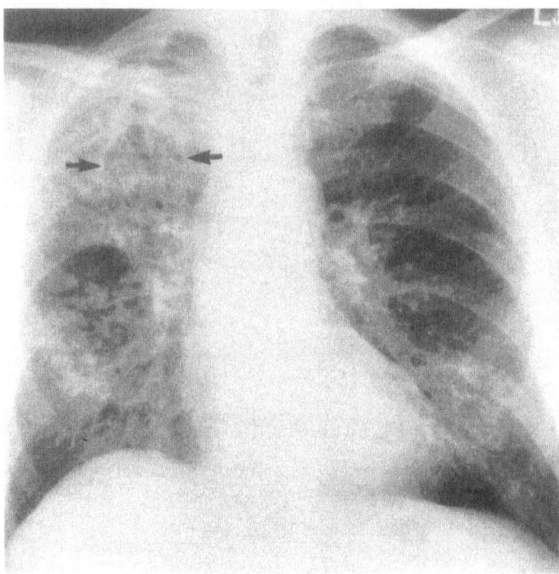

Figure 4. Chest X-ray with changes of aspiration pneumonia bilaterally with cavitation in the right upper lobe (arrowed). Note atypical site with right upper lobe predominance.

has been reported in patients with RA, SLE, idiopathic thrombocytopenic purpura (ITP) and Coombs-positive haemolytic anaemia. However, in a series of 20 patients whose neutropaenia was unrelated to treatment, serious respiratory infections were unusual, and only one patient developed pneumonia and respiratory failure [16].

On a more prosaic note, aspiration pneumonia can be a feature of several autoimmune disorders (Figure 4). In polymyositis, symmetrical weakness of the pharyngeal muscles permits aspiration of food or stomach contents and is a poor prognostic sign in patients with this disease. Difficulty in swallowing is a frequent presenting feature of myasthenia gravis, and a tracheostomy is more often required to protect the airway from the inhalation of food than for weakness of the intercostal muscles and diaphragm. Aspiration pneumonia may also occur in patients with diabetes mellitus as a result of hyperglycaemic, hyperosmolar coma and its attendant delay in gastric emptying.

3. Differential Diagnosis of Diffuse Pulmonary Infiltrates

Pneumonia remains the most common cause of diffuse pulmonary infiltrates in patient with autoimmune disease. Opportunitistic infections are more frequent in patients with autoimmune disease and need not be due to treatment. However, similar radiological appearances may occur as a result

Table 1. Differential diagnosis of pulmonary infiltrates in autoimmune lung disease

Rate of onset of symptoms	Radiographic appearance	
	Diffuse	Focal/nodular
Rapid	*Pneumocystis carinii*[1] *Cytomegalovirus*[1] *Mycoplasma* (pulmonary oedema) (pulmonary haemorrhage) (leukoagglutination)	Gram-negative bacilli[2] *S. aureus*[2] *Aspergillus*[2] (pulmonary infarction)
Subacute	*Cytomegalovirus*[1] *Mycoplasma* (drug-induced) (SLE pneumonitis) (pulmonary eosinophilia) *Strongyloides*[1]	*Aspergillus*[2] *Cryptococcus*[1] *Legionella*[1] (bronchiolitis obliterans with organizing pneumonia) (non-specific interstitial pneumonitis) (septic emboli) (Wegener's granulomatosis) (rheumatoid nodules) (lung abscess)
Chronic	(pulmonary fibrosis)	*Nocardia*[1] *Cryptococcus*[1] Tuberculosis (recrudescence of Wegener's granulomata or rheumatoid nodules)

[1] Associated with impaired T-cell immunity, e.g. due to high-dose steroids.
[2] Neutropaenia, e.g. due to penicillamine, gold, azathioprine.
  Brackets denote non-infectious causes of radiographic appearances.

of the disease process (Table 1). Pneumonia is defined pathologically by the presence of an inflammatory infiltrate in the alveoli of the lung. An infection of the lower respiratory tract usually presents with fever, breathlessness, purulent sputum and occasionally pleuritic pain. Radiographically, alveolar shadowing with air bronchograms or reticulonodular infiltrates are characteristic of infection (Figure 5). Resolution of fever is one of the first signs of successful treatment, and a persistent high temperature should alert the cinician to an alternative diagnosis, as much as to the need to exclude bronchial obstruction, inadequate antibiotic treatment or progressive infection, such as an empyema or lung abscess.

3.1. Pneumocystis carinii *Pneumonia* (PCP)

Pneumocystis carinii pneumonia was initially described in young malnourished children but later became associated with immunodeficiency or immunosuppressive treatment before its present major role in defining

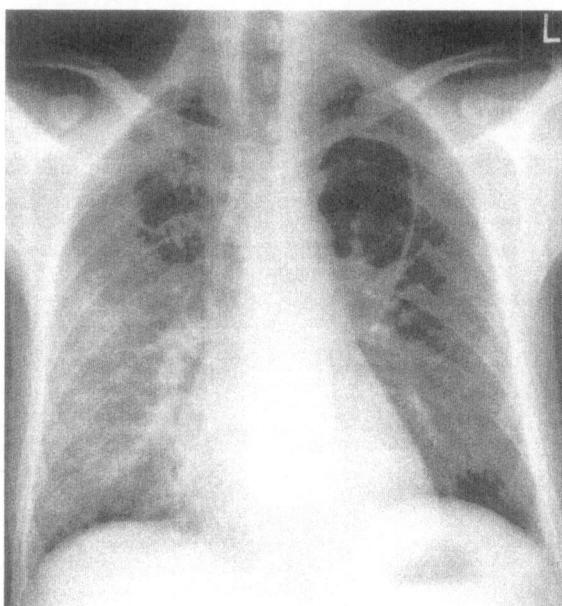

Figure 5. Radiograph with coarse reticular nodular infiltrates due to infection with *Pseudomonas aeruginosa*.

acquired immunodeficiency syndrome (AIDS) in patients infected with the human immunodeficiency viruses (HIV) [17]. Patients with autoimmune diseases are at a low risk of PCP. Lymphopaenia is the main risk factor associated with PCP in patients with SLE (Figure 6) [18]. Only two in a series of 34 patients with PCP and autoimmune disease in the absence of HIV infection were not receiving immunosuppressive treatment and both had SLE, one with an associated lymphopaenia and the other with very active disease [19]. The remainder had received treatment with corticosteroids (mean dose of 1.2 mg/kg/day) for the previous 2 months, and 24 of these 32 had also been treated with additional immunosuppressive agents. In Wegener's granulomatosis, PCP is usually associated with drug-induced lymphopaenia [20]; death from PCP was especially associated with methotrexate and glucocorticoid therapy [21, 22].

Patients with PCP experience breathlessness and cough and have a respiratory rate and hypoxaemia which is usually out of proportion to the degree of radiographic infiltration. The classic radiographic features include a perihilar and basal reticular infiltrate or ground-glass shadowing. High-resolution CT demonstrates the characteristic central ground-glass shadowing and cystic air spaces well. Lymphadenopathy and pulmonary nodules are uncommon. Upper-lobe pneumonia is a well-recognized presentation. Most patients have a lymphopaenia and treatment with high-dose trime-

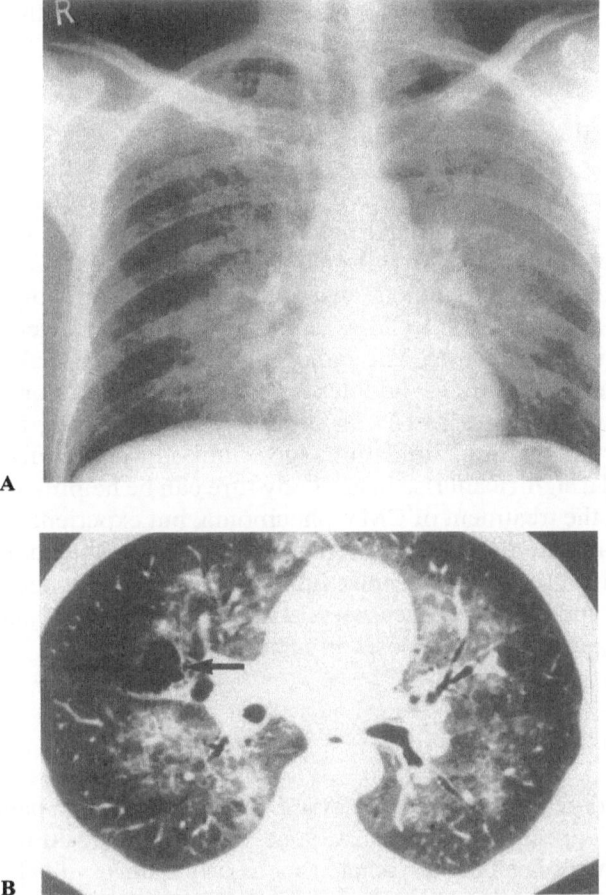

Figure 6. *Pneumocystis carinii* pneumonia. (A) Chest X-ray with a typical perihilar, fine reticular infiltrate and ground-glass shadowing. (B) HRCT of the same patient with central ground-glass shadowing, thickening of interlobular septae and a large air space typical of *Pneumocystis carinii* (arrowed).

thoprim-sulphamethoxazole can be initiated on clinical suspicion, as the cysts may be recovered by bronchoalveolar lavage for several days after the start of treatment [23]. Patients with PCP have a greater risk of pneumothorax and fatal haemorrhage from transbronchial biopsy [23]. Pentamidine, clindamycin and primaquine, dapsone and trimethoprim combined and atovaquone have all been used with success in the treatment of PCP. Many of these drugs are secreted via the kidneys, and dose-related adjustments are required where the creatinine clearance is low. Corticosteroids are helpful in severe disease, especially in patients with respiratory failure ($pO_2 < 8$ kPa).

Hydroxychloroquine might be protective, as withdrawal of this treatment has been associated with the development of PCP [24].

3.2. Cytomegalovirus *Pneumonia*

Pneumonia due to *Cytomegalovirus* (CMV) is an important disease associated with immunosuppression and has most commonly been described in patients following bone marrow transplantation or with AIDS. Systemic features are common and include myalgia, arthralgia and fatigue. Definitive diagnosis is difficult, as CMV, in common with other herpesviruses, causes a persistent infection. The radiographic findings are also variable, including reticular infiltrates, nodules or alveolar consolidation (Figure 7). Bronchoalveolar lavage (BAL) can be helpful in obtaining material for culture and cytological examination; IgM antibody is produced early in infection, and a significant rise in antibody titre can be helpful. Ganciclovir is effective in the treatment of CMV pneumonia, but experience of patients with CMV pneumonia following bone marrow transplantation has suggested that the use of intravenous immunoglobulin with the drug may improve outcome [25, 26]. Foscarnet is also effective in CMV pneumonitis. Both drugs require modified doses in renal impairment.

3.3. *Mycoplasma*

Although *Mycoplasma* pneumonia is a frequent respiratory pathogen, the pathogenesis appears to involve immune complex deposition, and IgM rheumatoid factor has been associated with early recovery [27].

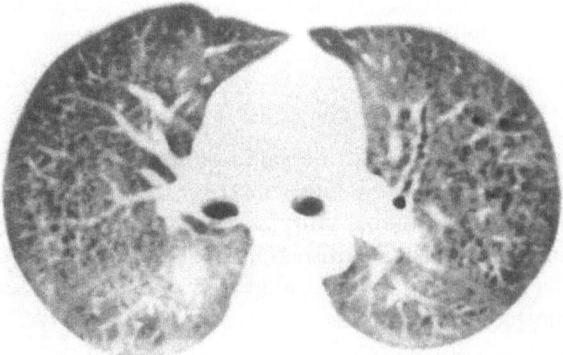

Figure 7. Cytomegalovirus pneumonia. HRCT with ground-glass shadowing, thickening of the interlobular septae and a nodule in the apical segment of the right lower lobe due to cytomegalovirus.

3.4. Differentiating Autoimmune Diffuse Infiltrates from Respiratory Infections

3.4.1. SLE pneumonitis: Patients with acute SLE pneumonitis have many features in common with bacterial pneumonia, except that the sputum is less frequently purulent and more often greenish. Clinical examination reveals consolidation in both pneumonia and SLE pneumonitis. The chest radiograph may show a reticular or ground-glass appearance because of the perivascular nature of the pathology and the relative absence of intra-alveolar material by comparison with bacterial pneumonia (Figure 8). A lung biopsy shows alveolar damage, interstitital oedema and hyaline membrane formation, with perivascular lymphocytic and plasma cell infiltrates. Active disease responds to corticosteroids and immunosuppression [28].

3.4.2. Pulmonary haemorrhage: Pulmonary haemorrhage (Figure 9) is usually of more rapid onset than a respiratory infection and is a rare but potentially fatal complication of SLE. Rapid diagnosis with high doses of corticosteroids and immunosuppression with azathioprine or cyclophosphamide is the treatment of choice [28].

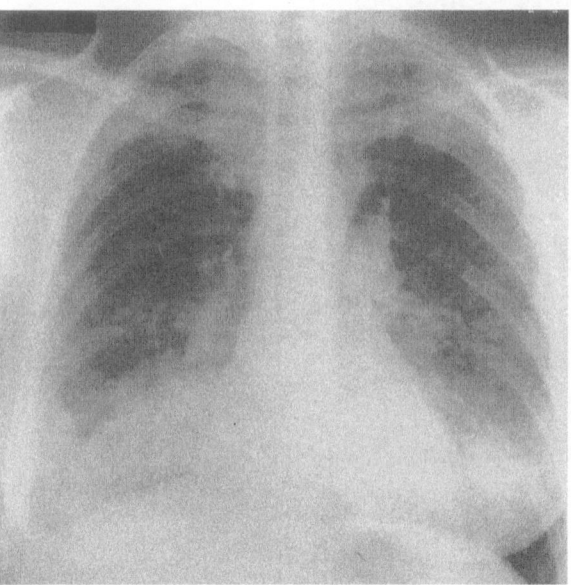

Figure 8. SLE pneumonitis. Chest X-ray with patchy, ill-defined opacities due to diffuse alveolar damage in SLE. Note that radiological differentiation from haemorrhage or infection may be difficult.

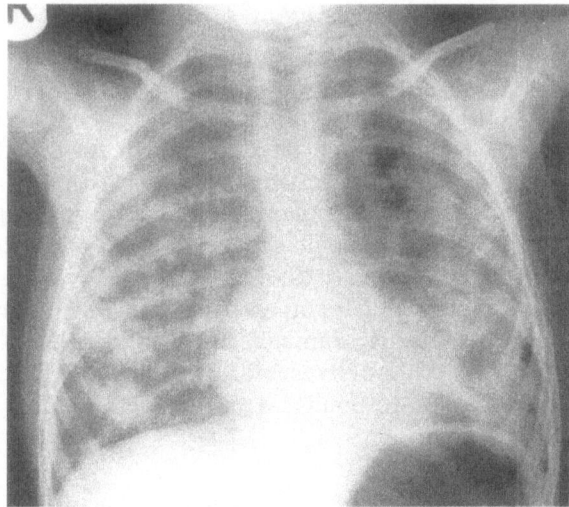

Figure 9. Chest X-ray of a child with extensive bilateral intrapulmonary haemorrhage, mimicking infection.

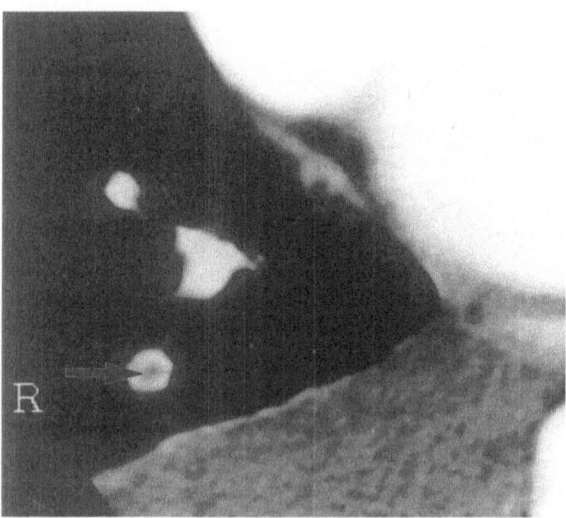

Figure 10. Helical CT pulmonary angiography demonstrating a small thrombus (arrowed) in a segmental artery in the right lower lobe with a pleural effusion.

3.4.3. Pulmonary emboli: Patients with SLE and lupus anticoagulant may experience breathlessness with transient lung infiltrates due to pulmonary emboli; treatment is again aimed at the underlying disorder. Helical pulmonary CT angiography is useful, as it directly visualizes the thrombus in the proximal pulmonary arteries (Figure 10).

3.4.4. Pulmonary oedema: Pulmonary oedema due to poor renal function (in autoimmune diseases, most commonly lupus nephritis) may be difficult to distinguish radiographically from pneumonia, but the absence of fever and the presence of other clinical features of fluid overload (e.g. tachycardia, raised jugular venous pressure, fourth heart sound) are most helpful.

3.4.5. Others: Diffuse infiltrates due to Wegener's granulomatosis (Figure 11) are a common presenting feature of the disease, but the more insidious onset more commonly suggests a pneumonia (Figure 12) due to an obstructing neoplasm [29]. Candidiasis has been associated with polymyositis/dermatomyositis [30].

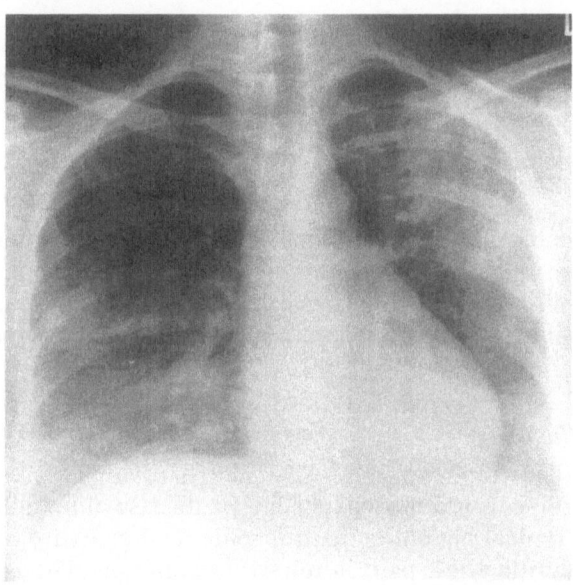

Figure 11. Wegener's granulomatosis. Radiograph with asymmetrical infiltrates due to Wegener's granulomatosis in the left upper lobe, anterior segment of the right upper lobe and right base.

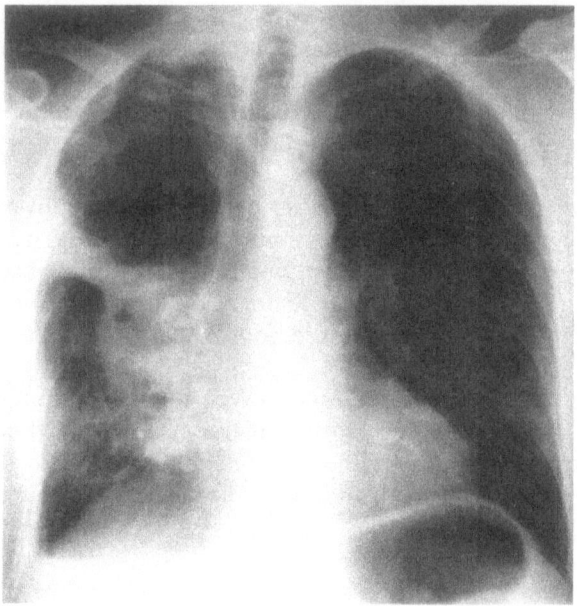

Figure 12. Wegener's granulomatosis. Radiograph demonstrating pneumonic changes distal to Wegener's involvement in the right middle lobe and anterior segment of the right upper lobe in a 64-year-old man.

4. Focal Infiltrates

4.1. Gram-Negative Bacillary Pneumonias

Gram-negative bacillary pneumonia usually occurs in debilitated patients, especially those with chronic renal failure (a common concomitant of certain autoimmune disease, including diabetes) or drug-induced neutropaenia. Combination therapy with a β-lactam and aminoglycoside is recommended.

4.2. Aspergillus

Invasive aspergillosis is almost exclusively a disease of immunosuppressed patients. The typical patient is neutropaenic, and apart from a dry cough and fever, pleuritic chest pain is relatively common. The most common radiographic finding is that of patchy focal consolidation. Local vascular invasion leads to haemorrhagic infarction. High-resolution CT may lead to early diagnosis by demonstrating nodules (areas of infarction) with a surrounding haemorrhagic halo (CT halo sign; Figure 13). A sequestrum of necrotic tissue giving the appearance of an "air crescent" on CT scanning

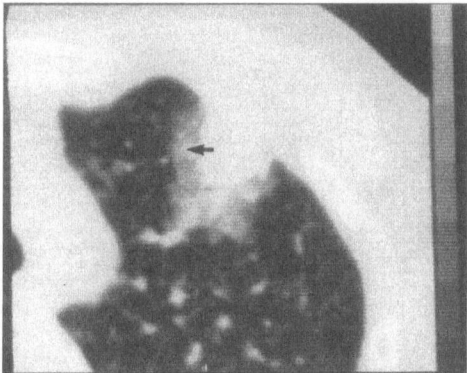

Figure 13. Invasive aspergillosis. A CT scan of a bone marrow transplant recipient, illustrating a nodule with a surrounding halo (arrowed, CT halo sign), typical of invasive aspergillosis.

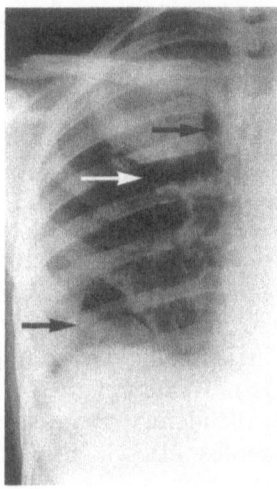

Figure 14. Chest X-ray demonstrating two "air crescents" (arrowed) due to retraction of infarcted lung in a bone marrow transplant recipient with invasive aspergillosis.

is seen late in the disease after retraction of infarcted lung (Figure 14) [31, 32]. The radiographic appearance of *Aspergillus* pneumonia is often sufficiently diagnostic to begin treatment with amphotericin, perhaps in combination with 5-fluorocytosine. Liposomal amphotericin is especially useful in patients with impaired renal function. Chronic necrotizing aspergillosis (Figure 15) may occur in patients with diabetes or receiving low-dose corticosteroids. The pulmonary infiltrates evolve more slowly and often cavitate. These lesions respond to medical treatment but may require surgical resection [33].

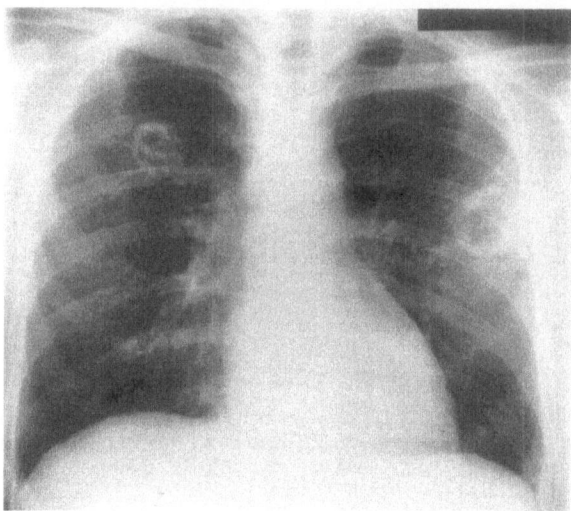

Figure 15. Radiograph showing bilateral chronic necrotizing aspergillosis in a young man (proven on percutaneous biopsy).

4.3. Cryptococcus

Cryptococcus neoformans is a saprophytic fungus that may be found in patients receiving therapeutic doses of corticosteroids and occasionally in patients with diabetes or uraemia [34]. Non-specific respiratory symptoms are common, but more than a third of patients may be asymptomatic. Radiographic appearances include single or multiple masses without hilar lymphadenopathy (Figure 16). Treatment in the absence of extrapulmonary dissemmination is not mandatory. Regimens which include amphotericin, flucytosine or imidazoles, often in combination are reported to be effective.

4.4. Nocardia

Nocardiosis has been reported in association with RA [35]. The organism is now an opportunist pathogen in patients with debilitating illnesses of almost any type. The chest radiograph most often has the appearance of tuberculosis, with both focal infiltrates and nodular shadowing which may cavitate (Figure 17). Clinical features are non-specific, and the diagnosis is made on sputum or histology. Treatment has traditionally been with sulphonamides, and the combination of trimethoprim and sulphamethoxazole is effective, although amikacin and imipenem are preferred treatments.

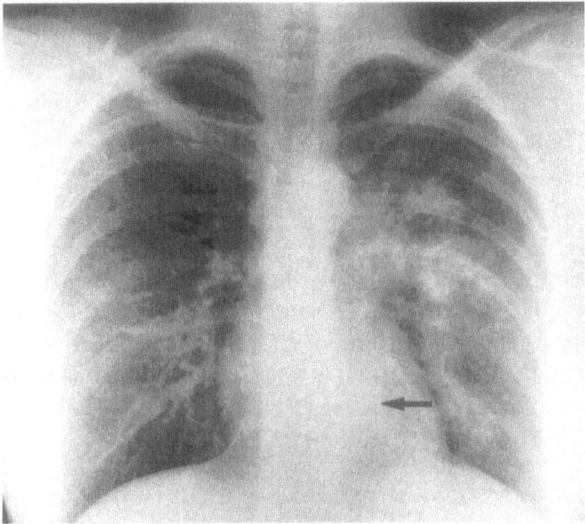

Figure 16. *Cryptococcus neoformans*. Radiograph illustrating multiple masses in a left peri-hilar distribution in a 38-year-old man with a further mass in the left lower lobe (arrowed) due to *Cryptococcus neoformans*. (Courtesy Prof. S. Spiro)

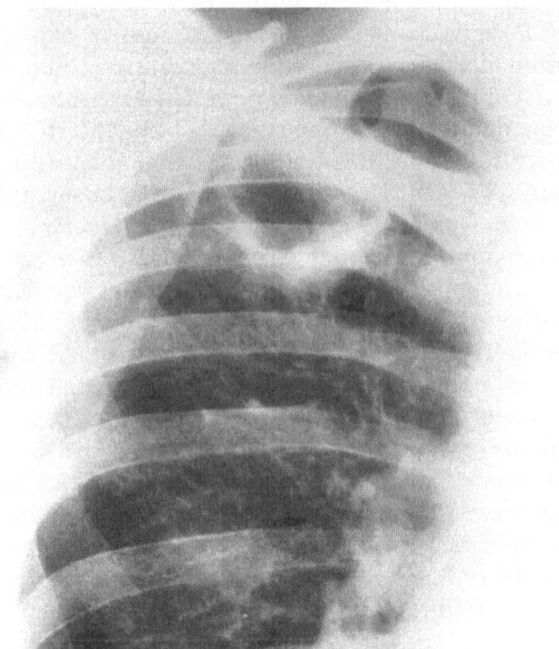

Figure 17. *Nocardia asteroides*. Radiograph with a cavitating lesion in the right upper lobe due to *Nocardia*, initially treated abroad as tuberculosis.

4.5. Phycomycetes

These fungi are rarer causes of infection compared with *Aspergillus*, invading the pulmonary vasculature and having a predilecton for the central nervous system.

4.6. Parasitic Infections

Parasitic infections, such as filariasis, may cause arthritis, myositis and vasculitis [36]. The diagnosis of "parasitic rheumatism" is suggested by a poor response to anti-inflammatory drugs and improvement following specific treatment. Paragonomiasis has been reported as an infrequent but treatable cause of haemoptysis in patients with SLE [37].

4.7. Bronchiolitis Obliterans and Bronchiolitis Obliterans Organizing Pneumonia

Bronchiolitis obliterans occurs especially in patients with RA [38, 39]. Treatment with gold or penicillamine has been implicated, although the condition may occur in RA patients not taking these drugs [40–42]. Patients are breathless, respiratory function tests show irreversible airways obstruction and a chest radiography may appear normal or with hyperinflated lungs. High-resolution CT demonstrates focal air trapping in expiration scans associated with bronchiectasis on occasion. Bronchiolitis obliterans organizing pneumonia (BOOP) is significantly rarer and describes an interstitial pneumonia associated with autoimmune disease [43–45]. BOOP has been found in patients with RA and SLE [39, 46] as well as other autoimmune rheumatic disorders [47, 48]. However, BOOP may occur following respiratory infections such as *Nocardia asteroides, Legionella* spp., *Cryptococcus* and human immunodeficiency virus [45, 49]. Patients present with non-specific but often long-standing symptoms, such as cough and breathlessness, and an influenza-like illness precedes the radiographic changes in approximately 30%. The chest radiograph is non-specific but typically shows bilateral patchy consolidation; ground glass, reticular shadowing or nodules may also occur and give a typical peripheral appearance on CT (Figure 18). Respiratory function tests have a restrictive pattern and a decreased carbon monoxide transfer factor (TLCO). BAL reveals large numbers of lymphocytes. The non-specific nature of the illness requires antibiotic treatment at first [46]. If the disease progresses clinically, a lung biopsy is required. In BOOP, there is a proliferative bronchiolitis and an intraluminal exudate of fibroblasts, mucopolysaccharides and inflammatory cells in the terminal bronchioli and alveoli. In RA, joint involvement usually precedes but may be concurrent with BOOP and women are particularly affected [39]. The role of corticosteroid treatment remains unclear:

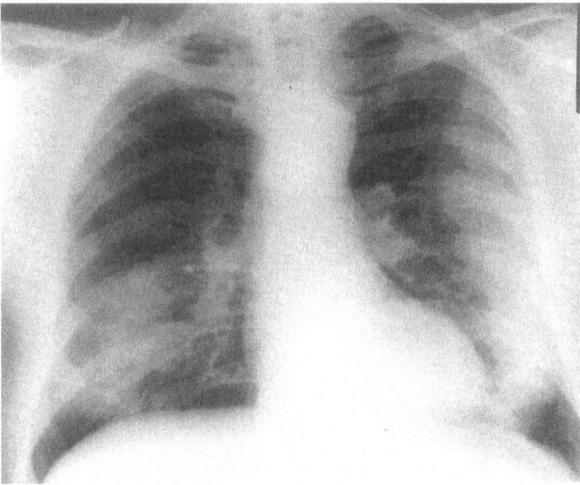

Figure 18. BOOP. Typical changes of bronchiolitis obliterans organising pneumonia with bilateral patchy consolidation which failed to respond to antibiotics. (Courtesy Prof. S. Spiro)

most patients with BOOP receive steroids and do well, but there have been no prospective trials of this treatment.

5. Lung Nodules

The vast majority of lung nodules are due to malignant disease; multiple nodules of similar size favour either infection or granulomatous disorders. Lung abscesses, fungal disease and tuberculosis may all be difficult to distinguish radiographically from rheumatoid nodules and Wegener's granulomatosis (Figure 19). However, it is most unusual for there to be rheumatoid nodules in the lungs without systemic features of RA; most patients have a positive rheumatoid factor and subcutaneous rheumatoid nodules [39]. Rheumatoid lung nodules occur in <1 % of patients with RA [42]. Although they are found predominantly in the upper lobes and may cavitate, calcification is rare, and there is no associated mediastinal lymph node enlargement (Figure 20). Nodules are as common as pulmonary infiltrates in patients with Wegener's granulomatosis, and as fever may occur in 25–50%, distinction from an infective cause can be a problem [29]. Examination of the sputum, the presence of extrapulmonary features of Wegener's granulomatosis and a positive antinuclear cytoplasmic antibody titre are the most helpful discriminators. Lymphocytic interstitial pneumonitis (pseudolymphoma) is rarely a diagnostic problem in view of its more benign course and is found mainly in patients with Sjögren's syndrome and SLE [28].

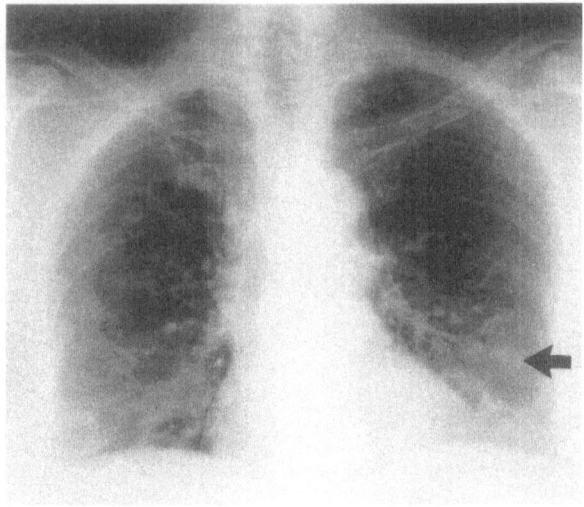

A

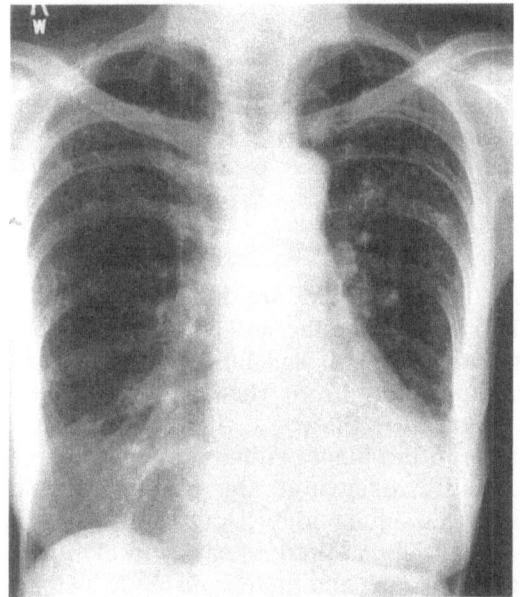

B

Figure 19. Characterising lung nodules may be difficult. (A) Radiograph with ill-defined nodules (arrowed) and basal bronchial wall thickening due to rheumatoid arthritis. (B) Radiograph with multiple nodules. The presence of some miliary nodules suggested active tuberculosis, which was confirmed. (C) Radiograph with reticular infiltrates and scattered nodules bilaterally (arrowed) due to *Cryptococcus*.

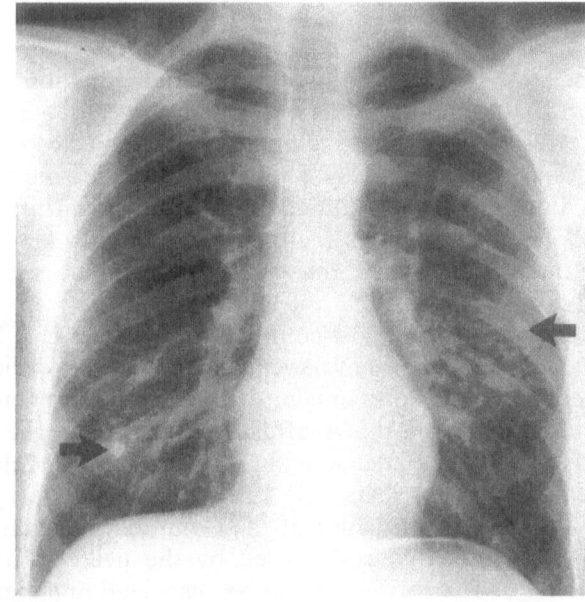

C

Figure 19. (continued)

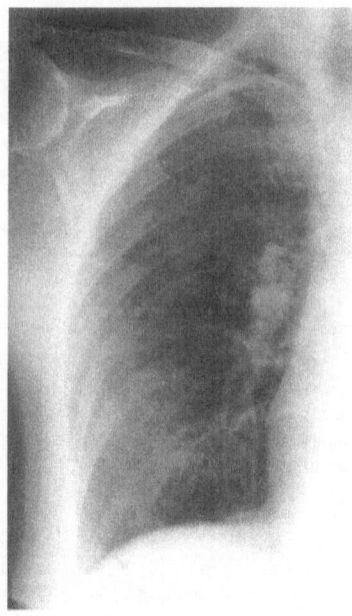

Figure 20. Methotrexate-induced pneumonitis. Radiograph of a patient with rheumatoid arthritis with methotrexate-induced pneumonitis. (Courtesy Prof. D. Isenberg). Note the fine reticular infiltrates and apical pneumothorax.

6. Pleural Effusions

Pleural lesions are found frequently at postmortem and at thoracotomy in all patients with autoimmune disease [49]. However, pleural thickening and pleural effusions are rarely clinical problems except in RA and SLE. Pleural aspiration and biopsy is the only definitive method to distinguish pleural fluid due to autoimmune disease from an infectious aetiology (Table 2). A pleural biopsy, either blind or during thoracoscopy, can yield granulomata, which make tuberculosis the more probable diagnosis.

Pleural involvement is the most common manifestation of lung disease in RA and occurs in about 5% of patients. Autopsies have shown significant involvement at frequencies greater than would be suspected clinically or by chest radiography [50]. In RA, effusions often occur when the disease is active and usually in patients with subcutaneous nodules, most of whom are men aged 40–60 years [39]. Empyema is not uncommon, or the exudate may be sterile, consisting of large numbers of white cells and fibrinoid debris or infective and caused by the necrosis of subpleural rheumatoid nodules. The former should be suspected in patients with RA who are debilitated, have a low serum albumin concentration, are receiving corticosteroids and who have a fever. The frequency of empyema in pleural effusions with RA recommends an active approach to diagnosis rather than blind treatment with corticosteroids.

Pleural disease is characteristic of SLE and occurs in 50–70% of patients during the course of their illness [50]. Patients usually complain of pain on breathing, breathlessness, cough and fever, and in contrast to patients with RA, they invariably have symptoms at the time the effusion is noted. Pleural effusions may also occur in patients with SLE as a result of

Table 2. Comparison between infectious and autoimmune pleural effusions

	Empyema	Post-pneumonic	TB	RA	SLE
Exudate[1] [51]	yes	yes	yes	yes	yes
Protein level	⩾30 g/l	>30 g/l	>30 g/l	⩾30 g/l	>30 g/l
Glucose [52]	low	low/normal	low	< 1.4 mM	≥ 4.4 mM
pH [50]	<7.2	<7.0	<7.2	<7.2	>7.35
Cell types	neutrophils > lymphocytes	neutrophils > lymphocytes	lymphocytes	lymphocytes	neutrophils and lymphocytes
% Rf + [53]		41	14	100	20
Other features	smell!	straw	straw	low complement immune complexes [50]	ANA + [54] low C′
	unilateral	unilateral	unilateral	uni/bilateral	uni/bilateral

[1] Exudate defined as (1) pleural fluid/serum protein ratio >0.5; (2) pleural fluid LDH >2/3 upper limit of serum LDH; or (3) pleural fluid/serum LDH >0.6 [49].

nephrotic syndrome and hypoalbuminaemia, pulmonary embolism, para-pneumonic effusions and uraemia.

Pleural effusions occur in Wegener's granulomatosis due to pulmonary infarction, heart failure, uraemia and bacterial infection of infarcted lung. A diagnostic aspirate is essential to discover the infrequent occasions where rupture of a nodule leads to a pyopneumothorax.

7. Drug Treatment – Cause or Mimic of Respiratory Infections?

7.1. Drug-Induced Neutropaenia

Neutropaenia is a relatively common response to penicillamine and gold and also occurs with agents which directly suppress the bone marrow such as azathioprine and cyclophosphamide. Pulmonary infections may be caused by coliforms, *Pseudomonas* spp. or *Aspergillus* (Table 3). The symptoms of fever confusion and breathlessness predominate, and sputum is usually scanty. Radiographic changes are minimal and may show only venous congestion; patchy pneumonia and abscesses occur later and often appear dramatically when the neutrophil count rises as a result of granulocyte transfusions or recovery of normal bone marrow function. In patients with neutropaenia, empirical treatment with a β-lactam and aminoglycoside is often the first course of action after sputum or bronchoalveolar lavage has been sent for microbiological examination. The CT scan may be especially helpful in differentiating fungal pneumonia from a Gram-negative bacilliary cause. The former shows a necrotizing pneumonia with the appearance of a pulmonary infarct often with nodules, whereas the latter is more diffuse, and microabscesses may be seen.

7.2. High-Dose Corticosteroids

Corticosteroids depress cell-mediated immunity in a dose-dependent fashion. The suppression of the inflammatory response allows infections to

Table 3. Respiratory infections associated with treatment of autoimmune disease

Neutropaenia e.g. penicillamine, gold, azathioprine	Impaired cell-mediated immunity e.g. high-dose steroids, methotrexate
Gram-negative bacilli	*Pneumocystis carinii*
esp. *Pseudomonas*	Tuberculosis
S. aureus	*Cryptococcus*
Aspergillus	*Nocardia*
Candida	*Legionella*
Mucormycosis	

progress insidiously and reach an advanced stage before clinical symptoms alert the physician. Common respiratory infections are listed in Table 3.

7.3. Methotrexate

Treatment of rheumatoid arthritis with disease-modifying drugs is recommended, and a combination of methotrexate, sulphasalzine and hydroxychloroquine appears especially helpful [55]. In surveys of the pulmonary effects of cytotoxic agents other than bleomycin, methotrexate was by far the most frequent cause of morbidity [56, 57], and close monitoring of all patients treated with this drug is recommended [58]. Patients with RA treated with methotrexate have an increased risk of infection (RR 1.43, 95% CI 0.96–2.14) when compared to other patients with RA [59]. Low-dose methotrexate therapy for RA has been associated with *P. carinii* pneumonia, cryptococcosis, nocardiosis, aspergillosis and cytomegalovirus pneumonia [60–64]. Pneumonia due to *P. carinii* was the most common infectious complication of methotrexate in one series, and the differential diagnosis lay with methotrexate-induced pneumonitis, rheumatoid lung disease and pulmonary emboli [65]. Methotrexate-induced pneumonitis (Figure 20) is a rare but potentially life-threatening complication of treatment [39]. The onset is insidious with a dry cough, breathlessness and fever. The chest radiograph may at first appear normal, but later there is a diffuse infiltrate and ground-glass appearance. Patients are hypoxic, and there may be a peripheral eosinophilia. Respiratory function tests may be normal but can show either an obstructive or a restrictive picture. BAL is helpful to exclude infection with bacteria or *P. carinii*. A lung biopsy shows a massive lymphocytic infiltrate and granuloma formation. Pre-existing lund disease may be a risk factor for methotrexate-induced pneumonitis.

7.4. Other Drugs

Sulphasalazine is associated with an allergic eosinophilic pneumonia more commonly than with respiratory infections [66]. Penicillamine may be associated with bronchiolitis and bronchitis [41], but can be a cause of pulmonary haemorrhage in patients with renal failure [67]. Gold salts may lead to hypogammaglobulinaemia, but respiratory infections as a consequence have not been reported [68, 69].

8. Respiratory Infections in the Pathogenesis of Autoimmune Disease

Respiratory infections might play a role in the pathogenesis of autoimmune disease. The periodicity of *Mycoplasma* infections reflected the incidence of juvenile rheumatoid arthritis over the years 1975–1992 [70]. However, exposure to *Mycoplasma* is so common that serological tests which might implicate this organism in the development of any autoimmune disease are almost impossible to interpret. Increased bacterial urease activity in faeces from patients with juvenile chronic arthritis has suggested a possible role for gut flora in the pathogenesis of this disorder [71]. Chronic Q fever has been associated with a syndrome with features of an autoimmune vasculitis [72]. *Chlamydia pneumoniae* has been found in patients with reactive arthritis with a suggestion that there may be progression to more chronic disease [73]. In a review of possible infections associated with juvenile chronic arthritis, the evidence for viral infections (rubella, influenza A, parvovirus B19, Coxsackie and Epstein-Barr virus) and bacteria (*Streptococcus, Borrelia burgdorferi*, enteric organisms and *Chlamydia*) was not convincing.

Infection may exert a non-specific effect in the initiation or exacerbation of autoimmune disease. Heat shock proteins (hsps) are induced as a response to stress in both bacterial and human cells. The identification of an epitope from hsp60 associated with the development of adjuvant arthritis in mice [74] led to studies of human immune responses to these proteins [75, 76]. The expression of these proteins is abnormal in patients with autoimmune disease, and over-expression of hsp90 and autoantibodies to it are raised specifically in patients with SLE [77–80]. The possibility that concurrent infection might be responsible for the abnormal expression of proteins to which autoantibodies may be found has been raised by finding that cytomegalovirus induces expression of the 60-kDa Ro antigen on human keratinocytes [81]. Interferon treatment has been associated with the development of SLE or lupus autoantibodies [82–84]. Mouse models have also shown the importance of tumour necrosis factor α (TNFα) in collagen-induced arthritis, raising the possibility that infections might be responsible for exacerbations of RA. Chimeric or humanized monoclonal antibodies TNF have been successful in treating RA [85, 86].

The associations between human lymphocyte antigens and autoimmune disease are well documented but alone are insufficient to induce such conditions [87, 88]. The identification of genes in murine models of autoimmune disease (e.g. apoptosis genes in models of SLE) will encourage the discovery of human equivalents. With the sequencing of the human genome in sight, the next few years should tell us how microbial factors might be involved in the initiation or exacerbation of autoimmune disease. The importance of the respiratory tract as a source of infection predicts an exciting time to examine the relationship between respiratory infection and autoimmune disease and for the design of new treatments.

References

1. Walker WC (1967) Pulmonary infections and rheumatoid arthritis. *Q J Med* 36: 239–251.
2. Suzuki A, Ohosone Y, Obana M, Mita S, Matsuoka Y, Irimajiri S, Fukuda J (1994) Cause of death in 81 autopsied patients with rheumatoid arthritis. *J Rheumatol* 21: 33–36.
3. Ginzler E, Diamond H, Kaplan D, Wiener M, Schlesinger M, Seleznick M (1978) Computer analysis of factors influencing the frequency of infection in systemic lupus erythematosus. *Arthritis Rheum* 21: 37–44.
4. Swaak AJG, Nossent JC, Bronsveld W, van Rooyen A, Nieuwenhuys EJ, Theuns L, Smeenk RJT (1989) Systemic lupus erythematosus, outcome and survival. *Ann Rheum Dis* 48: 447–454.
5. Bresnihan B (1989) Outcome and prognosis in systemic lupus erythematosus. *Ann Rheum Dis* 48: 443–445.
6. Fairfax AJ, Haslam PL, Pavia D, Sheahan NF, Bateman JRM, Agnew JE, Clarke SW, Turner-Warwick M (1981) Pulmonary diseases associated with Sjögren's syndrome. *Q J Med* 50: 279–295.
7. Solanki T, Neville E (1992) Bronchiectasis and rheumatoid arthritis: Is there an association? *Br J Rheumatol* 31: 691–693.
8. McMahon MJ, Swinson DR, Shettare S, Wolstenholme R, Chattopadhyay C, Smith P, Johns P, Crosby NH (1992) Bronchiectasis and rheumatoid arthritis: A clinical study. *Ann Rheum Dis* 52: 776–779.
9. Shadick NA, Fanta CH, Weinblatt ME, O'Donnell W, Coblyn JS (1994) Bronchiectasis: A late feature of severe rheumatoid arthritis. *Medicine* (Baltimore) 73: 161–170.
10. Walport MJ (1993) Systemic lupus erythematosus. In: Lachman PJ, Peters KD, Rosen FS, Walpert MJ (eds) *Clinical aspects of immunology*, 5th ed. Boston: Blackwell Scientific Publications, 1161–1204.
11. Eriksson P, Almroth G, Denneberg T, Lindstrom FD (1994) IgG2 deficiency in primary Sjögren's syndrome and hypergammaglobulinaemia purpura. *Clin Immunol Immunopathol* 70: 60–65.
12. Jimenez A, Alvarez-Deforno R, Garcia Rodriguez MC, Ferreira A, Lopez-Trascasa M, Forstan F (1991) Autoantibodies in patients with IgA and IgG2 deficiency. *APMIS* 99: 327–332.
13. Bahr GM, Sattar MA, Stanford J, Shaaban MA, Al-Shimali B, Siddiqui Z, Gabrul M, Al-Saffor M, Shahin A, Chugh TD, Prok GAW, Behbehani K (1989) HLA-DR and tuberculin tests in rheumatoid arthritis and tuberculosis. *Ann Rheum Dis* 48: 63–68.
14. Jacob CO (1992) Tumor necrosis factor α in autoimmunitiy: Pretty girl or old witch. *Immunol Today* 13: 122–125.
15. Barada FA, O'Brien W, Horowitz DA (1982) Defective monocyte cytotoxicity in rheumatoid arthritis. *Arthritis Rheum* 25: 15–21.
16. Hartman KR, Wright DG (1991) Identification of autoantibodies specific for the neutrophil adhesion glycoproteins CD11b/CD18 in patients with autoimmune neutropaenia. *Blood* 78: 1096–1104.
17. Nouza M (1992) *Pneumocystis carinii* pneumonia after 40 years. *Infection* 20: 113–117.
18. Porges AJ, Beattie SL, Ritchlin C, Kimberley RP, Chrittian CL (1992) Patients with systemic lupus erythematosus at risk for *Pneumocystis carinii* pneumonia. *J Rheumatol* 19: 1191–1194.
19. Godeau B, Coutant-Perronne V, Thi Huong DL, Guillevin L, Magadur G, de Bandt M, Dellion S, Rossert J, Rostoker G, Pretto SC, et al. (1994) *Pneumocystis carinii* pneumonia in the course of connective tissue disease: Report of 34 cases. *J Rheumatol* 21: 246–251.
20. Godeau M, Mainarde J-L, Roudot-Thoraval F, Machinella E, Guillevain L, Huong Du LT, Jarrousse B, Remy P, Schaeffer A, Pierre J-C (1995) Factors associated with *Pneumocystis carinii* pneumonia in Wegener's granulomatosis. *Ann Rheum Dis* 54: 991–994.
21. Hoffman GS, Leavitt RY, Kerr GS, Fauci A (1992) The treatment of Wegener's granulomatosis with glucocorticoids and methotrexate. *Arthritis Rheum* 35: 1322–1329.
22. Jarrousse B, Guillevin L, Bindi P, Leclerc P, Gilson B, Remy P et al. (1993) Increased risk of *Pneumocystis carinii* pneumonia in patients with Wegener's granulomatosis. *Clin Exp Rheumatol* 11: 615–621.

23. Miller RF, Leigh TR, Collins JV, Mitchell DM (1990) Tests giving an aetiological diagnosis in pulmonary disease in patients infected with the human immunodeficiency virus. *Thorax* 45: 62–65.
24. Podrebarac TA, Joraisas A, Karsh J (1996) *Pneumocystis carinii* pneumonia after discontinuation of hydroxycloroquine in two patients with systemic lupus erythematosus. *J Rheumatol* 23: 199–200.
25. Emmanuel D, Cuningham I, Jules-Elysee K, Brochstein JA, Kernan NA, Laver J, Stoter D, White DA, Fels A, Polsky B et al. (1988) Cytomegalovirus pneumonia after bone marrow transplantation successfully treated with the combination of ganciclovir and high-dose intravenous immune globulin. *Ann Intern Med* 109: 777–782.
26. Reed EC, Bowden RA, Dandliker PS, Lilleby KE, Meyers JD (1988) Treatment of cytomegalovirus pneumonia with ganciclover and intravenous cytomegalovirus immunoglobulin in patients with bone marrow transplants. *Ann Intern Med* 109: 783–788.
27. Mizutani H, Mizutani H (1986) Immunoglobulin M rheumatoid factor in patients with mycoplasmae pneumonia. *Am Rev Respir Dis* 134: 1237–1240.
28. Pines A, Kaplinsky N, Olchovsky D, Rozenman J, Frankl O (1985) Pleuro-pulmonary manifestations of systemic lupus erythematosus: Clinical features of its subgroups. *Chest* 88: 129–135.
29. Hoffman GS, Kerr GS, Leavitt RY, Hallahan CW, Lebovics RS, Travis WD, Rottem M, Fauci AS (1992) Wegener granulomatosis: An analysis of 158 patients. *Ann Intern Med* 116: 488–498.
30. Dickey BF, Myer AR (1984) Pulmonary disease in polymyositis/dermatomyositis. *Sem Arthritis Rheum* 14: 60–76.
31. Curtis AMcB, Smith GJW, Ravin CE (1979) Air crescent sign of invasive aspergillosis. *Radiology* 133: 17–21.
32. Kuhlman JE, Fishman EK, Siegelman SS (1985) Invasive pulmonary aspergillosis in acute leukemia: Characterisitc findings in CT, and CT halo sign, and the role of CT in early diagnosis. *Radiology* 157: 611–614.
33. Pennington JE (1994) Opportunistic fungal pneumonias: *Aspergillus, Mucor, Candida, Torulopsis*. In: Pennington JE (ed.). *Respiratory infections: Diagnosis and management*, 3rd. New York: Raven Press, 533–549.
34. Levitz SM (1991) The ecology of *Cryptococcus neoformans* and the epidemiology of cryptococcosis. *Rev Infect Dis* 13: 1163–1169.
35. Gruberg L, Thaler M, Rozenman J, Bank I, Pras M (1991) *Nocardia asteroides* infection complicating rheumatoid arthritis. *J Rheumatol* 18: 459–461.
36. McGill BE (1995) Rheumatic syndromes associated with parasites. *Ballière's Clin Rheum* 9: 201–203.
37. Kraus A, Guerra-Batista G, Chavarria P (1990) Paragonomiasis: An infrequent cause of hemoptysis in systemic lupus erythematosus. *J Rheum* 17: 244–246.
38. Geddes DM, Corrin B, Brewerton DA, Davis RJ, Turner-Warwick M (1977) Progressive airway obliteration in adults and its association with rheumatoid disease. *Q. J Med* 46: 427–444.
39. Anaya J-M, Diethelm L, Ortoz LA, Gutierrez M, Citera G, Welsh RA, Espinoza LR (1995) Pulmonary involvement in rheumatoid arthritis. *Sem Arthritis Rheum* 24: 242–254.
40. O'Duffy JD, Luthra HS, Unni KK, Hyatt RE (1986) Bronchiolitis in a rheumatoid arthritis patient receiving auranofin. *Arthritis Rheum* 29: 556–559.
41. Epler GR, Snider GL, Gaensler EA, Cathcart ES, FitzGerald MX, Carrington CB (1979) Bronchiolitis and bronchitis in connective tissue disease: A possible relationship to the use of penicillamine. *JAMA* 242: 528–532.
42. Shannon TM, Gale ME (1992) Noncardiac manifestations of rheumatoid arthritis in the thorax. *J Thorac Imag* 7: 19–29.
43. Geddes DM (1991) BOOP and COP. *Thorax* 46: 545–547.
44. Costabel U, Guzman J (1991) BOOP: What is old, what is new? *Eur Respir J* 4: 771–773.
45. Epler G (1992) Bronchiolitis obliterans organizing pneumonia: Definition and clinical features. *Chest* 102: 2S–6S.
46. Gammon RB, Bridges TA, Al-Nazir H, Alexander CB, Kennedy JL (1992) Bronchiolitis obliterans organizing pneumonia associated with systemic lupus erythematosus. *Chest* 102: 1171–1174.

47. Katzenstein AA, Myers JL, Prophet WD, Corley LS, Shin MS (1986) Bronchiolitis obliterans and usual interstitial pneumonia: A comparative clinicopathologic study. *Am J Surg Pathol* 10: 373–381.
48. Tazelaar HD, Viggiano RW, Pickersgill J, Colby TV (1990) Interstitial lung disease in polymyositis and dermatomyositis: Clinical features and prognosis as correlated with histologic findings. *Am Rev Respir Dis* 141: 727–733.
49. Carey CF, Mueller L, Fotopoulos CL, Dall L (1991) Bronchiolitis obliterans-organizing pneumonia associated with *Cryptococcus neoformans* infection. *Rev Infect Dis* 131: 253–254.
50. Joseph J, Sahn SA (1993) Connective tissue diseases and the pleura. *Chest* 104: 262–270.
51. Light RW, MacGregor MI, Luchsinger PC, Ball WC (1972) Pleural effusions: The diagnostic separation of transudates and exudates. *Ann Intern Med* 77: 507–513.
52. Halla JT, Schrohenloher RE, Volanakis JE (1980) Immune complexes and other laboratory features of pleural effusions: A comparison of rheumatoid arthritis, systemic lupus erythematosus and other diseases. *Ann Intern Med* 92: 748–752.
53. Levine H, Szanto M, Grieble HG, Bach GL, Anderson TO (1968) Rheumatoid factor in nonrheumatoid pleural effusions. *Ann Intern Med* 69: 487–492.
54. Khare V, Baethge B, Lang S, Wolf RE, Campbell Jr GD (1994) Antinuclear antibodies in pleural fluid. *Chest* 106: 866–871.
55. O'Dell JR, Haire CE, Erikson N, Drymallski W, Palmer W, Eckhoff J, Garwood V, Maloley P, Klassen LW, Wees S, Klein H, Moore GF (1996) Treatment of rheumatoid arthritis with methotrexate alone, sulfasalazine and hydroxychloroquine or a combination of all three. *N Engl J Med* 334: 1287–1289.
56. Hanrahan PS, Scrivens GA, Russell AS (1989) Prospective long term follow-up of methotrexate therapy in rheumatoid arthritis: Toxicity, efficacy and radiological progression. *Br J Rheumatol* 28: 147–153.
57. Twomey KJ, Matthay RA (1990) Pulmonary effects of cytotoxic agents other than bleomycin. *Clin Chest Med* 11: 31–54.
58. American Colege of Rheumatologists *Ad Hoc* Committee on Clinical Guidelines (1996) Guidelines for monitoring drug treatment in rheumatoid arthritis. *Arthritis Rheum* 39: 723–731.
59. van der Veen MJ, van der Heide A, Kruize AA, Bijlsma JW (1994) Infection rate and use of antibiotics in patients with rheumatoid arthritis treated with methotrexate. *Ann Rheum Dis* 53: 224–228.
60. Woolner A, Mohle-Boetane J, Lambert RE, Perruquet JL, Raffin TA, McGuire JL et al. (1991) *Pneumocystis carinii* pneumonia complicating low dose methotrexate therapy for rheumatoid arthritis. *Thorax* 46: 205–207.
61. Altz-Smith M, Kendall LG Jr, Stamm AM (1987) Cryptococcosis associated with low dose methotrexate for rheumatoid arthritis. *Am J Med* 83: 179–181.
62. Cornellissen JJ, Bakker LJ, van der Veen MJ, Rozenberg-Arska M, Bijlsma JWJ (1991) *Nocardia asteroides* pneumonia complicating low dose methotrexate treatment of refractory rheumatoid arthritis. *Ann Rheum Dis* 50: 642–644.
63. O'Reilly S, Hartley P, Jeffers M, Casey E, Clancy L (1994) Invasive aspergillosis associated with low dose methotrexate therapy for rheumatoid arthritis: A case report of treatment with itraconazole. *Tubercle Lung Dis* 75: 153–155.
64. Clare B, Brousse C, Mariette X, Bennet P, Bisson M (1991) Cytomegalovirus pneumonia in a patient with rheumatoid arthritis treated with low dose methotrexate and prednisone. *Ann Rheum Dis* 50: 67.
65. Barrera P, Laan RFJM, van Riel PLCM, Dekhuijzen PNR, Boerbooms AMTh, van der Putte LBA (1994) Methotrexate-related pulmonary complications in rheumatoid arthritis. *Ann Rheum Dis* 53: 434–439.
66. Jordan A, Cowan RE (1988) Reversible pulmonary disease and eosinophilia associated with sulphasalazine. *J Roy Soc Med* 81: 233–235.
67. Turner-Warwick M (1981) Adverse reactions affecting the lung: Possible association with D-penicillamine. *J Rheumatol* 8 (Suppl 7): 166–168.
68. Tizman ECS, Gottlieb NL (1987) Adverse reactions with oral and parenteral gold preparations. *Med Toxicol* 2: 177–189.
69. Haskard DO, MacFarlane D (1988) Adult acquired combined immune deficiency in a patient with rheumatoid arthritis on gold. *J Roy Soc Med* 81: 548–549.

70. Oen K, Fast M, Postl B (1995) Epidemiology of juvenile rheumatoid arthritis in Manitoba, Canada, 1975–1992. Cycles in incidence associated with *Mycoplasma*. *J Rheumatol* 22: 745–750.
71. Malin M, Yerronen P, Mykkänen H, Salmenen S, Isolaurc E (1996) Increased bacterial urease activity in faeces in juvenile chronic arthritis: Evidence of altered intestinal microflora? *Br J Rheumatol* 35: 689–694.
72. Kayser K, Wiebel M, Schulz V, Gabius HJ (1995) Necrotizing bronchitis, angiitis and amyloidosis associated with chronic Q fever. *Respiration* 62: 114–116.
73. Braun J, Laitko S, Treharne J, Eggens U, Wu P, Distler A, Sleper J (1994) *Chlamydia pneumoniae*: A new causative agent of reactive arthritis and undifferentiated oligoarthritis. *Ann Rheum Dis* 53: 100–105.
74. van Eden W, Thole JER, van der Zee R, Noordzij A, van Embden JDA, Hensen EJ, Cohen IR (1988) Cloning of the mycobacterial epitope recognised by T lymphocytes in adjuvant arthritis. *Nature* 331: 171–173.
75. Lamb JR, Bal V, Mendez-Semperio P, Mehlert A, So A, Rothbard J, Jundal S, Young RA, Young DB (1989) Stress proteins may provide a link between the immune response to infection and autoimmunity. *International Immunology* 1: 191–196.
76. Kiessling R, Grönberg A, Ivanyi J, Söderström K, Ferm M, Kleinau S, Nilsson E, Klareskog L (1991) Role of hsp60 during autoimmune and bacterial inflammation. *Immunol Rev* 121: 89–111.
77. Lehner T, Lavey E, Smith R, van der Zee R, Mizushia Y, Shinnick T (1991) Association between the 65 kD heat shock protein of *Streptococcus sanguis* and the corresponding antibodies in Behçet's syndrome. *Infect Immun* 59: 1434–1441.
78. Dhillon V, McCallum S, Wilks D, Twomey B, Latchman D, Isenberg D (1993) The differential expression of heat shock proteins in rheumatic disease. *Br J Rheumatol* 32: 883–892.
79. Conroy SE, Faulds GB, Wiliams W, Latchman DS, Isenberg DA (1994) Detection of autoantibodies to the 90 kDa heat shock protein in systemic lupus erythematosus and other autoimmune diseases. *Br J Rheumatol* 33: 923–926.
80. Conroy SE, Tucker LB, Latchman DS, Isenberg DA (1996) Incidence of anti-hsp90 and 70 antibodies in children with SLE, juvenile dermatomyositis and juvenile chronic arthritis. *Clin Exp Rheum* 35: 99–104.
81. Zhu J (1995) Cytomegalovirus infection induces expression of 60 kD/Ro antigen in human keratinocytes. *Lupus* 4: 396–406.
82. Schilling PJ, Kurzock R, Kantarjian H, Gutterman JU, Talpaz M (1991) Development of systemic lupus erythematosus after interferon therapy for chronic myelogenous leukaemia. *Cancer* 68: 1536–1537.
83. McSweeney EN, Addison IE, Worman CP, Isenberg DA, Goldstone AH (1993) Autoantibody induction in patients treated with recombinant alpha interferon. *Br J Haematol* 45: 81.
84. Flores A, Olivé A, Felon E, Jena X (1994) Systemic lupus erythematosus following interferon therapy. *Br J Rheumatol* 33: 787.
85. Elliott MJ, Maini RN, Feldmann M, Kalden JR, Antoni C, Smolen JS et al. (1994) Randomised double-blind comparison of chimeric monoclonal antibody to tumour necrosis factor-α (cA2) versus placebo in rheumatoid arthritis. *Lancet* 344: 1105–1110.
86. Rankin ECC, Choy EHS, Kassimos D, Kingsley GH, Sopwith AM, Isenberg DA, Panayi GS (1995) The therapeutic effects of a humanized anti-tumour necrosis factor alpha antibody (CDP 571) in rheumatoid arthritis. *Brit J Rheumatol* 34: 334–342.
87. Theofilopoulos AN (1995) The basis of autoimmunity. Part II. Genetic disposition. *Immunol Today* 16: 150–159.
88. Wicks I, McColl G, Harrison L (1994) New perspectives on rheumatoid arthritis. *Immunol Today* 15: 553–556.

Autoimmune Aspects of Lung Disease
ed. by D.A. Isenberg and S.G. Spiro
© 1998 Birkhäuser Verlag Basel/Switzerland

CHAPTER 6
Human Immunodeficiency Virus and the Lung

Carlo Agostini, Rosaria Sancetta and Gianpietro Semenzato

Department of Clinical and Experimental Medicine, University School of Medicine, Padua Hospital, Padua, Italy

1. Introduction

The primary function of the immune system is to maintain the integrity of the host by eliminating microbial infringements without clinical sequelae. The lung has the capacity to initiate and regulate immune responses against microbial invasion and neoplastic transformation. Mechanical mechanisms and innate host defences are important to avoid infections of the lung, but the respiratory tract is also equipped with an extraordinary repertoire of immunologically competent cells capable of eliciting protective effector functions [1–3]. Among these, the major initiators and regulators of the pulmonary immune system are alveolar macrophages (AMs), dendritic cells (DCs) and pulmonary T cells which, interacting with each other either

Table 1. Immunologic abnormalities commonly observed in the lungs of patients with HIV infection

---

- T-cell alveolitis sustained by CD8⁺ CTL with HIV-specific and NK-like cytotoxic activities
- Increase in the number of pulmonary γ/δ TCR cells
- Progressive loss in the number of pulmonary CD4 T-cells
- Recruitment, proliferation and activation of AMs
- Local hyperproduction of macrophage-derived cytokines (including IL-1, IL-6, IL-8, IL-15, IFN-γ, TNF-α, GM-CSF, IP-10 and MIP-1α)
- Accumulation of neutrophils in patients with opportunistic infections

---

directly or via cytokines, activate a variety of alloreactive responses to clear foreign antigens [1–3].

Much of the information on the immunopathogenetic mechanisms taking place in the lung has been acquired thanks to the recovery of cells from the lung microenvironment through bronchoalveolar lavage (BAL). A striking example of this is the impetus given by BAL to research into the inflammatory events taking place in the lungs of patients with human immunodeficiency virus (HIV) infection. Numerous studies have demonstrated the spread of HIV into the pulmonary parenchyma and the appearance of local HIV-specific immune responses which attempt to eradicate the virus from the respiratory tract [4–11]. Other studies have concentrated on the role of cytokines and specific receptors for such cytokines in the pathogenesis of the pulmonary disease associated with HIV infection (Table 1).

The goal of this chapter is to summarize the current concepts concerning the contribution of lung immunocompetent cells in host defences against HIV, including recent findings suggesting that intercellular communications between AMs and pulmonary cytotoxic T lymphocytes (CTL) lead to the accumulation of HIV-specific effector cells in the lung microenvironment. The cell pattern of HIV infection in the lung will be highlighted, and recent findings on the role of the retrovirus in weakening pulmonary host defenses and its spreading into the lower respiratory tract will be indicated.

2. Pulmonary Defences and HIV Infection

A distinctive feature of the lung is the organization of the lymphoid tissue that can be functionally subdivided into two major components [3], lymphoid cells arranged in organized aggregates or follicles which are located throughout the bronchial tree. These structures are equipped with B-cell germinal centers surrounded by T-cells, macrophages and DCs and represent a site of secondary lymphoid differentiation; and diffuse lymphoid tissue consisting of scattered lymphocytes which interplay with

AMs and DCs in the induction of effector functions related to both cellular and humoral immunity.

Lymphocytes and AMs diffusely distributed throughout the bronchial and alveolar mucosa may be obtained by BAL. The vast majority of BAL cells obtained in a healthy, non-smoking individual are AMs, which account for more than 90% of the cells within the alveolar spaces [12]; lymphocytes represent the second most numerous alveolar population (5–10%), while polymorphonucleates (PMN) are rare (1–3%) [13]. In general, AMs, DCs and T-cells expressing surface molecules and secretory molecules determine the type and direct the magnitude of immune response to sites of pulmonary inflammation. However, other cells are involved in lung immunity. Endothelial and epithelial cells might contribute to immune events by co-operating with accessory cells in the presentation of antigen to pulmonary effectors and by producing immunomodulatory molecules, including interleukin (IL)-1 and interferon-γ (IFN-γ) [14].

In striking contrast to the peripheral CD4 lymphopenia, HIV may cause marked increases in the number of CD8 lymphocytes in peripheral blood along with CD8 infiltration in the lung [11, 15–19]. An increased number of pulmonary CD45R0 T-cells are retrieved from BAL both in the early stages of HIV infection and in patients with full-blown AIDS and severe T-cell depletion, suggesting that immune function in the lung is regulated differently than in the peripheral blood [17]. An increase in AMs is also non-specific, since this phenomenon has been demonstrated in HIV-seropositive individuals with and without lung infections. By contrast, the neutrophil number is usually normal in asymptomatic patients but can increase in patients with AIDS and opportunistic infections [16, 18].

2.1. Pulmonary Lymphocytes

2.1.1. Compartmentalization of lymphocytes in the lung: Many studies have shown that HIV-infected individuals may develop an alveolitis, comprised mostly of CD8$^+$CTL [11, 15, 20–23]. Consistent with data obtained on cells retrieved from BAL, a common immunohistological finding is the presence of a diffuse CD8$^+$ T-cell infiltration of the lung parenchyma. While lung CD8$^+$ lymphocytes dramatically increase, CD4 helper T-cells are virtually absent both in BAL and biopsy specimens, even if remarkable differences are detectable in the absolute number of lung CD4 cells among patients at different disease stages [17]. The proportion of lung B-cells is generally superimposable in HIV-infected patients and controls (less than 5% of BAL lymphocytes). B-cells do not show an abnormal expression of B-related markers (CD19, CD20, CD23) but *in vitro* produce increased amounts of immunoglobulins. As a consequence, high concentrations of immunoglobulins [24], including antibodies specific to HIV, and immune complexes may be detected in the BAL fluid of HIV-infected patients. There are also reports suggesting that AMs may influence the local release of immunoglobulins by the *in situ* production of IL-6 [25].

2.1.2. Progressive loss of lung CD4⁺ T-cells impairs local immunity: A distinctive feature of the pulmonary involvement in patients with AIDS is the decline of lung CD4 cells. Since this process is accompanied by an impairment of the local immunocompetence, which sets the stage for the development of opportunistic infections, most studies have systematically explored the mechanisms leading to the progressive depletion of lung CD4 cells (reviewed in [11]). The maintenance of the CD4 T-cell population within the lung requires the continuous traffic of T-cells through the lung. In fact, physiologically dead lung T-cells are replaced by a mechanism of tissue homeostasis occurring through the cellular recruitment of T-cells from the secondary follicles. In this scenario it has been hypothesized that cell-to-cell contact between infected and uninfected CD4 T-cells and a high local concentration of HIV in the follicular DC network of lymph node germinal centers contribute to enhance the rate of infection of CD4⁺ cells trafficking in the pulmonary secondary lymphoid tissue [26]. Since cytoplasmic HIV-DNA can be demonstrated in almost all BAL specimens [27, 28], it is tempting to speculate that the quantitative defect of CD4⁺ lung T-cells may be at least in part the result of the well-known direct cytopathic effect of the accumulation of cytoplasmic retroviral DNA.

As specified in detail in the following paragraphs, HIV-specific CTL accumulate in the lung of HIV-infected individuals [11, 15, 20−23]. It is thought that local CTL activity may cause the progressive clearance of pulmonary HIV-infected CD4⁺ cells. Furthermore, there are data indicating that a dysregulation of the apoptosis control system takes place in HIV-infected patients [29], suggesting that the process of activation-induced cell death might influence the progressive loss of lung CD4⁺ cells. Syncytia formation between HIV-infected AMs and uninfected T-cells has been claimed as an additional cause for the depletion of CD4⁺ T-cells in the pulmonary microenvironment.

2.1.3. Role of lung CD8⁺ T-cells in the immune response against HIV: Current functional and phenotypic evidence indicates that lymphocyte alveolitis is mainly due to the compartmentalization of three functionally distinct populations of CTL: major histocompatibility (MHC)-restricted CTL with anti-HIV activity, T-cells with NK-like activity; and a discrete subset of $V_\delta 2^+$ γ/δ T-cell receptor (TCR) cells [11, 15, 20−23, 30−32].

Perhaps the best understood phenomenon is the antigen-driven oligoclonal accumulation of HIV-specific CTL. The demonstration that CD8 CTL are recruited to the lung parenchyma in response to the presence of HIV proteins and HIV-infected cells was provided for the first time by Plata et al. [20], who documented that BAL CTL lyse HIV-infected autologous

AMs. The lysis of AMs is MHC-restricted because anti-HLA-A,B,C mAbs are able to completely inhibit the CTL activity [21–23]. Taken together, these data indicate that a major component of the alveolitis is due to MHC-restricted CTL which are able to recognize and attack HIV structural proteins on the surface of infected cells.

A relatively high number of lung T-cells expressing CD56 NK-associated markers and provided with NK-like activity accumulate in the alveolar spaces of HIV-infected patients [15]. Interestingly, this cellular component of alveolitis is largely negative for CD16 and does not seem to take part in host defences against HIV. Rather, it contributes to resistance against pulmonary pathogens. The importance of NK killing in controlling the infectivity of opportunistic infections varies during the different phases of HIV disease. In particular, various studies indicate that a progressive decline of NK activity can be documented during the course of HIV disease [15]. The variance, which has been involved in the development of opportunistic infections, probably depends on the altered production of cytokines, including IL-2 and IL-12, which are known to potentiate innate immunity (see below).

Very little is known about the role of pulmonary $V_{\delta}2^+$ TCR cell expansion in the lung of patients with AIDS. There are several reports suggesting that γ/δ T-cells may recognize either classical MHC molecules and MHC-related gene products or highly conserved antigens, including heat shock proteins [33]. Through the recognition of different sets of antigens with respect to those recognized by TCR α/β cells, γ/δ T-cells could provide an alternative line of host defence against opportunistic infections [34]. In addition, it is possible that γ/δ cells may be involved in maintaining AMs in a primed state. To verify this hypothesis, a correlation between the presence of γ/δ cells in the BAL and the production of cytokines by AMs should be assessed. The recently suggested possibility [35] that γ/δ T-cells may provide antiviral activities should be investigated.

2.1.4. Regulation of pulmonary inflammation in the HIV lung: Studies examining the mechanisms leading to the development of T-cell alveolitis have shown that a definite number of T-cells present in the BAL of HIV-infected individuals express the cell-cycle-related Ki67 antigen, supporting the concept that these cells proliferate *in situ* [4]. However, recent information indicates that the interactions between cytokine receptors and their ligands might define regulatory networks which contribute to the lymphocyte proliferation in the pulmonary microenvironment. In particular, four cytokines, IL-2, IL-15, tumor necrosis factor α (TNF-α) and macrophage inflammatory protein (MIP-1α), have been involved in the development of T alveolitis [11, 25, 36–41].

IL-2 is regarded as an essential growth factor in initiating and promoting CTL proliferation. In fact, the early phases of HIV infection are characterized by a pulmonary compartmentalization of the IL-2 production [36, 37].

Other findings are consistent with the hypothesis that IL-2 might act as a growth factor for CTL. In particular, BAL CD8+ cells from patients with HIV infection and T-cell alveolitis express the p75, p64 and, to some extent, p55 chains of the IL-2 receptor (CD122, TUGh4 and CD25, respectively) [42]. Furthermore, over 90% of BAL CD8 cells efficiently bind IL-2. Considering the fact that the binding of IL-2 to its receptors initiates the cell-cycle progression leading to T-cell replication and that HIV *per se* may upregulate IL-2 secretion [43], these data emphasize the potential role of the IL-2/IL-2R system in the mechanisms leading to the activation and amplification of the pulmonary inflammatory process during early HIV infection. It is also possible that IL-2 binding might be important in regulating the potential capabilities of CTL.

Since the number of Th1 cells (i.e. the cell source of IL-2) progressively declines during the course of HIV disease, it is conceivable that other cytokines replace IL-2 in promoting the HIV-specific CTL infiltrate when a starvation of IL-2 occurs as a consequence of the low number of CD4 T-cells [11]. Recently, we and others addressed the question of whether other cytokines besides IL-2 are involved in the pathogenesis of CTL alveolitis. Two reasonable candidates were TNF-α, a cytokine which is able to provide co-stimulatory proliferative signals for lung T-cells [39] and is released in high amounts in the lungs of these patients [38, 40] and IL-15, a newly discovered cytokine, which induces activation and proliferation of T and NK cells [44–47] and promotes the proliferation and differentiation of preactivated normal and leukemic B-cells [48].

In order to determine the regulatory networks which TNF-α defines in the HIV lung, we extensively evaluated the interactions between some members of the TNF-receptor (TNF-R) and TNF-ligand (TNF-L) super-families in the pulmonary microenvironment [39]. We demonstrated that CD120b (i.e. the type-2 receptor for TNF) is highly expressed by T-cells retrieved from the BAL of patients with AIDS. Furthermore, they express the CD70/CD27L molecule and could be induced to proliferate by co-stimulation with IL-2 and TNF-α. In parallel, AMs from individuals with T-cell alveolitis abundantly express members of the TNF-L superfamily, including mTNF and CD30L. Thus, TNF compartmentalization may represent a crucial step in the expansion of the CTL pool in the lung. Inasmuch as the biologic functions of CD120b and CD70 (BAL CD8 cells of HIV-infected patients bear both molecules at high density) include a co-stimulatory signal for generation of CTL, the role of TNF-R and TNF-L in the regulation of the CTL function remains to be investigated.

More recent data indicate that cytokine IL-15 [44] is a key molecule responsible for initiating and maintaining T-cell alveolitis. *In vitro* studies have shown that IL-15 stimulates CD8+ T-cells to exhibit long-term memory-CTL activity against infected target cells [49], favors the recruitment of T-cells at sites of inflammation in different organs [50, 51], including the lung. Furthermore, it induces the proliferative activity of circulating lymphocytes in HIV-infected individuals in response to HIV-specific antigens [52]. All the above effects of IL-15 are mediated *via* binding with the β and γ chains of the IL-2R system [44]. In particular, the fact that IL-15 favours migration and activation of T-cells at sites of inflammation [50, 51] makes it an attractive candidate to investigate mechanisms promoting host CTL immune response against HIV and regulating the superscript development of CD8[+] T-cell infiltrate. Our preliminary data confirm this hypothesis. In fact, AMs from patients with AIDS and high-intensity CD8 T-cell alveolitis express high levels of IL-15 mRNA and membrane/cytoplasmic IL-15, while AMs from healthy subjects do not. Furthermore, IL-15, both alone and in co-operation with IL-2 and TNFα, triggers the proliferation of BAL T-cells, and the proliferative activity of IL-15 is signalled through the β and γ chains of the IL-2R system.

Viewing the above data as a whole, it is tempting to postulate that in the early phases of the disease (i.e. when the number of CD4 T-cells is within the normal range), the compartmentalization of IL-2 represents the crucial step in the expansion and activation of the pulmonary CTL pool. By contrast, in patients with full-blown AIDS, AMs directly drive the development of the lymphocyte alveolitis, via the release of IL-15 and TNF-α. Additional molecules are likely to be involved in proliferative signals for lung CTL, including IL-12, which is produced by AMs of patients with HIV infection (our preliminary data). Provided its ability to activate NK and T-cells, this cytokine helps the shift of uncommitted T helper cells towards a cellular type 1 (Th1) response and represents a key molecule in initiating resistance to microbial infections [53]. IL-12 might also represent an additional factor that induces the local growth of the intra-alveolar CTL pool.

Two final considerations are needed to interpret the mechanisms underlying the development of CTL alveolitis in patients with AIDS. Adhesion molecules facilitate the interaction of lymphocytes with the cellular and extracellular matrix components [54], and the expression of these molecules (CD54, CD102 and CD106) on pulmonary endothelium is induced by inflammatory mediators locally released following HIV infection [55]. It is therefore conceivable that the heightened expression of these molecules may result in the recruitment of HIV-specific effector cells from secondary lymphoid tissues to the inflamed pulmonary parenchyma. It will be also intriguing to assess whether a dysregulation of the physiological cell death mechanism, and in particular of the bcl_2 and Fas-L/Fas control systems on activated CD8[+] lung T-cells [56, 57], may ultimately lead to abnormal control of the T-cell immune response in the pulmonary microenvironment.

2.1.5. The TCR repertoire of HIV-specific CTL: Two different chain combinations of the TCR are used by T-cells for antigen recognition. In fact, four distinct TCR-related antigen-binding chains (α, β, γ and δ) are expressed as mutually exclusive heterodimers, i.e. the TCR α/β and TCR γ/δ receptors [58]. The use of mAbs that have specificity for defined variable

(V) regions together with DNA molecular analysis of the α/β or the γ/δ TCR genes allows us to verify whether the cell population we are dealing with is made up of cells consistently undergoing an identical TCR rearrangement (monoclonal expansion), cells belonging to a limited number of clones (oligoclonal expansion) or a body of cells that are different from each other (polyclonal expansion).

Utilizing molecular biology procedures, we recently evaluated the repertoire of the TCR of lavage and blood T lymphocytes from HIV-infected patients. Analysis of the usage of β-chain constant region segments (Cβ1 vs. Cβ2) and variable elements (Vβ) by BAL T-cells has suggested that the TCR repertoire may be restricted in the HIV lung, confirming a pattern of growth in the lung which is consistent with a TCR oligoclonality. Specifically, we showed a quantitative skewing in the use of Vβ chain regions of the TCR by lung CD8$^+$ T-cells, with an overexpression of T-cells bearing some Vβ region segment products (Vβ2, Vβ3, Vβ7 and Vβ9), whose percentage may comprise up to 30% of BAL lymphocytes [59]. Interestingly, these cells show an *in vitro* hyporesponsiveness to superantigenic molecules, resembling T lymphocytes that, following stimulation with their cognate antigen, behave as exhausted cells.

Different mechanisms could account for the limited use of the TCR repertoire in the lung. One hypothesis is that microbial and/or HIV protein(s) drive an oligoclonal expansion of T-cells using particular Vα or Vβ regions. Previous studies in humans have shown that T-cells expressing certain V genes are stimulated preferentially by specific superantigens [60]. However, the discovery that retrovirus-derived superantigens are involved in the pathology of murine retrovirus infection [61] suggests the attractive hypothesis that HIV-encoded superantigens may contribute to the pathogenesis of T-cell alveolitis by activating or deleting relevant T-cell subsets. In addition, given the known similarities between HIV proteins and several known enterotoxins [61], it is also possible that bacterial products released during opportunistic infections might drive T-cell selection by inducing either expansion or reduction of HIV-specific T-cells bearing discrete Vβ gene products.

2.1.6. Importance of CTL efficiency decline in HIV disease: As discussed in the previous paragraphs, the high number of HIV-specific CTL which supply the respiratory tract should confer a resistant state against the spread of HIV into the surrounding microenvironment. Nevertheless, an impairment of lung CTL efficiency can be demonstrated along the clinical course of HIV disease, and the loss of this function leads to an inability to control the development of opportunistic infections [11].

BAL studies have been particularly useful in explaining the downregulation of HIV-specific and NK-like CTL activity. Current data emphasize the role of HIV infection of lung CD8$^+$ T-cells in the fall in lytic activity ([62], see below). Other factors which have been involved in the loss of CTL response in the lung include [11]: the decrease and functional impairment of CD4+ T-cells; the progressive inability to release cytokines which are essential for the effectiveness of CTL (including IL-2 and TNF-α); the inappropriate secretion of inhibitory cytokines (TGF-β, IL-10); the emergence of HIV variants; the production of soluble inhibitors [63]; and the alteration of the Th1/Th2 regulatory networks in the lung. Moreover, since there is a short region of sequence homology between *Fas* and gp120 HIV protein [64], it is possible that anti-gp 120 antibodies might cross-react with *Fas* to transmit an apoptosis-inducing signal. This phenomenon would contribute to the progressive loss of cytotoxic activity by lung CD8+ T-cells, which are equipped with increased amounts of CD95 molecules [29].

The shifts of the Th1/Th2 regulatory networks may be also important in determining the progressive impairment of local immunocompetence. It has been suggested that following HIV infection, Th1 cells responsible for cell-mediated immune responses producing IFN-γ, IL-2 and TNF-β, switch to Th2 cells with a concomitant release of IL-10, IL-6 and IL-4 [65]

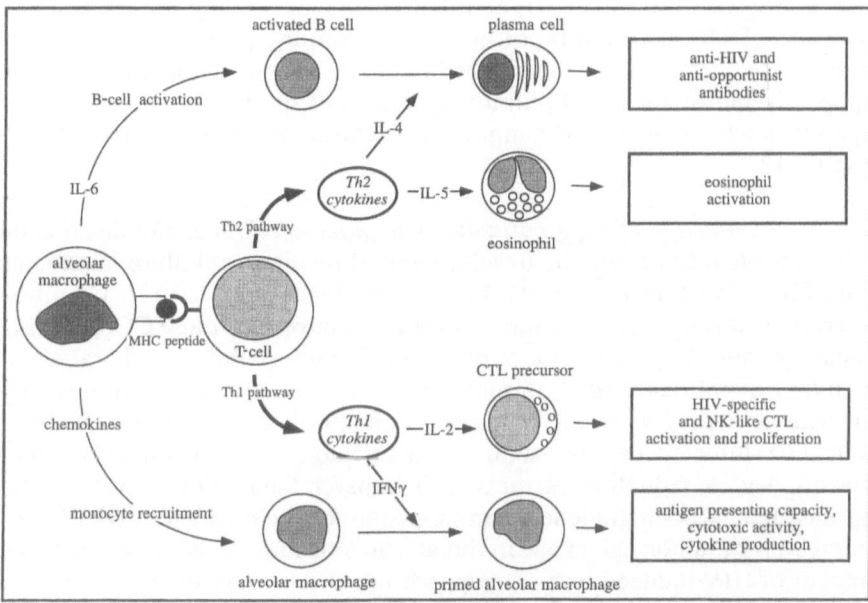

Figure 1. Acting as APCs in the uptake and processing of HIV peptides, alveolar macrophages acquire a series of properties related to their functional properties including the ability to release a set of biological mediators of the immune response, such as IFN-γ and IL-12. At least in the early phases of HIV disease, pulmonary macrophage-derived IFN-γ and IL-12 predominantly promote a Th1-like pulmonary inflammatory response, which in turn favors the development of the CD8 alveolitis and elicits further activation of the macrophage component of the alveolitis. As the disease progresses, a loss of the pulmonary Th1-like response takes place, with a relative preservation of the Th2-like function. This perturbation is likely to play a role in the loss of the local protective cell-mediated responses to HIV and intracellular pathogens.

(Figure 1). This shift in the balance of immunoregulatory cells could cause a progressive loss of protective cell-mediated response against pathogens of the lung. In fact, Th1 cells mediate resistance to several intracellular microorganisms which colonize the lung in HIV disease. However, it is important to mention that conflicting data have been reported on the Th1 versus Th2 switch during HIV infection [66], and it is at present largely unknown whether such an imbalance actually occurs in the lung in response to HIV and opportunistic infections.

It would also be important to address the issue of the putative role of AMs in the differentiation of T-cells [11, 67–70]. Experiments to define the mechanisms controlling the differentiation of Th cells have demonstrated that the B7/CD28 co-stimulatory pathway is involved in the initial commitment of naive Th cells. In particular, it has been suggested that the B7-2 (CD86) ligand expression on antigen-presenting cells (APC) plays a critical role, since it is able to initiate a Th2 response, while B7-1 (CD80) is more important in the maintenance of Th1 response [71]. Inasmuch as human AMs express CD80 ligands following activation with proinflammatory cytokines [including TNF-α and granulocyte-macrophage colony-stimulating factor (GM-CSF)] and that T-cells accounting for alveolitis in ILD are CD28$^+$, it would be of interest to examine whether HIV may influence the expression of these co-stimulatory ligands in the lung, causing apoptosis and/or anergy of pulmonary Th1 cells or allowing the release of cytokines which alter the dynamics of Th differentiation, including TGFβ and IL-12.

2.1.7. The damage of lung epithelia is immune-mediated: Studies related to the events influencing the development of respiratory failure in patients with HIV infection have been recently published [9, 72, 73]. Common alterations throughout the course of HIV infection are a low CO diffusing capacity caused by impairment of the exchanging ability of the alveolar capillary membrane and abnormal oxygenation that is present in virtually all patients with *Pneumocystis carinii* pneumonia after exercise. In addition, HIV-infected patients with no identifiable lung infections or neoplasms have a reduction in mean CO transfer factor (TL$_{CO}$) values and accelerated ^{99m}Tc-diethylene triamine penta-acetate clearance (DPTA-Cl). Interestingly, abnormal TL$_{CO}$, in the absence of lung disease, represents a marker of HIV-induced immunosuppression and is therefore a predictor of rapid progression to AIDS [74].

Since HIV may spread to epithelial cells [75], to explain the pathogenesis of lung damage it has been postulated that lung epithelium represents a potential target for CTL which during immune-mediated response against HIV are recruited from the blood to the interstitium and then to the epithelial surface. The finding that HIV-seropositive individuals with no evidence of lung disease may have a high intensity alveolitis associated with a reduction in pulmonary function confirms this hypothesis. As a matter of fact, a strong correlation exists between the degree of CD8$^+$ T-cell alveolitis and the value of epithelia permeability, as determined by the DPTA-Cl; abnormalities of K_{CO} and PaO_2 are also independently associated with the increase in the absolute number of alveolar CD8$^+$ T-cells. As discussed in the following sections, it is now clear that other soluble molecules may contribute to lung damage, including macrophage-derived cytokines [76] and neutrophil-derived enzymes.

2.2. Alveolar Macrophages

2.2.1. Macrophage alveolitis is a common finding in HIV-infected patients:
The prominent cell population obtained from the alveoli of healthy individuals are AMs, which are peculiar among the mononuclear phagocytes in different body compartments because they are located strategically at the air–tissue interface and are exposed regularly to inhaled antigen [12]. Most AMs arise from circulating monocytes which, originally formed in the bone marrow, pass into the peripheral blood and migrate through the alveolar walls into the lungs [77], where they differentiate into mature AMs under the influence of vitamin D metabolites and other unknown stimuli. The usually slow daily rate of monocyte recruitment can considerably increase during inflammatory processes. It is believed that expression of molecules involved in leukocyte-endothelial cell recognition (CD11a/CD18, CD49a and CD62L), the consequent binding of monocytes to tissue-specific vascular adhesion molecules and the release of type-IV collagenase might play a role in determining the compartmentalization of monocytes into sites of pulmonary inflammation [77]. Local epithelial regulatory factors with the potential to regulate leukocyte homing [14] and production of chemoattractant monokines are likely to cooperate in this phenomenon. Furthermore, it is known that the local release of macrophage growth factors may also induce the self-renewal of the resident macrophage pool in lung diseases characterized by a macrophage alveolitis. In particular, GM-CSF plays a crucial role in controlling the number and the activity of macrophage cells.

In most patients with HIV infection an increased number of circulating monocytes differentiate into AMs. In fact, a high percentage of AMs show a monocyte-like phenotypic pattern, providing indirect evidence of a heightened redistribution of monocytes from the peripheral blood to the lung. Furthermore, chemoattractant cytokines (such as TNF-α, IL-1, IL-8, IP-10, RANTES and other chemokines) are locally released, and it is possible that uncharacterized inhibitors of monocytic mobility may help to immobilize monocytes in the pulmonary foci of inflammation, thus perpetuating the macrophage alveolitis [67, 70].

As reported above, it is known that the release of growth factors may induce the expansion of the local macrophage pool. Not surprisingly, macrophage alveolitis partly derives from self-replicating pools of resident

AMs. In particular, the colony-stimulating factors (CSFs), like GM-CSF, play a crucial role in controlling the number of AMs in HIV infection [78]. An enhanced number of AMs express the cell-cycle-related Ki67 antigen, synthesize GM-CSF, bear GM-CSF receptor and enter the proliferative phase of the cell cycle following stimulation with this CSF. According to this data, AMs could themselves be responsible for the growth and differentiation of the macrophage pool.

2.2.2. Expression of surface antigens by AMs during HIV infection: AMs isolated from the lungs of patients with HIV infection are phenotypically heterogeneous. Under physiological conditions, AMs express class II MHC-related determinants (HLA-DR, -DP and -DQ) and show high-affinity receptors for the Fc portion of IgG (CD64 and CD32), and complement (CD11b, CD35, CD11c). Furthermore, a small subset (< 5%) react with the CD4 determinants, i.e. the main receptor for HIV. The control of AM function is achieved through a fine balance of inhibitory and activating signals which dictate the expression of the above molecules. Following activation, AMs bear increased levels of activation markers, cytokine receptors and adhesion molecules involved in cell-to-cell or cell-to-endothelium contact [55, 70, 79, 80].

Variation in expression of surface markers related to the differentiation or state of activation occurs within AMs of HIV-infected individuals. At least in the early phase of HIV infection, AMs strongly increase the surface density of molecules related to their functional activation. In fact, they show an increased expression of class II MHC antigens and other activation markers [55, 79, 80]. These cells also bear high levels of adhesion molecules and others involved in cell-to-cell contact (CD11a/CD18, CD44, CD49, CD54 and CD58), cytokine receptors (IL-2-R, CSF-R, TNF-R and TNF-L), high-affinity receptors for the Fc portion of IgG (CD64), IgE (CD23) and complement (CD11b). A discrete number of AMs express CD14, an antigen to some extent specific for monocytes; this supports the above-mentioned concept that the recruitment of circulating monocytes plays a critical role in the accumulation of pulmonary macrophages. Finally, it has been suggested that increased expression of the CD4 molecule sets the stage for the high susceptibility of AMs to retroviral infection [11].

2.2.3. Immunoregulatory role of AMs: Numerous studies have examined the cytokine networks in the lungs of HIV-infected patients, attempting to learn what determines the immune response against HIV and other microbial agents (reviewed in [11]). A wide range of macrophage-derived cytokines is locally released, including TNF-α, IL-1, IL-6, IL-8, IL-12, IL-15, IFN-γ, IP-10, GM-CSF and MIP-1α) (Figure 2). The interrelationship between cytokines and their receptors results in a network of effects which alters the functional capabilities of AMs.

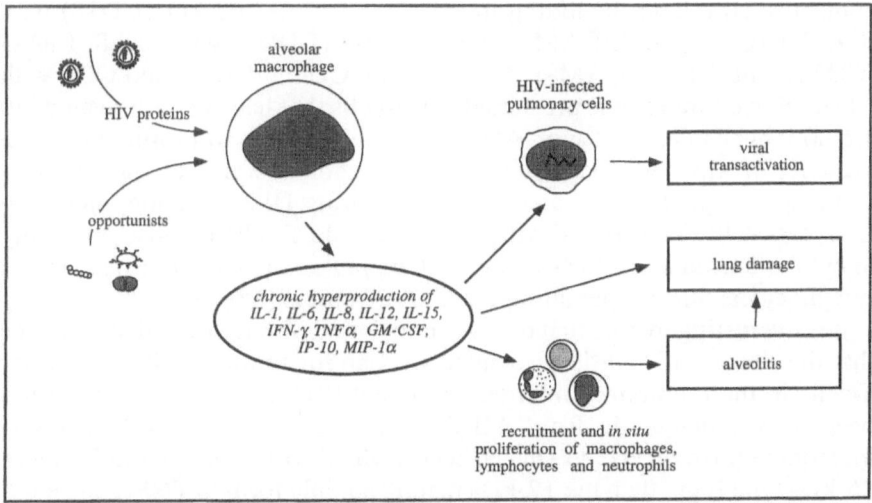

Figure 2. The chronic release of macrophage-derived molecules not only favors the development of the CD8 alveolitis but also directly contributes to the decline in pulmonary function and to the reactivation of virulent HIV strains. The cytokine-induced damage of the pulmonary microenvironment could lead to an enhanced susceptibility to serious opportunistic infections; the latter, in turn, may induce further *in situ* production of cytokines.

Releasing toxic oxygen metabolites, activated AMs directly participate in the intracellular killing of pulmonary opportunists. Furthermore, they initiate the T cell immune response against invading microorganisms. In fact, the eradication of several intracellular pathogens, including bacteria, clamydiae, fungi and protozoa needs effective AM-T-cell co-operation. The pathogen is ingested by endocytosis and degraded, and part of its molecule is transported to the cell membrane and bound to the class II MHC molecules, i.e. the structures which physically present non-self antigens to the TCR. Acting as professional APCs, AMs release biological mediators relevant to the expansion of effector mechanisms which account for the clearance of invading microorganisms.

The APC capacity of AMs in patients with AIDS was investigated systematically. Twigg et al. [68–70] have shown that, while normal AMs are poor APCs for priming T-cells even when they express class II MHC molecules, macrophages obtained from the lungs of HIV-infected individuals strongly promote the proliferative activity of allogeneic T-cells. To explain these functional changes it has been proposed that AMs recently recruited from the peripheral blood, and thus similar to circulating monocytes in phenotype and function, are responsible for the increased APC capacity. It is likely that the increased expression of molecules involved in cell-to-cell communication is involved in this behavior. More specifically, multiple counter-receptors might contribute to establishing AM-T-cell contact in HIV lung, including interaction of LFA-1 (CD11a/CD18) with ICAM-1 (CD54) and ICAM 2 (CD102), B7 (CD80) with CD28, LFA-3 (CD58) with CD2, VCAM-1 (CD106) with CD49d/CD29, and CD5 with CD72. Furthermore, it is presumed that T-cells that have been activated but are no longer in contact with AMs might still be able to proliferate in the presence of AM-derived T-cell stimulatory cytokines. In fact, most biological response modifiers secreted by AMs during HIV infection, including IL-1, GM-CSF, TNF-α and MIP-1α might hold T-cells in close proximity to cytokine-producing AMs and/or initiate *per se* the local proliferation of lymphocytes, thus perpetuating the CTL alveolitis [68–70].

It is interesting to note that data in animal models have provided evidence that the release of TNF is associated with an infiltration of inflammatory T-cells in the pulmonary microenvironment [81]. As report above, it has been shown that AMs from AIDS patients express the 26-kDa transmembrane form of TNF-α (mTNFα) [39]. TNF-α is synthesized first as a 26-kDa type II gp, then the 17-kDa mature soluble form of TNF-α is generated by cleavage of this precursor molecule. While the soluble 17-kDa TNF-α exerts its effect by the binding of TNF-Rs, mTNFα, an integral polypeptide containing a hydrophobic portion, is believed to be involved in direct cell contact-dependent interactions. Since AM-T-cell contact initiates the proliferative activity of T-cells in HIV-seropositive individuals, mTNF expression might be crucial in maintaining AM-T-cell adherence and thus the development of T-cell alveolitis.

2.2.4. Involvement of macrophage-derived cytokines in lung damage: Macrophage-derived cytokines are thought to be involved in lung injury. In particular, because TNF-α is able to alter the lung endothelium, causing oedema and interstitial damage, it is possible that, in addition to the T-cell cytotoxicity, the chronic release of this molecule may directly contribute to decline in pulmonary function [11]. In this regard, the release of cytokines, inducing damage of alveolar epithelial cells, could also enhance the probability that opportunistic infections colonize the pulmonary tissue, further favoring the decline in pulmonary function. As recently suggested by Dalgleish et al. [82], it is possible that reducing TNF-α levels could be beneficial in HIV-mediated disease. BAL analysis of pulmonary immunocompetence could represent an invaluable tool to monitor an immunotherapeutic strategy against TNF-α-mediated complications in HIV disease.

Cytokine hyperproduction may also dictate HIV replication and spreading throughout all of the compartments of the lung [11]. As reported in detail below, cells belonging to the monocyte-macrophage lineage are infected by HIV *in vivo* [83–87], and in turn cytokines spontaneously released in the lungs of HIV-infected patients, such as IL-2, GM-CSF, TNF-α and IL-6, may potentiate HIV replication following both transcriptional or post-transcriptional pathways [11]. Thus, the pulmonary dissemination of HIV could be initiated by some of the cellular factors which participate in host defense against HIV infection. The relationship between virus burden and cytokine expression has also been examined by Sierra-Madero et al. [87], who provided the demonstration that macrophages express increased levels of mRNA for TNF-α, IL-1β and IL-6 during early and late stages of HIV disease, regardless of virus load. Interestingly, IL-13, a cytokine secreted by activated T-cells, is able to downregulate cytokine production by AMs [88] and protect AMs from productive HIV infection [89]; but whether this anti-inflammatory molecule is released *in vivo* by pulmonary T-cells during HIV-related ILD (interstitial lung disease) still remains elusive.

2.3. Polymorphonuclear Cells

2.3.1. Pulmonary compartmentalization of neutrophils: Polymorphonucleates (PMNs) represent a second line of host defenses against many bacterial and fungal infections. Only a very small proportion of PMNs are found in the alveoli or interstitial lung tissues of normal non-smokers (less than 5%). By contrast, pulmonary compartmentalization of PMNs may occur in acute or chronic lung inflammation and involves the interaction between homing surface receptors which rolling neutrophils are equipped with (CD62, CD11a/CD18 complex and CD49 antigens) and molecules expressed by cytokine-stimulated endothelial cells (CD54, CD62P and CD106) [13]. In this regard, it is known that the migration of PMNs to the sites of inflammation is initiated and driven by chemotactic factors for PMNs, including IL-1, IL-8, GM-CSF and TNF-α [11, 90]. Interestingly, recent evidence suggests that activated neutrophils *per se* are able to release IL-1, IL-8, IFN-γ and TNF-α, further heightening the ongoing inflammatory response [91].

BAL studies suggest a role for PMNs in pulmonary defences during opportunistic infections. In a subset of patients with AIDS, infectious inflammatory processes of the airway are associated with a high-intensity neutrophilic alveolitis and the presence of nonspecific indicators of inflammation in cell-free BAL fluid [16, 17]. In addition, patients with severe opportunistic infections and a high neutrophil BAL count show a high protein concentration and the presence of α_2-globulin in the BAL fluid [92]. Moreover, BAL fluid levels of chemokines strongly correlate with the neutrophil count and, as discussed in detail below, individuals with BAL neutrophilia have a poor prognosis [93, 94]. These findings validate the concept that in an attempt to control respiratory tract infections PMNs are recruited into the lung.

2.3.2. Neutrophil products may derange alveolar structures: What is the role of PMNs in lung injury? Benfield et al. [94] have shown that assessment of BAL fluid levels of IL-8 is a sensitive method for the clinical follow-up of respiratory illness in subjects with HIV infection. In fact, a significant correlation between changes in IL-8 levels and differences in the alveolar arterial oxygen pressure gradient can be observed in some patients. The finding that HIV-seropositive individuals with increased amounts of IL-8 in BAL fluid and neutrophil alveolitis have a reduction in TL_{CO} supports the suggestion that local accumulation of PMNs plays a role in the progressive decline of pulmonary function. In particular, it is currently thought that neutrophil-derived oxygen metabolites and proteases may be directly toxic to epithelial cells.

PMNs degranulate in response to appropriate activation signals. It is possible that immune responses elicited by pathogens trigger extracellular degranulation of neutrophils, thus contributing significantly to injure alveolar structures [11]. As a matter of fact, the increase in neutrophils and high molecular weight protein levels in patients with AIDS correlates to gas-exchange abnormalities and improves as the opportunistic infections resolves. This supports the hypothesis that neutrophil products released in response to opportunistic infections could be directly toxic to epithelial cells.

3. Pathogenesis of HIV Infection of Pulmonary Cells

3.1. Pulmonary Cells as Target Cells for HIV Infection

Much of the information on this topic has been acquired through the studies in lymphoid tissues [95]. After primary infection, the retrovirus disseminates throughout the body and is compartmentalized in secondary lymphoid tissues. Extracellular virions are trapped in the follicular dendritic cell network, which represents a continuous source of infection for lymphoid cells. With the onset of AIDS, the dissolution of the follicular dendritic cell network in the lymph nodes leads to the inability to trap extracellular virions and favors HIV redistribution outside the secondary to tertiary lymphoid tissues. Since the lung can be considered as an important lymphoid organ, it is not surprising that HIV spreads early to the resident cell populations of the lung (Table 2).

Therefore, the migratory process of infected T-cells originating from secondary lymphoid tissues can explain the establishment of HIV infection in pulmonary tissues. The demonstration that cell-free virus is carried by the microcirculation provides additional information to elucidate the pathways followed by HIV to infect the lung [96]. It is conceivable that free

Table 2. Characteristics of lung infection by HIV

- Secondary lymphoid follicles are a reservoir for HIV
- HIV genome may be detected in AMs, CD4+ and CD8+ BAL T-cells, and lung fibroblasts from the early stages of HIV infection
- Highly monocytotropic HIV clones can be isolated from BAL
- HIV strains evolve independently within the lung and blood microenvironments

---

extracellular virion may cross the alveolocapillary membrane, entering the lung parenchyma and infecting resident cells. The infection and/or integration of the HIV genome has also been shown in non-lymphoid pulmonary cell populations, including AMs [83–86, 97–99]. Thus it is possible that blood CD4+ monocytes that harbor the provirus may enter the lung, where they differentiate into latently infected AMs. Finally, recent observations implicate CC-chemokine receptors (CC-CKR) in HIV infection of target cells [100]. Since CXC-chemokines (such as IL-8 and IP-10) and CC-chemokines (such as MIP-1α and MCP-1) are released actively in the lung [101], the influence of the expression of CC-CKR by pulmonary cells on the viral burden in the respiratory tract should be investigated.

3.1.1 HIV infection of pulmonary macrophages: Pulmonary macrophages, the most numerous alveolar cell population, were the first cell type shown to be infected by HIV. HIV genome in AMs retrieved from the BAL of HIV-infected patients was detected definitively by several groups (reviewed in [11]). Although AMs are infected latently by HIV *in vivo*, at resting conditions they are not a site for viral replication [86]. Conversely, HIV replication in AMs is enhanced by incubation with cytokines which are released spontaneously in the lungs of HIV-infected patients [102]. Entry of infectious HIV into AMs requires interaction with cell surface CD4, since the soluble CD4 blocks infection of pulmonary AMs [103].

HIV clones derived from BAL have been well characterized. It has been shown that they are highly monocytotropic [104], in addition, AM infection by monocytotropic HIV variants appears to increase with disease progression. More recently, it has been demonstrated that HIV strains from BAL cells, but not from peripheral blood cells, contain V3 domain nucleotide sequences with a great degree of homogeneity in the C-terminal region and a highly conserved, negatively charged amino acid motif [105]. This suggests that the V3 loop C-terminal structure is involved in the ability of BAL HIV strains to infect AMs. Through a comparative analysis of V3-domain nucleotide sequences in cells of monocyte/macrophage lineage recovered from the lung and the peripheral blood, Itescu et al. [105] demonstrated that strains infecting AMs have evolved further from a presumed ancestral species than those infecting blood monocytes. It is possible that, as the disease progresses, viral strains in lung and blood microenvironments are not in a state of unrestricted bidirectional traffic but, instead, evolve independently. Conceivably, the local hyperproduction of cytokines and the generalized immune activation which occurs following pulmonary opportunistic infections [106, 107] are factors which do not play a bystander's role in this phenomenon (Figure 2).

3.1.2. HIV infection of lung T-cells: Although pulmonary lymphocytes expressing CD4 receptor are the principal cell targets for HIV, we demonstrated an unexpected *in vivo* infectivity of HIV towards the pulmonary CD8 cell compartment [62]. When proviral load on pulmonary T-cell subsets was assessed using the DNA-PCR technique, most of the BAL proviral DNA was found in the under-represented CD4 T-cell subset, but polymerase chain reaction (PCR) analysis directly performed on the CD8 cell subset showed that this population also carries detectable amounts of HIV DNA. And as recently demonstrated, circulating CD8[+] T-cells may be infected by the virus [108].

These findings have crucial implications for understanding the pattern of HIV infection and the pathways of viral spreading to lymphoid cells. We believe that repeated contacts occurring in the lung microenvironment between activated HIV-specific CTL and relevant targets could ultimately lead to the infection of CD8 cells. This hypothesis is supported by *in vitro* studies showing that HIV may be transmitted through cell-to-cell contact between persistently infected CD4 cells and CD8 CTL [109, 110]. An additional, and not necessarily alternative, hypothesis is that pulmonary HIV-specific CTL derive from T-cell precursors that transiently co-express both CD4 and CD8 determinants in secondary follicles where trapped extracellular virions are present [11].

A related issue is whether HIV infection of CD8 cells significantly contributes to the progressive fall in lytic activity of lung CTL. It is conceivable that the proportion of CD8[+] T-cells which harbor HIV infection varies during the different phases of HIV disease, perhaps under the influence of abnormal triggering signals. Further longitudinal studies on a series of patients with HIV infection are needed to define whether the intensity of viral burden in CD8 cells plays a role in the progressive loss of *in situ* cytotoxic activity and, ultimately, in the progression of pulmonary disease. Furthermore, the pattern of HIV infection within CD8[+] T-cells bearing different Vβ region segments should be investigated to determine whether HIV infection results in the loss and/or expansion of T-cell subsets expressing discrete Vβ region segments.

4. Model for Pulmonary Immunity in HIV Infection

A model can be proposed summarizing the results of studies which have elucidated the molecular and cellular basis of pulmonary host response against HIV. AMs and lung fibroblasts can be infected by the etiologic agent of AIDS. The intra-alveolar presence of HIV evokes a discrete CTL immune response which is considered the major tool for the clearance of retroviral infections. AMs are not bystander cells in the host defense mechanisms against HIV, since they release a broad array of mediators of inflammation, such as monokines, proinflammatory cytokines, chemokines and growth factors. Repeated contacts occurring in the pulmonary microenvironment between HIV-specific CTL, AMs presenting HIV antigen(s) and infected targets lead to the infection of the CD8 cell compartment. HIV infection of CD8 cells and the decline of CD4 cells contribute to the progressive fall of the *in situ* HIV-specific and NK-like CTL activities, favoring the appearance of opportunistic infections and the progression of pulmonary disease. As a consequence of the presence of opportunistic infections in the pulmonary tract, AMs continuously release cytokines that, besides influencing the activation state of other immunocompetent cells, facilitate the spread of virulent HIV strains and, in some patients, the development of respiratory failure. Thus, cells and cell by-products that are involved in the pathogenesis of intrapulmonary inflammatory lesions may paradoxically favor the dissemination of HIV into the lung and the progression of pulmonary disease.

In conclusion, we would like to emphasize the importance of the use of BAL analysis in patients with HIV infection. The present knowledge of the complex network of interactions between cellular components of the pulmonary immune system largely arises from the evaluation of cell populations retrieved from the BAL fluid. One hope is that this technique will ultimately prove valuable to clinicians challenged by the need to manage patients with HIV infection. Since the early 1990s, the prognostic utility of morphological and immunologic evaluations of BAL cell populations in determining the mortality risk in HIV infection have been taken into consideration. There are data suggesting that the risk of death is increased in HIV-seropositive individuals with opportunistic infections and BAL neutrophilia [18]. Furthermore, recent data suggest that levels of soluble markers related to the degree of the T-cell alveolitis (including sCD8) are elevated both in peripheral blood [111] and BAL [112] of HIV-infected patients and can provide indication of pulmonary disease progression. Nevertheless, these studies were based on the analysis of data obtained from selected groups of individuals. Since the number of patients was small, it was impossible to evaluate how the changes in individual BAL parameters alter patients' prognosis in HIV infection. Furthermore, other markers, such as viral burden or cytokine levels in BAL fluid, should be considered. Larger multicentric co-operative studies, in which BAL data can be correlated with demographic, clinical and immunologic variables of HIV infection, will permit the selection of patients who are at risk of death, and thus represent the most likely candidates to benefit from intervention with therapeutic agents capable of preventing pulmonary complications or reducing the retroviral load in the pulmonary tract.

Acknowledgements

The authors wish to thank their colleagues from the Department of Clinical and Experimental Medicine who contributed to the original studies discussed in this chapter; Drs. P. Cadrobbi and A. Cipriani from the Divisions of Infectious Diseases and Pulmonary Medicine of Padua Hospital, who contributed to this project by allowing the study of their patients and performing the bronchoscopy; and Prof. A. De Rossi from the Institute of Oncology for her contribution in virologic analyses. We also wish to thank Martin Donach for his help in preparing the manuscript. This chapter was supported by a grant from the Ministero della Sanità, Istituto Superiore di Sanità (MS/ISS), Progetto AIDS 1996/1997 (Rome, Italy).

160   C. Agostini, R. Sancetta and G. Semenzato

References

1. Agostini C, Chilosi M, Trentin L, Zambello R, Semenzato G (1993) Pulmonary immune cells in health and disease: Lymphocytes. *Eur Respir J* 6: 1378–1401.
2. Skerret SJ (1994) Host defenses against respiratory infection. *Med Clin North Am* 78: 941–951.
3. Lipscomb MF, Bice DE, Lyons CR, Schuyler MR, Wilkes D (1994) The regulation of pulmonary immunity. *Adv Immunol* 59: 369–454.
4. Agostini C, Trentin L, Zambello R, Semenzato G (1993) HIV-1 and the lung. Infectivity, pathogenic mechanisms and cellular immune response taking place in the lower respiratory tract. *Am Rev Respir Dis* 147: 1038–1041.
5. Mayaud CM, Cadranel J (1993) HIV in the lung: Guilt or not guilt. *Thorax* 48: 1191–1195.
6. Davis L, Beck JM, Shellito J (1993) Update: HIV infection and pulmonary host defenses. *Semin Respir Infect* 8: 75–85.
7. Newbury RL, Beck JM (1995) Immunology of the lung in HIV-infected individuals. *Sem Respir Crit Care Med* 16: 161–172.
8. Robinson DS, Mitchell DM (1995) Lung immunology in HIV infection. In: Walters EH, du Bois RM (eds). *Immunology and management of interstitial lung diseases*. London: Chapman & Hall, 255–269.
9. Semenzato G, Agostini C (1995) HIV-related interstitial lung disease. *Curr Opin Pulmon Med* 1: 383–381.
10. Semenzato G, De Rossi A, Agostini C (1993) Human retroviruses and their etiological link to pulmonary diseases. *Eur Respir J* 6: 925–932.
11. Agostini C, Zambello R, Trentin L, Semenzato G (1996) HIV and pulmonary immune responses. *Immunol Today* 17: 359–364.
12. Lohman-Matthes ML, Steinmuller C, Franke-Ullmann G (1994) Pulmonary immune cells in health and disease: Pulmonary macrophages. *Eur Respir J* 7: 1678–1689.
13. Sibille Y, Marchandise FX (1993) Pulmonary immune cells in health and disease: Polymorphonuclear neutrophils. *Eur Respir J* 6: 1659–1671.
14. Thompson AB, Robbins RA, Romberger DJ (1995) Immunological functions of the pulmonary epithelium. *Eur Respir J* 8: 127–149.
15. Agostini C, Zambello R, Trentin L, Feruglio C, Masciarelli M, Siviero F, Poletti V, Spiga L, Gritti F, Semenzato G (1990) Cytotoxic events taking place in the lung of patients with HIV-1 infection: Evidence for an intrinsic defect of the MHC-unrestricted killing partially restored by the incubation with rIL-2. *Am Rev Respir Dis* 142: 516–522.
16. Agostini C, Zambello R, Trentin L, Poletti V, Spiga L, Gritti F, Cipriani A, Salmaso L, Cadrobbi P, Semenzato G (1991) Prognostic significance of the evaluation of bronchoalveolar lavage populations in patients with HIV-1 infection and pulmonary involvement. *Chest* 100: 1601–1606.
17. Guillon JM, Autran B, Denis M, Fouret P, Plata F, Mayaud CM, Akoun GM (1988) Human immunodeficiency virus-related lymphocytic alveolitis. *Chest* 94: 1264–1270.
18. Mason GR, Hashimoto CH, Dickman PS, Foutty LF, Cobb CJ (1989) Prognostic implications of bronchoalveolar lavage neutrophilia in patients with *Pneumocystis carinii* pneumonia and AIDS. *Am Rev Respir Dis* 139: 1336–1342.
19. Agostini C, Cipriani A, Cadrobbi P, Semenzato G (1995) The pulmonary immune system and HIV infection. In: Semenzato G (ed). *AIDS and the lung. Eur Respir Mon* 1: 89–124.
20. Plata F, Autran B, Martins LP, Wain-Hobson S, Raphael M, Mayaud C, Denis M, Guillon JM, Debre P (1987) AIDS-virus specific cytotoxic T lymphocytes in lung disorders. *Nature* 328: 348–351.
21. Autran B, Plata F, Guillon JM, Joly P, Mayaud C, Debré P (1990) HIV-specific cytotoxic T lymphocytes directed against alveolar macrophage in HIV-1 infected patients. *Res Virol* 141: 131–136.
22. Autran B, Sadat-Sowti B, Hadida F (1991) HIV-1 specific cytotoxic T lymphocytes against alveolar macrophages: Specificities and downregulation. *Res Virol* 142: 113–116.
23. Hoffenbach A, Langlade-Demoyen P, Dadaglio G, Vilmer E, Michel F, Mayaud C, Autran B, Plata F (1989) Unusually high frequencies of HIV-specific cytotoxic T lymphocytes in humans. *J Immunol* 142: 452–462.

24. Young KR, Rankin JA, Naegel GP, Paul ES, Reynolds HY (1985) Bronchoalveolar lavage cells and proteins in patients with acquired immunodeficiency syndrome: An immunological analysis. *Ann Intern Med* 103: 522–533.

25. Trentin L, Garbisa S, Zambello R, Agostini C, Caenazzo C, Di Francesco C, Cipriani A, Francavilla E, Semenzato G (1992) Spontaneous production of IL-6 by alveolar macrophages of HIV-1 seropositive patients. *J Infect Dis* 166: 731–737.

26. Pantaleo G, Graziosi C, Demarest JF, Cohen OJ, Vaccarezza M, Gantt K, Muro-Cacho C, Fauci AS (1994) Role of lymphoid organs in the pathogenesis of human immunodeficiency virus (HIV) infection. *Immunol Rev* 140: 105–130.

27. Landay AL, Schade SZ, Takefman DM, Kuhns MC, McNamara AL, Rosen RL, Kessler HA, Spear GT (1993) Detection of HIV-1 provirus in bronchoalveolar lavage cells by polymerase chain reaction. *J AIDS* 6: 1721–1726.

28. Rose RM, Krivine A, Pinkston P, Gillis JM, Huang A, Hammer SM (1991) Frequent identification of HIV-1 DNA in bronchoalveolar lavage cells obtained from individuals with the acquired immunodeficiency syndrome. *Am Rev Respir Dis* 143: 850–854.

29. Agostini C, Zambello R, Sancetta R, Cerutti A, Milani A, Tassinari C, Facco M, Cipriani A, Trentin L, Semenzato G (1991) Expression of TNF-receptor superfamily members by lung T lymphocytes: A putative role in the maintenance of the T-cell alveolitis in patients with interstitial lung disease. *Am J Respir Critical Care Med* 153: 1359–1367.

30. Agostini C, Zambello R, Trentin L, Cerutti A, Bulian P, Crivellaro C, Semenzato G (1994) γ/δ T cell receptor subsets in the lung of patients with HIV-1 infection. *Cell Immunol* 153: 194–205.

31. Perrella O, Perrella A, Soscia E, Marinelli A, Minnini V, Guerriero S, Briante R, Finelli L (1994) What is the role of T-lymphocytes with gamma/delta receptors in *Pneumocystic carinii* pneumonia in AIDS patients? *AIDS* 8: 395–396.

32. Kagi MK, Fierz W, Grob PJ, Russi EW (1993) High proportion of gamma-delta T-cell receptor positive T-cells in bronchoalveolar lavage and peripheral blood of HIV-infected patients with *Pneumocystis carinii* pneumonias. *Respiration* 60: 170–177.

33. Moretta L, Ciccone E, Ferrini S, Pelicci PG, Mingari MC, Zeromski J, Bottino C, Grossi C, Moretta A (1991) Molecular and cellular analysis of human T lymphocytes expressing $\gamma\delta$ T-cell receptor. *Immunol Rev* 120: 117–135.

34. Kaufmann SHE (1996) γ/δ and other unconventional T lymphocytes: What do they see and what do they do? *Proc Natl Acad Sci USA* 93: 2272–2279.

35. Wallace M, Bartz SR, Chang WL, Mackenzie DA, Pauza CD, Malkovsky M (1996) γ/δ T lymphocyte responses to HIV. *Clin Exp Immunol* 103: 177–184.

36. Spain BA, Soliman DM, Sidner RA, Twigg HL (1995) Enhanced proliferation and IL-2 secretion by lung lymphocytes from HIV-infected subjects. *Am J Physiol* 269: L498–L506.

37. Biglino A, Forno B, Pollono AM, Ghio P, Albera C (1993) Alveolar immune mediators in HIV-related pneumonia: Different role of IL-2 and IL-1 in inducing lung damage. *Chest* 103: 439–443.

38. Agostini C, Zambello R, Trentin L, Garbisa S, Francia di Celle P, Bulian P, Onisto M, Poletti V, Spiga L, Raise E, et al. (1991) Alveolar macrophages from patients with AIDS and AIDS-related complex constitutively synthesize and release tumor necrosis factor alpha. *Am Rev Respir Dis* 143: 195–201.

39. Agostini C, Zambello R, Trentin L, Cerutti A, Enthammer C, Facco M, Milani A, Sancetta R, Garbisa S, Semenzato G (1995) Expression of TNF receptors by T-cells and membrane TNF-α by alveolar macrophages suggests a role for TNF-α in the regulation of the local immune responses in the lung of HIV-1-infected patients. *J Immunol* 155: 2928–2938.

40. Israel-Biet D, Cadranel J, Beldjord K, Andrieu M, Jeffrey A, Even P (1991) Tumor necrosis factor producton in HIV-seropositive subjects: Relationship with lung opportunistic infections and HIV expression in alveolar macrophages. *J Immunol* 147: 490–494.

41. Denis M, Ghadirian E (1994) Alveolar macrophages from subjects infected with HIV-1 express macrophage inflammatory protein-1α (MIP-1α): Contribution to CD8+ alveolitis. *Clin Exp Immunol* 96: 187–192.

42. Zambello R, Trentin L, Benetti R, Cipriani A, Crivellaro C, Cadrobbi P, Agostini C, Semenzato G (1992) Expression of a functional p75 interleukin 2 receptor on lung lymphocytes from patients with HIV-1 infection. *J Clin Immunol* 12: 371–377.

43. Westendorp MO, Li-Weber M, Frank RW, Krammer PH (1994) Human immunodeficiency virus type 1 *tat* upregulates interleukin-2 secretion in activated T-cells. *J Virol* 68: 4177–4185.

44. Tagaya Y, Bamford RN, DeFilippis AP, Waldmann TA (1996) IL-15: A pleiotropic cytokine with diverse receptor/signaling pathways whose expression is controlled at multiple levels. *Immunity* 4: 329–336.

45. Giri JG, Ahdieh M, Eisenman J, Shanebeck K, Grabstein KH, Kumaki S, Namen A, Park LS, Cosman D, Anderson D (1994) Utilization of the β and γ chains of the IL-2 receptor by the novel cytokine IL-15. *EMBO J* 13: 2822–2830.

46. Grabstein KH, Eisenmann J, Shanebeck K, Rauch C, Srinivasan S, Fung V, Beers C, Richardson J, Schoenborn MA, Ahdieh M, et al. (1994) Cloning of a T-cell growth factor that interacts with the β chain of the interleukin-2 receptor. *Science* 264: 965–968.

47. Zambello R, Facco M, Trentin L, Sancetta R, Tassinari C, Perin A, Milani A, Pizzolo G, Rodeghiero F, Agostini C, et al. (1997) IL-15 triggers the proliferation and the cytotoxicity of granular lymphocytes in patients with lymphoproliferative disease of granular lymphocytes. *Blood*. In press.

48. Trentin L, Cerutti A, Zambello R, Sancetta R, Tassinari C, Facco M, Adami F, Rodeghiero F, Agostini C, Semenzato G (1996) IL-15 promotes the growth of leukemic cell of patients with B-cell chronic lymphoproliferative disorders. *Blood* 87: 3327–3335.

49. Khan IA, Kasper LH (1996) IL-15 augments CD8+ T-cell-mediated immunity against *Toxoplasma gondii* infection in mice. *J Immunol* 157: 2103–2108.

50. Agostini C, Trentin L, Facco M, Sancetta R, Cerutti A, Tassinari C, Cimarosto L, Adami F, Cipriani A, Zambello R, et al. (1996) Role of IL-15, IL-2 and their receptors in the development of T-cell alveolitis in pulmonary sarcoidosis. *J Immunol* 157:910–917.

51. McInnes IB, Al-Mughales J, Field M, Leung BP, Huang F, Dixon R, Sturrock RD, Wilkinson PC, Liew FY (1996) The role of interleukin-15 in T-cell migration and activation in rheumatoid arthritis. *Nature Med* 2: 175–178.

52. Seder RA, Grabstein KH, Berzofsky JA (1995) Cytokine interactions in human immunodeficiency virus infected individuals: Roles of interleukin (IL)-2, IL-12, and IL-15. *J Exp Med* 182: 1067–1078.

53. Gazzinelli RT (1996) Molecular and cellular basis of interleukin-12 activity in prophylaxis and therapy against infectious diseases. *Mol Med Today* 2: 258–267.

54. Mulligan MS, Vaporciyan AA, Warner RL, Jones ML, Foreman KL, Miyasaak M, Todd RF III, Ward PA (1995) Compartmentalized roles for leukocytic adhesion molecules in lung inflammatory injury. *J Immunol* 154: 1350–1363.

55. Agostini C, Trentin L, Zambello R, Bulian P, Garbisa S, Cipriani A, Cadrobbi P, Semenzato G (1993) Alveolar macrophages from patients with HIV-1 infection express accessory molecules, activation markers, and release increased amounts of biological response modifiers. *Chest* 102S: 108–112.

56. Akbar AN, Salmon M, Savill J, Janossy G (1993) The role of bcl-2 in T-cell memory a "balancing act" between cell death and survival. *Immunol Today* 14: 256–260.

57. Lenardo MJ (1996) Fas and the art of lymphocyte maintenance. *J Exp Med* 183: 721–724.

58. Moss PAH, Rosenberg WMC, Bell JI (1992) The human T-cell receptor in health and disease. *Ann Rev Immunol* 10: 71–96.

59. Trentin L, Zambello R, Facco M, Sancetta R, Cerruti A, Milani A, Tassinari C, Crivellaro C, Cipriani A, Agostini C, et al. (1996) Skewing of the T-cell repertoire in the lung of patients with HIV-1 infection. *AIDS* 10: 729–736.

60. Gascoigne NRJ (1993) Interaction of the T-cell receptor with bacterial superantigens. *Sem Immunol* 5: 13–19.

61. Bisset LR, Fierz W (1992) Areas of sequence homology between several staphylococcal exotoxin "superantigens" and the HIV-1 *pol* protein. *AIDS Res Human Retroviruses* 8: 1543–1545.

62. Semenzato G, Agostini C, Ometto L, Zambello R, Trentin L, Chieco-Bianchi L, De Rossi A (1995) CD8+ T lymphocytes in the lung of AIDS patients harbor human immunodeficiency virus type 1. *Blood* 85: 2308–2314.

63. Sadat-Sowti B, Parrot A, Quint L, Mayaud C, Debre P, Autran B (1994) Alveolar CH8$^+$/CD57$^+$ lymphocytes in human immunodeficiency virus infection produce an inhibitor of cytotoxic function. *Am J Respir Crit Care Med* 149: 972–980.
64. Szawlowski PWS, Hanke T, Randall RE (1993) Sequence homology between HIV-1 gp120 and the apoptosis mediating Fas protein. *AIDS* 7: 1018–1025.
65. Clerici M, Shearer GM (1993) Th2 switch is a critical step in the etiology of HIV infection. *Immunol Today* 14: 107–111.
66. Romagnani S (ed.) (1996) Th1 and Th2 cells in health and disease. *Chem Immunol* 63: 1–218.
67. Agostini C, Sancetta R, Cerutti A, Semenzato G (1995) Alveolar macrophages as a cell source of cytokine hyperproduction in HIV-related interstitial lung disease. *J Leukoc Biol* 58: 495–500.
68. Twigg HL, Lipscomb MF, Yoffe B, Barbaro DJ, Weissler JC (1989) Enhanced accessory cell function by alveolar macrophages from patients infected with human immunodeficiency virus and its potential role for depletion of CD4$^+$ cells in the lung. *Am J Respir Cell Mol Biol* 1: 391–400.
69. Twigg HL, Soliman DM (1994) Role of alveolar macrophage-T-cell adherence in accessory cell function in human immunodeficiency virus-infected individuals. *Am J Respir Cell Mol Biol* 11: 138–146.
70. Twigg HL, Iwamoto GK, Soliman DM (1992) Role of cytokines in alveolar macrophage-T-cell adherence in accessory cell function in HIV-infected individuals. *J Immunol* 149: 1462–1469.
71. Thompson CB (1995) Distinct roles for the costimulatory ligands B7-1 and B7-2 in T helper cell differentiation. *Cell* 81: 979–980.
72. Agostini C, Semenzato G (1994) Does bronchoalveolar lavage analysis provide a tool to monitor disease progression or predict survival in patients with HIV-1 infection? *Thorax* 49: 848–851.
73. Meignan M, Guilon JM, Denis M, Joly P, Rosso J, Carette MF (1990) Increased lung epithelia permeability in HIV-infected patients with isolated cytotoxic T lymphocytic alveolitis. *Am Rev Respir Dis* 141: 1241–1248.
74. Nieman RB, Fleming J, Coker RJ, Harris JR, Mitchell DM (1993) Reduced carbon monoxide transfer factor (TLCO) in human immunodeficiency virus type I (HIV-I) infection as a predictor for faster progression to AIDS. *Thorax* 48: 481–485.
75. Phillips DM, Bourinbaiar AS (1992) Mechanisms of HIV spread to epithelia. *Virology* 186: 261–267.
76. Buhl R, Jaffe HA, Holroyd K (1993) Activation of alveolar macrophages in asymptomatic HIV-infected individuals. *J Immunol* 150: 1019–1028.
77. Agostini C, Garbisa S, Trentin L, Zambello R, Fastelli G, Onisto M, Semenzato G (1989) Pulmonary alveolar macrophages from patients with active sarcoidosis express type IV collagenolytic proteinase: An enzymatic mechanism for influx of mononuclear phagocytes at sites of disease activity. *J Clin Invest* 84: 605–612.
78. Agostini C, Trentin L, Zambello R, Bulian P, Caenazzo C, Cipriani A, Cadrobbi P, Garbisa S, Semenzato G (1992) Release of GM-CSF by alveolar macrophages in the lung of HIV-1 infected patients: A mechanism accounting for macrophage and neutrophil accumulation. *J Immunol* 149: 3379–3385.
79. Lipman MCI, Johnson MA, Bray DH, Poulter LH (1995) Changes to alveolar phenotype in HIV infected individuals with normal CD4 counts and no respiratory disease. *Thorax* 50: 777–781.
80. Bohnet S, Braun J, Dalhoff K (1994) Intercellular adhesion molecule-1 (ICAM) is up-regulated on alveolar macrophages from AIDS patients. *Eur Respir J* 7: 299–304.
81. Dubinett SM, Huang M, Lichtenstein A, McBride WH, Wang J, Markovitz G, Kelley D, Grody WW, Mint LE, Dhanani S (1994) Tumor necrosis factor-α plays a central role in interleukin-2-induced pulmonary vascular leak and lymphocyte accumulation. *Cell Immunol* 157: 170–179.
82. Dalgleish AG (1995) The immune response to HIV: Potential for immunotherapy. *Immunol Today* 16: 356–358.
83. Clarke JR, Krishnan V, Bennet J, Mitchell D, Jeffries DJ (1990) Detection of HIV-1 in human lung macrophages using the polymerase chain reaction. *AIDS* 4: 1133–1136.

84. Plata F, Garcia-Pons F, Ryter A, Lebargy F, Goodenow MM, Quan Dat HQ, Autran B, Mayaud C (1990) HIV-1 infection of lung alveolar fibroblasts and macrophages in humans. *AIDS Res Human Retroviruses* 6: 979–986.
85. Rich EA, Chen ISY, Zack JA, Leonard ML, O'Brien WA (1992) Increased susceptibility of differentiated mononuclear phagocytes to productive infection with human immunodeficiency virus-1 (HIV-1). *J Clin Invest* 89: 176–183.
86. Lebargy F, Branellec A, Deforges L, Bignon J, Bernaudin JF (1994) HIV-1 in human alveolar macrophages from infected patients is latent *in vivo* but replicates after *in vitro* stimulation. *Am J Respir Cell Mol Biol* 10: 72–78.
87. Sierra Madero JG, Toossi Z, Hom DL, Finegan CK, Hoenig E, Rich EA (1994) Relationship between load of virus in alveolar macrophages from human immunodeficiency virus type 1-infected persons, production of cytokines and clinical status. *J Infect Dis* 169: 18–27.
88. Yanagawa H, Sone S, Haku T, Mizuno K, Yano S, Ohmoto Y, Ogura T (1995) Contrasting effect of interleukin-13 on interleukin-1 receptor antagonist and proinflammatory cytokine production by human alveolar macrophages. *Am J Respir Cell Mol Biol* 12: 71–76.
89. Denis M, Ghadirian E (1994) Interleukin-13 and interleukin-4 protect bronchoalveolar macrophages from productive infection with human immunodeficiency virus type 1. *AIDS Res Hum Retroviruses* 10: 795–802.
90. Strieter RM, Chensue SW, Basha MA, Standiford TJ, Lynch JP III, Baggiolini M, Kunkel SL (1990) Human alveolar macrophage gene expression of interleukin-8 by tumor necrosis factor-α, lipopolysaccharide and interleukin-1β. *Am J Respir Cell Mol Biol* 2: 321–326.
91. Cassatella ML (1995) The production of cytokines by polymorphonuclear neutrophils. *Immunol Today* 16: 21–26.
92. Sadaghdar H, Huang ZB, Eden E (1992) Correlation bronchalveolar lavage findings to severity of *Pneumocystis carinii* pneumonia in AIDS: Evidence for the development of high-permeability pulmonary edema. *Chest* 102: 63–69.
93. Lipschik GY, Doerfler ME, Kovacs JA, Travis WD, Andrawis VA, Lawrence MG (1993) Leukotriene B4 and interleukin-8 in human immunodeficiency virus-related pulmonary disease. *Chest* 104: 763–769.
94. Benfield TL, Vestbo J, Junge J, Nielsen TL, Jensen AB, Lundgren JD (1995) Prognostic value of interleukin-8 in AIDS-associated *Pneumocystis carinii* pneumonia. *Am J Respir Crit Care Med* 151: 1058–1062.
95. Donaldson YK, Bell JE, Ironside JW, Brettle RP, Robertson JR, Busuttil A, Simmonds P (1994) Redistribution of HIV outside the lymphoid system with onset of AIDS. *Lancet* 343: 383–385.
96. Piatak M, Saag MS, Yang LC, Clark SJ, Kappes JC, Luk KC, Hahn BH, Shaw GM, Lifson JD (1993) High levels of HIV-1 in plasma during all stages of infection determined by competitive PCR. *Science* 259: 1749–1754.
97. Clarke JR, Gates AJ, Coker RJ J, Douglass JA, Williamson JD, Mitchell DM (1994) HIV-1 proviral DNA copy number in peripheral blood leukocytes and bronchoalveolar lavage cells of AIDS patients. *Clin Exp Immunol* 96: 182–186.
98. Pinkston P, Pelettier N, Arena C, Schock J, Garland R, Rose RM (1995) Quantitative culture of HIV-1 from bronchoalveolar lavage cells. *Am J Respir Crit Care Med* 152: 254–259.
99. Sei S, Kleiner DE, Kopp JB, Chandra R, Klotman PE, Yarchoan R, Pizzo PA, Mitsuya H (1994) Quantitative analysis of viral burden in tissues from adults and children with symptomatic human immunodeficiency virus type 1 infection assessed by polymerase chain reaction. *J Infect Dis* 170: 325–333.
100. Bates P (1996) Chemokine receptors and HIV-1: An attractive pair? *Cell* 86: 1–3.
101. Strieter RM, Standiford TJ, Huffnagle GB, Colletti LM, Lukacs NW, Kunkel SL (1996) "The good, the bad and the ugly": The role of chemokines in models of human disease. *J Immunol* 156: 3583–3586.
102. Agostini C, Semenzato G (1996) Immunologic effects of HIV in the lung. *Clin Chest Med* 17: 633–645.
103. Potash MJ, Zeira M, Huang ZB et al. (1992) Virus-cell membrane fusion does not predict infection of alveolar macrophages by human immunodeficiency virus type 1 (HIV-1). *Virology* 188: 864–868.

104. Schuitemaker H, Koot M, Kootstra NA et al. (1992) Biological phenotype of human immunodeficiency virus type 1 clones at different stages of infection: Progression of disease is associated with a shift from monocytotropic to T-cell-tropic virus populations. *J Virol* 66: 1354–1360.
105. Itescu S, Simonelli PF, Winchester RJ, Ginsberg HS (1994) Human immunodeficiency virus type 1 strains in the lungs of infected individuals evolve independently from those in peripheral blood and are highly conserved in the C-terminal region of the envelope V3 loop. *Proc Natl Acad Sci USA* 91: 11378–11382.
106. Goletti D, Weissman D, Jackson RW, Graham NMH, Vlahov D, Klein RS, Ortona L, Cauda R, Fauci AS (1996) Effect of *Mycobacterium tuberculosis* on HIV replication: Role of immune activation. *J Immunol* 157: 1271–1278.
107. Vanham G, Edmonds K, Qing L, Hom D, Toossi Z, Jones B (1996) Generalized immune activation in pulmonary tuberculosis: Co-activation with HIV infection. *Clin Exp Immunol* 103: 30–34.
108. Livingstone WJ, Moore M, Innes D, Bell JE, Simmonds P (1996) Frequent infection of peripheral blood CD8-positive T-lymphocytes with HIV-1. *Lancet* 348: 649–654.
109. De Maria A, Colombini S, Schnittman SM, Moretta L (1994) CD8+ cytolytic T lymphocytes become infected *in vitro* in the process of killing HIV-1-infected target cells. *Eur J Immunol* 24: 531–537.
110. De Maria A, Pantaleo G, Schnittman SM, Grenhouse JJ, Baseler M, Orenstein JM, Fauci AS (1991) Infection of CD8+ T lymphocytes with HIV: Requirement for interaction with infected CD4+ cells and induction of infectious virus from chronically infected CD8+ cells. *J Immunol* 146: 2220–2229.
111. Agostini C, Semenzato G, Vinante F, Sinicco A, Trentin L, Zambello R, Zuppini B, Zanotti R, Siviero F, Veneri D, et al. (1989) Increased levels of soluble CD8 molecule in the serum of patients with acquired immunodeficiency syndrome (AIDS) and AIDS-related disorders. *Clin Immunol Immunopathol* 50: 146–151.
112. Willsie SK, Herndon BL, Miller L, Dew M (1996) Soluble versus cell-bound CD4, CD8 bronchoalveolar lavage: Correlation with pulmonary diagnoses in human immunodeficiency virus-infected individuals. *J Leukoc Biol* 58: 813–816.

Autoimmune Aspects of Lung Disease
ed. by D.A. Isenberg and S.G. Spiro
© 1998 Birkhäuser Verlag Basel/Switzerland

CHAPTER 7
Lung Cancer: Immunological Disturbances and Clinical Implications

Tariq Sethi

Respiratory Medicine Unit, Department of Medicine (RIE), University of Edinburgh Royal Infirmary, Edinburgh, Scotland, UK

1. Introduction

Lung cancer is the most frequently occurring malignancy in the developed world, and its incidence is expected to rise even further over the next 20 years, with an increasing number of cases unrelated to smoking [1]. The epidemic proportions of lung cancer are contrasted sharply with the general failure of conventional treatment. Novel approaches to the treatment of these tumours are needed urgently.

Recent advances in immunology have provided insights into the relationship between host resistance and the clinical course of lung cancer. A decline in host resistance was suggested initially by increased susceptibility to infections, poor wound healing and the debilitating nature of lung cancer [2, 3]. These symptoms are often disproportionate to the patient's tumour burden and are analogous to immunodeficiency disorders [4, 5]. It seems probable that immunological surveillance plays a part in controlling the growth of tumours once initiated. Patients with transplanted kidneys have a higher than expected risk of developing malignant lymphomas and malignant neoplasms transferred from kidney grafts from affected donors. The increased risk is thought to be due to the continuous immunosuppressive therapy administered to the recipients to weaken or abolish the immunological reaction against the foreign kidney [5].

Several areas of immunological function are impaired in patients with lung cancer in comparison with normal subjects, and the degree of impairment seems to correlate with the stage of the disease. This has been demonstrated using a variety of measures of the cell-mediated immune response: anergy in delayed hypersensitivity skin testing, delayed rejection of cultured cell allografts, relative lymphopaenia in the peripheral blood and diminished *in vitro* proliferative responses to the lymphocyte mitogen phytohaemagglutinin [6–8]. Multiple studies using intradermal antigens have suggested that anergy in delayed hypersensitivity skin testing correlated directly with a poor prognosis [9]. Thus, impaired immune function might be the cause of poor survival in lung cancer patients. In addition, the retrospective observation that empyema (associated with enlarged reactive lymph nodes) following surgical resection for lung cancer was associated with improved survival over uninfected controls suggested that augmentation of the immune system may provide a novel type of therapeutic option [10–11].

Pathologists have long recognised that lung cancers are heavily infiltrated by lymphoid cells [12]. Eight case reports of spontaneous remission have been identified in the literature [13]. Despite this low frequency, remission of lung cancer has been cited as evidence for tumour immunoreactivity. The fact that carcinomas with the greatest amount of necrosis (e.g. small-cell lung cancer) demonstrate the least amount of stromal reaction and that there is a correlation between tumour differentiation and the amount of mononuclear cellular infiltrate suggests that this is a tumour-specific immune response rather than just a non-specific simple inflammatory reaction to necrotic tissue [14]. Studies examining the tumour-infiltrating lymphocyte population within and around non-small-cell lung cancers have not shown any deficit of particular effector cell types (T-cells, B-cells or natural killer cells). Also, lung cancers are able to stimulate antibody production, as evidenced by the generation of monoclonal antibodies to surface antigens and antibody-mediated paraneoplastic syndromes. However, tumours continue to grow despite the presence of all the necessary immunoeffectors. I will therefore examine the apparent functional capacity of each effector arm to elucidate possible mechanisms by which lung cancers escape immune surveillance and the novel clinical implications of this greater understanding of the host immune response to lung cancers.

2. Humoral Immune Response to Lung Cancer

Lung cancers are able to generate an antibody response both *in vitro* and *in vivo* and are thus able to elicit an immune response and reveal in some way that the cancer is non-self. These antibodies could potentially be the first signals to initiate host immune effector responses.

2.1. Host Antibody Response

Paraneoplastic syndromes are common in patients with lung cancer and may be the presenting findings or first signs of recurrence. In addition, these syndromes may mimic metastatic disease and, unless detected, lead to inappropriate palliative rather than curative treatment. Often the paraneoplastic syndrome may be relieved by successful treatment of the tumour. Paraneoplastic neuronal disorders primarily result from anti-small cell lung cancer antibodies which cross-react with neuronal antigens. Neurologic/myopathic syndromes are seen in only 1% of patients but are dramatic and include the Eaton-Lambert myasthenic syndrome associated with small cell cancer. Peripheral neuropathies, subacute cerebellar degeneration, cortical degeneration and polymyositis are uncommon, occurring in less than 1% of patients, as are renal manifestations of nephrotic syndrome or glomerulonephritis.

These antibody responses to lung cancer have not been studied in great detail, and most of these studies are from small numbers of patients; however, taken together they illustrate a few basic principles.

1. Lung cancers can induce antibodies, and this is due to a lung cancer antigen-driven process [15].
2. In patients presenting with paraneoplastic neuronal disorders as a feature of small cell lung cancer, there is both clinical and serological heterogeneity. Patients with a given clinical syndrome may have different antineuronal antibodies, and patients with given autoantibody specificity have different clinical presentations [16–19].
3. At autopsy perivascular inflammatory infiltrates and deposits of anti-small-cell lung cancer antibodies which cross-react with neuronal antigens can be found in the central nervous system, suggesting that these anti-small cell lung cancer antibodies are responsible for the patient's clinical syndrome [16, 17].

Immune complexes have been noted in patients with lung cancer [20]. Nephrotic syndrome is occasionally associated with, and may even be the presenting feature of, lung cancers. It may disappear following resection of the tumour, and its reappearance may be the first indication of the presence of metastasis. Renal biopsy usually shows a membraneous glomerulonephropathy, and occasionally antibodies reacting with the cancer cells have been eluted in the deposits or immune complexes containing tumour-associated antigens including chorioembryonic antigen. Concentrations of immunoglobulins (IgA and IgG) have been found to be increased in the bronchial washings of patients with lung cancer. Indeed, the increases in immunoglobulin concentration were noted only in washings obtained from the lung that was involved with the tumour and not in the washings obtained from the contralateral tumour-free lung. The predominant immunoglobulin class accounting for the increased levels is IgA [21]. Despite this ability to generate antibodies to lung cancer–associated antigens derived from lung cancer cells, there is only sparse evidence that the host immune response relies on the generation of antibodies to fight lung cancer.

A number of animal studies using Calmette-Guérin bacillus (BCG) (subcutaneous), levamisole (oral) or *Corynebacterium parvum* (intrapleural) showed that these non-specific stimulants of the immune system could inhibit tumour growth. Multiple clinical trials aimed at boosting the host immune response to lung cancer, using BCG and other immunostimulants, were carried out. Although there were occasional positive results, most studies failed to demonstrate a significant difference between BCG and placebo. In most cases, these trials were plagued by uncertainty regarding the route of antigen administration. Systemic administration of BCG also resulted in toxicity despite occasional positive results. In phase I and II trials these antigen non-specific immunostimulants did not affect the natural history of lung cancer [22–23]. In addition, a prospective randomised study to evaluate the effect of adjuvant immunotherapy with intrapleural *Streptococcus pyogenes* in lung cancer patients after resection failed to demonstrate any beneficial effect on patient survival [24]. This probably refutes the earlier promise suggested by the retrospective study of post-surgical resection empyema.

2.2. Monoclonal Antibodies

With the development of monoclonal antibody techniques, the search for tumour-associated antigens in lung cancer has intensified, the progress of which has been reviewed by Souhami [25]. Monoclonal antibodies have been used to make earlier diagnoses, for staging, for pathologic differentiation and therapeutically for specific targeting of cytotoxic agents.

In screening studies, sputum cytology in high-risk populations has not been shown to facilitate the detection and cure of lung cancer. Lung cancer did not invariably develop in patients who demonstrated moderate or greater cellular atypia. In a retrospective review of sputum samples from such patients after staining with monoclonal antibodies specific for either small-cell or non-small-cell lung cancer, positive immunostaining was noted in 14 of the 22 patients who eventually had lung cancer, showing a sensitivity of 64% and a specificity of 88%. Many of the false negative immunostained samples were obtained 4–5 years before cancer was eventually detected, whereas true positive samples were obtained during the 2 years before the diagnosis of lung cancer. When only immunopositive staining was considered, the sensitivity of the assay improved to 91% [26]. The application of immunohistologic assessment of sputum samples may improve diagnostic sensitivity, but large-scale trials would be needed before the true clinical effect can be determined.

p53 is a oncogenic nuclear protein which causes cell cycle arrest in the G0/G1 transition in response to DNA-damaging agents, allowing the cell time to initiate repair. Failing this, p53 initiates programmed cell death (apoptosis). The induction of apoptosis by p53 following genotoxic insult may act as a defence mechanism to protect the propagation of cells that have sustained mutation. Abrogation of this p53 pathway is the most common specific mutation in human cancer and may be central to progression of the disease and to its response to treatment by radiation and chemotherapy. p53 alteration usually involves missense mutations that stabilise the p53 protein, which in turn accumulates, inducing a humoral response early in tumour development. p53 antibodies may therefore be useful as a precocious marker of p53 alteration before clinical manifestation of lung cancer [27].

Resolving whether a solitary pulmonary nodule on a chest X-ray represents a benign or malignant process remains a common clinical problem. It was hoped that measurement of tumour-associated antigen levels might distinguish benign from malignant lesions. In general, the specificity of measurements of tumour-associated antigens is poor when a single antigen is considered. However, this may improve when used in combination with other assays, for example, a panel of tumour-associated antigens or changes in hormonal levels that have also been noted to be increased in patients with lung cancer. Though monoclonal antibodies for chromogranin and neuron-specific enolase are not entirely specific, more recent data suggests that some nerve cell adhesion molecule monoclonal antibodies have good specificity for small-cell lung cancer. The ability of these lymphoid monoclonal antibodies to discriminate between small-cell and non-small-cell lung cancer may prove useful in the immunohistochemical diagnosis of lung cancers [28].

Monoclonal antibodies have also been used in staging patients with lung cancer [29]. The monoclonal antibody to the epidermal growth factor (EGF) receptor has been shown to effectively block the binding of EGF, transforming growth factor α (TGF-α) and inhibit the growth *in vitro* of non-small-cell lung cancer cell lines [30]. A phase I trial using this EGF monoclonal antibody in patients with unresectable squamous cell carcinoma shows that this antibody can be safely administered to patients and can localise efficiently to metastases even at relatively low doses.

Ricin A chain immunotoxins directed against a variety of the common cell surface antigens associated with small-cell lung cancer exerted selective toxic effects on small-cell lung cancer cell lines. The potency of the cytotoxic effects matched or exceeded that previously reported for ricin A chain immunotoxins directed against identical or similar antigens on other types of carcinomas, suggesting that small-cell lung cancer may be uniquely sensitive to this type of immunotoxin [31].

The immune system can recognise differentiation antigens that are expressed selectively on malignant cells and their normal cell counterparts. However, it is uncertain whether immunity to differentiation antigens can effectively lead to tumour rejection. A recent mouse model system suggests that passive immunisation with a mouse monoclonal antibody can induce protection and rejection of both subcutaneous tumours and lung metastases, including established tumours [32]. Also, monoclonal antibodies to the integrin $\alpha_v \beta_3$ can promote tumour regression by inducing apoptosis of angiogenic blood vessels, thereby inhibiting neovascularisation, in an *in vivo* angiogenesis model [33].

Despite the promise to date, no lung cancer monoclonal antibody has been found that is entirely tumour-specific. Also, cancer cells are heterogeneous and may undergo phenotypic changes with maturation *in vivo* and *in vitro*. Thus, monoclonal antibodies generated against a unique tumour at a particular moment are unlikely to remain sensitive in the detection of that tumour. This lack of absolute specificity of these antibodies, however, does not imply that they may not be clinically useful. It may be that panels of monoclonal antibodies will be more useful in a clinical setting than any one individual monoclonal antibody.

3. Cellular Immune Response to Lung Cancer

The cell-mediated immunologic response to lung cancer involves monocytes/macrophages and lymphocytes (natural killer cells, lymphokine-activated killer cells and cytotoxic T-cells). Augmentation of these cellular responses may have a therapeutic role in the treatment of lung cancer (Table 1).

3.1 Macrophages

Bronchoalveolar lavage commonly yields several million cells, the majority of which are macrophages. Tissue histochemistry of the alveolar spaces typically reveals alveolar macrophages with few lymphocytes and rare granulocytes. The functional role of macrophages has been implicated by the association of macrophages with control of *Mycobacteria tuberculosis* infections. Furthermore, skin testing and the delayed-type hypersensitivity response have been correlated with macrophage reactivity and host resistance to tuberculosis. Skin testing also correlated with lung cancer prognosis, suggesting an association between immunologic response and prognosis. Ninety-three percent of patients who failed to react to a dinitrochlorobenzene skin test were inoperable or had an early recurrence, whereas 92% of those who reacted remained free of disease for 6 months after operation [34]. Alveolar macrophages obtained from patients with lung cancer appear to have normal activation capabilities, as indicated by chemiluminescence techniques and normal phagocytic ability [35–36]. However, the cytotoxic function of alveolar macrophages obtained from patients with lung cancer is controversial, normal [37] in some studies and

Table 1. Therapeutic modulation of cellular immunity in lung cancer

Treatment	Route	Animal	Cellular response	Tumour response	Ref.
GM-CSF	Intraperitoneal	Mouse	↑ MØ	Inhibited tumour growth in post-op period	[41]
IL-2	Intrapleural	Human	↑ Lymphocyte nos ↑ LAK cells ↑ Cytotoxic T-cells	9/11 malignant pleural effusions disappeared	[56]
	Systemic	Human	↑ Cytotoxic T-cells	No tumour response	[58]
IL-2 + TNFα	Systemic	Human	↑ NK cell activity ↑ LAK cells	4/16 regressed + 7/16 stabilised for 3 mos	[55]
IL-2 + Tumour-derived LAK	Intrapleural	Human	Mononuclear cells recruited	12/18 malignant pleural effusions disappeared	[57]
	Systemic	Human	Mononuclear cells recruited	5/7 ↓ tumour size but not > 50%	[59]

GM-CSF: granulocyte-macrophage colony-stimulating factor; LAK: lymphokine-activated killer; IL-2: interleukin-2; MØ: macrophage; NK: natural killer; TNFα: tumour necrosis factor α; nos: numbers.

decreased in others [38]. In support of the latter observation, one group noted reduced cytostatic capability in alveolar macrophages from patients with lung cancer which returned to normal after treatment of these macrophages with interferon-γ [39].

In summary, macrophages are found within lung cancers. These macrophages have cytostatic capability, the extent of which may correlate with remission of disease; however, it is unclear whether the major role of alveolar macrophages is cytotoxic or immunomodulatory [40]. In this respect granulocyte-macrophage colony-stimulating factor (GM-CSF) is interesting because it induces macrophage tumourocidal activity *in vitro*. In a murine carcinoma model, GM-CSF-stimulated macrophages showed increased superoxide anion cytotoxicity, phagocytosis and interleukin-6 and tumour necrosis factor-α production. GM-CSF also inhibited tumour growth, and this effect persisted during the post-operative period, suggesting a possible therapeutic role in the treatment of cancers, particularly following primary resection [41].

3.2. Lymphocytes

Several developments in immunology have suggested that lymphocytes rather than macrophages may be the dominant effector cell in solid tumour immunity.

Natural killer cells are thought to be a first line of defence in the immune response to viral infections. In addition, they have been considered the first responders in the host immunosurveillance network that may act against the microscopic growth of tumours. Natural killer cell activity is low in the peripheral blood of patients with lung cancer but characteristically returns to normal after surgical excision of the cancer [42]. In addition, two other studies have shown that natural killer cell activity is decreased in lymphocytes taken directly from lung cancers [43, 44].

Detailed phenotypic immunohistochemical characterisation of cells infiltrating solid tumours has demonstrated that the majority of these cells are lymphocytes. Most of these tumour-infiltrating lymphocytes express CD4 and CD8 cell surface molecules, typical of cytotoxic T lymphocytes [45, 46]. Only a minority of the cells are mononuclear phagocytes. Furthermore, the study of selected solid tumours has suggested that an increased number of infiltrating T-cells correlates with improved prognosis [45, 46]. These cytotoxic T lymphocytes are likely effectors in autologous lymphocyte cytotoxicity assays. Two studies have shown that patients who have autologous lymphocyte cytotoxicity live longer than those lacking such a response; in one of these studies the mean disease-free time was 52 months in those with autologous tumour killing versus 7 months in those without it. In this same study other immune functions were intact in patients with or without autologous lymphocyte cytotoxicity. Thus, the prognostic difference was apparently not due to a generalised reduction in the immune response. In both studies natural killer cell activity did not predict the outcome.

The discovery of T-cell growth factor (interleukin-2) and the eventual cloning of the interleukin-2 gene permitted detailed *in vitro* studies of T-lymphocyte function. The role of cytokines such as interleukin-1, interleukin-2 and interferon-γ in immune responses to lung cancer has not been fully elucidated. Concentrations of interleukin-2 are increased in the bronchoalveolar lavage fluid obtained from patients with lung cancer; however such increases are also noted in other patients with non-malignant pulmonary disease [47]. The treatment of peripheral blood mononuclear cells with interleukin-2 results in the logarithmic expansion of lymphocytes *in vitro* [48]. Some of these expanded cells demonstrate antigen non-specific cytolytic activity – so-called lymphokine-activated killer cells [49]. Antigen-specific cytotoxic T lymphocytes are also expanded with interleukin-2 treatment. The addition of interferon-γ to tumour-infiltrating lymphocytes incubated with interleukin-2 has been shown to improve the lymphokine-activated killer cell activity of these lymphocytes [50, 51].

In vitro studies have demonstrated that a subset of T lymphocytes are able to bind efficiently and kill tumour target cells. This process can be repeated many times by an individual cytotoxic T lymphocyte and is referred to as the lytic cycle. These functional characteristics are consistent with a role as the primary mediators of tumour resistance [52]. T-lymphocyte binding to the tumour target cell requires both expression of the appropriate target antigen on the tumour cell and recognition by the antigen's specific T-cell receptor. This physical interaction of the T-cell receptor and the appropriate antigen triggers cytotoxic T-lymphocyte activation, resulting in a rise in intracellular concentration of calcium and the exocytosis of lytic granules, resulting in the destruction of the target cell [53]. In addition to triggering lysis of the target cell, activation of the T lymphocyte results in the proliferation of the activated cytotoxic T lymphocyte. The cellular progeny express an identical antigen-specific receptor, resulting in clonal expansion. The process of antigen-dependent cytotoxic T-lymphocyte proliferation plays an important role in expanding the pool of potentially reactive cytotoxic T lymphocytes. Clonally expanded memory T-cells migrate throughout the blood and lymphatic systems, concentrating in organs that are potential entry sites for pathogens, e.g. lung, gut and skin. Detailed studies of lymphocyte circulation have suggested overlapping recirculation patterns, and lung-associated lymphocytes may be found in skin and gut tissue; however, the majority will be found in lung- or bronchus-associated lymphoid tissue [54]. Lymphoid recirculation has been proposed as an explanation not only for systemic immunity but also for organ-selective patterns of cancer metastases.

The cytolytic potential of cytotoxic T lymphocytes combined with the T-lymphocyte ability to recirculate and provide systemic immunity emphasised the strategic advantages of cytotoxic T lymphocytes over other immune cells. The availability of human interleukin-2 provided an opportunity for the growth of cytotoxic T lymphocytes *ex vivo* and systemic treatment *in vivo*, and thus a mechanism for exploiting the functional potential of cytotoxic T lymphocytes as a novel therapy for lung cancer. A series of interleukin-2 clinical trials followed.

A phase I trial that used a combination of interleukin-2 and tumour necrosis factor-α was conducted in 16 patients with stage IIIB or IV non-small-cell lung cancer. Both natural killer cell and lymphokine killer cell activity *in vitro* increased during therapy. The tumour regressed in 4 patients, and disease stabilised in 7 patients for 3 months [55]. The side effects from treatment with interleukin-2 (fever, chills, malaise, diarrhoea, vomiting, hypotension, oedema and rash) were experienced by all patients. Side effects related to systemic administration of interleukin-2 can be minimised by pleural installation, which has been done successfully by two separate groups. In one, the administration of only interleukin-2 led to disappearance of a malignant effusion in 9 of 11 patients [56]. In the other, interleukin-2 and pleural effusion-derived lymphokine-activated killer cells were administered intrapleurally to 18 patients; the pleural fluid disappeared in 12 of them. Side effects were mild, but the benefits in terms of survival remain uncertain [57]. The interleukin-2 data on lung cancer were particularly disappointing, and the results of these trials were similar to those obtained in BCG studies. Although mononuclear cells appeared to be recruited into the tumour, interleukin-2 treatment only rarely resulted in tumour cell death [58]. Therapies that use only interleukin-2 are non-specific. When host lymphocytes, particularly those infiltrating the tumour are used, greater tumour specificity is the aim. One such approach has focused on lymphokine-activated killer cells derived from tumour-infiltrating lymphocytes. One study using 7 patients with metastatic adenocarcinoma of the lung showed that when tumour-infiltrating lymphocytes were extracted and infused after 1–4 months in culture with interleukin-2, 5 of the patients had a decrease in size of the tumour, but the reductions noted were never more than 50% [59]. Results of systemic administration of interleukin-2 and lymphokine-activated killer cells have been unsuccessful in patients with lung cancer. Nevertheless, these approaches still constitute passive immunotherapy, because the immune response is being augmented by extrinsic factors such as interleukin-2.

Peripheral blood lymphocytes from patients with lung cancer and also from otherwise healthy smoking control patients can generate lymphokine-activated killer cell activity. However, this activity against autologous tumour targets is less in tumour-infiltrating lymphocytes than in peripheral lymphocytes obtained from the same patient or from control patients. In addition, cell-mediated autoimmunity plays a central role in dermatomyositis, a diffuse autoimmune rheumatic disorder associated with malignancy in males over 50. Lymphocytes sensitised to tumour antigens cross-react with antigens predominantly on skin and muscle cells, mediat-ing inflammatory changes. These can appear 1–2 years before the clinical presentation of the tumour. This seems to imply that though lung cancer can activate cell-mediated immunity, there is some *in situ* functional deficiency.

4. Escape from Cell-Mediated Immunity

Recent observations suggest a number of possible ways by which lung cancers escape the host immune response. Both small-cell and squamous cell lung cancers appear to secrete immunomodulatory factors that down-regulate the immune response. Lung cancers may interfere with normal maturation of lymphocytes. Patients with lung cancer show a decrease in both CD4/CD8 ratio and the CD3 population of peripheral blood lympho-cytes [60]. These lymphocytes have increased lymphocytotoxicity against cultured lung cancer cell lines; however, this enhanced cytotoxicity de-creases as the stage of cancer advances [61]. The plasma concentration of soluble interleukin-2 receptors is increased in patients with lung cancer in comparison with normal subjects, and lower plasma levels of soluble interleukin-2 receptor correlates with improved therapeutic response [62]. Yet there does not seem to be a correlation between interleukin-2 pro-duction and stage of disease [63].

   Alveolar macrophages are thought to play a pivotal role in the pulmonary immune response, but their function does not always involve activation and cytolysis. They can attenuate the lymphoproliferative response of lymphocytes to antigens and inhibit natural killer cell activity [64, 65]. The tumour-infiltrating lymphocytes from patients with lung cancer may also fail to activate macrophages adequately. For example, peripheral mono-cytes from lung cancer patients express C3b receptors to a lesser extent than do monocytes from normal subjects. This abnormality is associated with decreased phagocytic capability after stimulation [66].

   The failure of the interleukin-2 trials may be due in part to the fact that the activation of cytotoxic T lymphocytes requires a substantially more complex cytokine microenvironment than that provided by interleukin-2 alone. Thus, systemic interleukin-2 treatment may be sufficient for the recruitment of lymphocytes and the proliferation of cytotoxic T lym-phocytes *ex vivo*, but it is insufficient for the development of cytotoxic T lymphocytes *in situ*. Recent data suggest that multiple cytokine signals must be present *in situ* to permit local amplification of the immune response [67]. The presence of cytokines *in situ* is the rationale behind the concept of genetically modifying cytotoxic T lymphocytes to secrete cytokines *in situ*.

4.1. Major Histocompatibility Antigen Class I Target Molecule

In addition to cytokine stimulation, cytotoxic T-lymphocyte activation also requires the interaction of the T-cell receptor and the tumour antigen. The best-characterised tumour-associated antigens have been variants of the major histocompatibility (MHC) antigen class I molecules. The MHC class I molecules are the dominant target molecules for cytotoxic T lymphocytes, both in tumour target killing and killing of virally infected cells, in addition to being the dominant transplantation antigen for both humoral and cellular immunity [52].

Early immunohistochemical studies showed that lung cancers express relatively low levels of MHC class I membrane molecules [68]. This low level of expression of MHC in lung cancer cells may therefore be below the recognition threshold and as a result too low to trigger cytotoxic T-lymphocyte-mediated tumour destruction, thus preventing subsequent clonal expansion. This proposed mechanism of escape from immune surveillance was tested by transfection of MHC class I gene products into a variety of tumour cell lines. After transfection, the tumour cell lines were tested against selected cytotoxic T-lymphocyte clones specific for the transfected gene product. A variety of experimental studies demonstrated that the level of cytotoxic T-lymphocyte-mediated killing of the tumour cells correlated with the level of MHC class I molecule expression. Furthermore, when MHC expression was increased by interferon-γ, the level of tumour target cell killing was restored [69]. These observations have encouraged efforts to use genetically modified cytotoxic T lymphocytes which secrete cytokines capable of both inducing the activation of other cytotoxic T lymphocytes and increasing the levels of MHC class I expression on tumour cells. Such manipulations have demonstrated promising results in a mouse tumour model system in which cytotoxic T lymphocytes transduced with interferon-γ showed enhanced *in vivo* antitumour efficacy against both metastatic and subcutaneous tumours [70].

Further detailed studies of the surface of lung cancer cell lines have suggested that lung cancers not only express low levels of MHC class I molecules but also other important surface molecules, e.g. ICAM-1 and LFA-3, which are believed to participate in the regulation of contact between cytotoxic T lymphocytes and the potential target cell [71, 72]. MHC class II molecules are thought to play an important role in T-cell activation and also in tumour development. The human lung adenocarcinoma cell line A549 is >95% negative for MHC class II antigen. Using anti-class II antibodies with interferon-γ, MHC class II antigen-positive cancer cells were selected from the A549 cell line. The class II antigen-positive cells had a flat morphology not observed in the parental A549 cells. Class II antigen expression in these flat cells was interferon-γ inducible, and there was a correlation between the inducibility and phenotypic changes. Induction of Class II antigen in this A549 subline restored contact inhibition and anchorage-dependent growth as well as loss of tumourigenicity in athymic mice [73].

In order to determine whether MHC class I molecules are sufficient to induce killing by antigen-specific cytotoxic T lymphocytes, Barbosa and colleagues transfected human MHC class I genes into mouse tumour cells. These cells expressed human MHC class I molecules at a density comparable to human cells, but in a cellular background that did not contain other human surface molecules. Crucially, human antigen-specific cytotoxic T lymphocytes were unable to kill these mouse tumour cells. The inability to recognise and lyse mouse tumour cells persisted despite extraordinary manipulations to make the cells immunogenic, including induction of high levels of MHC class I molecules, replacement of mouse β_2 macroglobulin with human β_2 macroglobulin and modification of MHC carbohydrate moieties to resemble mouse carbohydrates. None of these alterations affected cytotoxic T-lymphocyte recognition of the MHC expression mouse tumour cell lines. Furthermore, the study of monkey cell lines suggested a phylogenetic restriction to cytotoxic T-lymphocyte-mediated killing of the cell, i.e. the same cytotoxic T-lymphocyte clone would kill human cells very efficiently, monkey cells less efficiently and mouse cells not at all despite all tumour cell lines expressing the same level of the serologically intact MHC class I molecule [74, 75]. It would thus seem that cytotoxic T-lymphocyte recognition of MHC class I molecules requires another factor not encoded in the MHC class I gene. A number of laboratories have demonstrated that this factor is not only associated with MHC class I but is bound to the outer domains of the molecule.

X-ray crystallography has demonstrated a cleft between the two outer domains of the MHC class I molecule which creates a cradle for peptide molecules [76]. Studies using fragments of viral proteins suggest that small, 8 to 12-amino acid, molecules appear to lie in the cleft. The association of the MHC class I molecule and the small peptide creates a composite antigen. The peptides appear to be derived from a variety of sources including viral, foreign or tumour-associated proteins [76] and would be too small to be immunogenic without an associated micromolecule [77], which could explain the failure of investigators to serologically define tumour-associated antigen in most human cancers. Mononuclear cells, in particular CD8+ lymphocytes, have antigen-specific receptors that bind to class I molecules and which also appear able to discriminate between different MHC class I-associated peptides [78]. It seems likely that the evolutionary role of cytotoxic T lymphocytes was the recognition of self MHC class I molecules plus peptide molecular complexes and the recognition of transplanted MHC class I molecules probably results from cross-reactivity of cytotoxic T lymphocytes directed against self MHC class I plus peptide molecular complexes [79]. The mechanisms by which cytotoxic T lymphocytes fail to recognise MHC class I plus tumour peptide molecular complexes are beginning to be defined. The low level of expression of MHC class I on typical lung cancers is likely to be below the cytotoxic T-lymphocyte threshold for activation; the low levels of accessory molecules further lower the activation threshold. In addition, the low levels of MHC expression minimise activation not only of cytotoxic T lymphocytes but also of other lymphocytes. As a consequence, there is a diminished lymphocyte proliferation and a hypocellular inflammatory response to the tumour. This suppressed inflammatory response further compromises the cytokine microenvironment essential for cytotoxic T-lymphocyte development.

5. Future Developments

It seems clear that novel therapeutic approaches should emphasise enhancement of specific tumour cytotoxicity rather than immune function in general. Thus, treatments have progressed from non-specific immune stimulation (e.g. BCG and levamisole hydrochloride) to the area of specific immune targeting using the host's own cells. Active immunotherapy stimulates the immune response by vaccination with tumour-associated antigens and the use of biologic response modifiers on host effectors. One approach has been to immunise patients who have non-small-cell lung cancer with autologous cryo-preserved irradiated tumour cells mixed with BCG [80]. In a pilot study, vaccinated patients had a delayed cutaneous reaction to autologous irradiated tumour cells after immunisation; patients with stage II or III disease had relapses regardless of whether they exhibited delayed cutaneous reactivity to autologous tumour cells. Unfortunately, this pilot study was too small, and no conclusion can be drawn about the effects of such immunisation on the long-term outcome of patients with non-small-cell lung cancer.

Another study has examined the influence of vaccination with lung cancer-associated antigen and Freund's complete adjuvant in patients with stage I or stage II lung cancer. Eighty-five patients with squamous cell cancer of the lung were randomised to either a control group or a specific immunotherapy group that received monthly doses of tumour-associated antigen emulsified with Freund's complete adjuvant or a non-specific immunotherapy group that received three monthly doses of only Freund's complete adjuvant. The 5-year survival at follow-up of these patients was 34% for the control group, 53% for the non-specific immunotherapy group and 75% for the specific active immunotherapy group [81]. These results are encouraging, but this study is the first such investigation, and further substantiation is required. This active immunity approach has been further refined by the use of liposome-encapsulated tumour cell membrane, using sized liposomes as adjuvants [82].

It is possible that antigen-specific immunostimulants could be developed. The cure of micrometastasis following surgery is a major goal of cancer immunotherapy. Thus, in the case of lung cancers, resection of the primary tumour could be followed by identification and/or isolation of specific tumour-associated peptides. These peptides could then be used as vaccines against metastatic disease. A recent study isolated tumour-associated antigen peptides MUT 1 and MUT 2 derived from a mutated connexin 37 GAP junction protein from a malignant murine lung carcinoma. Synthetic MUT 1 or MUT 2 induces effective antitumour cytotoxic T lymphocytes. These peptide vaccines protect mice from spontaneous metastasis and reduce metastatic loads in mice carrying pre-established micrometastases of the lung carcinoma cells. Tumour-specific immunity was primarily mediated by CD8$^+$ T-cells. This provides early evidence that peptide therapy may be effective in treatment of residual tumours and provides a rationale for the development of peptide vaccines as a modality for cancer therapy [83]. A peptide vaccine could be combined with an appropriate immunostimulant. This would result in an increase in stimulated circulating cytotoxic T lymphocytes with a low threshold for activation. The increased number of lymphocyte precursors would also ensure a rich cytokine microenvironment *in situ*. In a further refinement, antibody cytokine fusion proteins have been developed that can target biologically active cytokines to various tumour sites, achieving local concentration sufficient to induce host immune responses leading to tumour elimination. A tumour-specific antibody lymphotoxin fusion protein has been shown to have antitumour activity on xenografted pulmonary metastases of human melanoma by a mechanism that functions in the absence of mature T-cells but requires B-cells and natural killer cells [84]. Experimental approaches involving gene therapy may be attractive in this clinical setting. The two basic types of genes have been transfected into lymphocytes, either those intended to induce immunity or those that are directly tumouricidal. Immunity-inducing genes that have been used in model (and some human) systems, include MHC molecules, co-stimulatory molecules and cytokines [85]. These are intended to induce effective systemic immune responses against tumour antigens which would not otherwise develop.

Clinical applications of immunology to lung cancer have occurred in many areas from screening to adjuvant therapy. It is to be hoped that, with increasing understanding of immune surveillance and further clarification of defects in the immunoregulatory network responsible for tumour growth and metastasis, the promising animal studies and early clinical trials will be developed to provide novel approaches to treating lung cancer.

References

1. Smyth JF, Fowlie SM, Gregor A, Crompton GK, Busutill A, Leonard RCF, Grant IW (1986) The impact of chemotherapy on small cell carcinoma of the bronchus. *Q J Med* 61: 969–976.
2. Hersh EM, Mavligit GM, Gutterman JU (1974) Immunotherapy as related to lung cancer: A review. *Semin Oncol* 1: 273–274.

3. Holmes EC (1976) Immunology and lung cancer. *Ann Thorac Surg* 21: 250–258.
4. Evans DA (1976) Immunology of bronchial carcinoma. *Thorax* 31: 493–506.
5. Gupta S (1986) Abnormality in immunoregulatory cells in human malignancies. *Adv Immun Cancer Ther* 2: 131–153.
6. Burdick JF, Wells SA Jr, Herberman RB (1975) Immunologic evaluation of patients with cancer by delayed hypersensitivity reactions. *Surg Gynecol Obstet* 141: 779–794.
7. DeMeester TR, Golomb HM, Dudek P, Hunter RL, Fang VS (1979) The relationship between immune reactivity, serum cortisol and stage of disease in patients with non-oat-cell bronchogenic carcinoma. *Surgery* 86: 130–137.
8. Marabella PC, Takita H (1975) Skin test with tumor extract in bronchogenic carcinoma: A preliminary study. *J Surg Oncol* 7: 299–301.
9. Bates SE, Suen JY, Tranum BL (1979) Immunoligical skin testing and interpretation: A plea for uniformity. *Cancer* 43: 2306–2314.
10. Ruckdeschel JC, Codish SD, Stranahan A, McKneally MF (1972) Postoperative empyema improves survival in lung cancer: Documentation and analysis of a natural experiment. *N Engl J Med* 287: 1013–1017.
11. McKneally MF (1982) Thoracic empyema after pulmonary resection for lung cancer. *Ann Thorac Surg* 33: 316–319.
12. Ioachim HL, Dorsett BH, Paluch E (1976) The immune response at the tumor site in lung carcinoma. *Cancer* 38: 2296–2309.
13. Bell JW (1970) Possible immune factors in spontaneous regression of bronchogenic carcinoma: Ten year survival in a patient treated with minimal (1,200 r) radiation alone. *Am J Surg* 120: 804–806.
14. Ioachim HL (1976) The stromal reaction of tumors: An expression of immune surveillance. *J Natl Cancer Inst* 57: 465–475.
15. Kuwana M, Fujii T, Mimori T, Kaburaki J (1996) Enhancement of anti-DNA topoisomerase I autoantibody response after lung cancer in patients with systemic sclerosis: A report of two cases. *Arthritis and Rheumatism* 39: 686–691.
16. Dropcho EJ (1996) Antiamphiphysin antibodies with small-cell lung carcinoma and paraneoplastic encephalomyelitis. *Ann Neurol* 39: 659–667.
17. Hersh B, Dalmau J, Dangond F, Gultekin S, Geller E, Wen PY (1996) Paraneoplastic opsoclonus-myoclonus associated with anti-Hu antibody. *Neurology* 44: 1754–1755.
18. Lennon VA, Kryzer TJ, Griesmann GE, O'Suilleabhain PE, Windebank AJ, Woppmann A, Miljanich GP, Lambert EH (1995) Calcium-channel antibodies in the Lambert-Eaton syndrome and other paraneoplastic syndromes. *N Engl J Med* 442: 1467–1474.
19. Takamori M, Takahashi M, Yasukawa Y, Twasa K, Nemoto Y, Suenaga A, Nagataki S, Nakamura (1995) Antibodies to recombinant synaptotagmin and calcium channel subtypes in Lambert-Eaton myasthenic syndrome. *J Neurol Sci* 133: 95–101.
20. Mandel MA, Dvorak KJ, Worman LW, DeCosse JJ (1976) Immunoglobulin content in the bronchial washings of patients with benign and malignant pulmonary disease. *N Engl J Med* 295: 694–698.
21. Paluch E, Ioachim HL (1979) Reactive antibodies in the bronchial washings of lung cancer patients. *Int J Cancer* 23: 42–46.
22. Holmes EC (1980) Immune adjuvant therapy in lung cancer. *Prog Exp Tumor Res* 25: 229–241.
23. Matthay RA (1982) Immunoadjuvant therapy for lung cancer: A critical review. *Clin Chest Med* 3: 423–441.
24. Lee YC, Luh SP, Wu RM, Lee CJ (1994) Adjuvant immunotherapy with intrapleural streptococcus pyogenes (OK-432) in lung cancer patients after resection. *Cancer Immunol Immunother* 39: 269–274.
25. Sonhami RL (1992) New perspectives in lung cancer. 3. The antigens of lung cancer. *Thorax* 47: 53–56.
26. Tockman MS, Gupta PK, Myers JD, Frost JK, Baylin SB, Gold EB, Chase AM, Wilkinson PH, Mulshine JL (1988) Sensitive and specific monoclonal antibody recognition of human lung cancer antigen on preserved sputum cells: A new approach to early lung cancer detection. *J Clin Oncol* 6: 1685–1693.
27. Lubin R, Zalcman G, Bouchet L, Tredanel J, Legros Y, Cazals D, Hirsch A, Soussi T (1995) Serum p53 antibodies as early markers of lung cancer. *Nat Med* 1: 702.

28. Ioachim HL, Pambuccian SE, Hekimgil M, Giancotti FR, Dorsett BH (1996) Lymphoid monoclonal antibodies reactive with lung tumors. *Am J Surg Pathol* 20: 64–71.
29. Kalofonas HP, Sivolapenko GB, Courtenay-Luck NS, Snook DE, Hooker GR, Winter R, McKenzie CG, Taylor-Papadimitriou JJ, Lavender PJ, Epenetos AA (1988) Antibody guided targeting of non-small cell lung cancer using 111In-labelled HMFG1 F(ab')2 fragments. *Cancer Res* 48: 1977–1984.
30. Modjtahedi H, Hickish T, Nicolson M, Moore J, Styles J, Eccles S, Jackson E, Salter J, Sloane J, Spencer L, et al. (1996) Phase I trial and tumour localisation of the anti-EGFR monoclonal antibody ICR62 in head and neck or lung cancer. *Br J Cancer* 73: 228–235.
31. Wawrzynczak EJ, Derbyshire EJ (1992) Immunotoxins to human small-cell lung cancer. *Cell Biophys* 21: 13–23.
32. Hara I, Takechi Y, Houghton AN (1995) Implicating a role for immune recognition of self in tumor rejection: Passive immunization against the brown locus protein. *J Exp Med* 182: 1609–1614.
33. Brooks PC, Montgomery AMP (1994) Integrin avb3 antagonists promote tumor regression by inducing apoptosis of angiogenic blood vessels. *Cell* 79: 1157–1164.
34. Eilber FR, Morton DL (1970) Impaired immunologic reactivity and recurrence following cancer surgery. *Cancer* 25: 362–367.
35. Hosker HSR, Corris PA (1991) Alveolar macrophage and blood monocyte function in lung cancer. *Cancer Detect Prev* 15: 103–106.
36. Gangemi JD, Olsen GN, Fechter C, Hightower JA, Baugess CT, Krech L (1985) Phagocytic activity of alveolar macrophages in patients with bronchogenic carcinoma. *Cancer Immunol Immunother* 20: 158–166.
37. Swinburne S, Moore M, Cole P (1982) Human bronchoalveolar macrophage cytotoxicity for cultured human lung-tumor cells. *Bri J Cancer* 46: 625–634.
38. Bordignon C, Avallone R, Peri G, Polentarutti N, Mangioni C, Mantovani A (1980) Cytotoxicity on tumour cells of human mononuclear phagocytes: Defective tumoricidal capacity of alveolar macrophages. *Clin Exp Immunol* 41: 336–342.
39. McDonald CF, Atkins RC (1990) Defective cytostatic activity of pulmonary alveolar macrophages in primary lung cancer. *Chest* 98: 881–885.
40. Takeo S, Yasumoto K, Nagashima A, Nakahashi H, Sugimachi K, Nomoto K (1986) Role of tumor-associated macrophages in lung cancer. *Cancer Res* 46: 3179–3182.
41. Hill AD, Redmond HP, Naama HA, Bouchier-Hayes D (1996) Granulocyte-macrophage colony-stimulating factor inhibits tumor growth during the postoperative period. *Surgery* 119: 178–185.
42. Lin C-C, Kuo Y-C, Huang W-C, Lin C-Y (1987) Natural killer cell activity in lung cancer patients. *Chest* 92: 1022–1024.
43. Pisani RJ, Krco CJ, Wold LE, McKean DJ (1989) Lymphokine-activated killer (LAK) cell activity in tumor-infiltrating lymphocytes from non-small cell lung cancer. *Am J Clin Pathol* 92: 435–446.
44. Moy PM, Holmes EC, Golub SH (1985) Depression of natural killer cytotoxic activity in lymphocytes infiltrating human pulmonary tumors. *Cancer Res* 45: 57–60.
45. Whiteside TL (1992) Tumor-infiltrating lymphocytes as antitumor effector cells. *Biotherapy* 5: 47–61.
46. Whiteside TL, Jost LM, Herberman RB (1992) Tumor-infiltrating lymphocytes: Potential and limitations to their use for cancer therapy. *Crit Rev Oncol Hematol* 12: 25–47.
47. Pitchenik AE, Guffee J, Stein-Streilein J (1987) Lung natural killer and interleukin-2 activity in lung cancer: A pulmonary compartment of augmented natural killer activity occurs in patients with bronchogenic carcinoma. *Am Rev Respir Dis* 136: 1327–1332.
48. Uchida A, Kariya Y, Okamoto N, Sugie K, Fugimoto T, Yagita M (1990) Prediction of postoperative clinical course by autologous tumor-killing activity in lung cancer patients. *J Natl Cancer Inst* 82: 1697–1701.
49. Fagan EA, Eddleston AL (1987) Immunotherapy for cancer: The use of lymphokine-activated killer (LAK) cells. *Gut* 28: 113–116.
50. Kradin RL, Bhan AK (1993) Tumor infiltrating lymphocytes. *Lab Invest* 69: 635–638.
51. Kradin RL, Kurnick JT, Lazarus DS, Preffer FI, Dubinett SM, Pinto CE, Gifford J, Davidson E, Grove B, Callahan RJ, et al. (1989) Tumour-infiltrating lymphocytes and interleukin-2 in treatment of advanced cancer. *Lancet* 1: 577–580.

52. Martz E (1977) Mechanism of specific tumor-cell lysis by alloimmune T lymphocytes: Resolution and characterization of descrete steps in the cellular interaction. *Contemp Top Immunobiol* 7: 301–361.
53. Mentzer SJ, Smith BR, Barbosa JA, Crimmins MA, Herrmann SM, Burakoff SJ (1987) CTL adhesion and antigen recognition are discrete steps in the human CTL-target cell interaction. *J Immunol* 138: 1325–1330.
54. Burnet FM (1959) *The clonal selection theory of acquired immunity*. London: Cambridge University Press.
55. Yang SC, Owen-Schaub L, Mendiguren-Rodriguez A, Grimm EA, Hong WK, Roth JA (1990) Combination immunotherapy for non-small cell lung cancer: Results with interleukin-2 and tumor necrosis factor-alpha. *J Thorac Cardiovasc Surg* 99: 8–12.
56. Yasumoto K, Mivazaki K, Nagashima A, Ishida T, Kuda T, Yano T, Sugimachi K, Nomoto K (1987) Induction of lymphokine-activated killer cells by intrapleural instillations of recombinant interleukin-2 in patients with malignant pleurisy due to lung cancer. *Cancer Res* 47: 2184–2187.
57. Li D, Wang Y, Tan X, Wang H, Yao X, Ba D (1990) A new approach to the treatment of malignant effusion. *Chinese Med J* (Engl) 103: 998–1002.
58. Mikulski SM, McGuire WP, Louie AC, Chirigos MA, Muggia FM (1979) Immunotherapy of lung cancer. I. Review of clinical trials in non-small cell histologic types. *Cancer Treat Rev* 6: 177–190.
59. Kradin RL, Boyle LA, Preffer FI, Callahan RJ, Barlai-Kovach M, Strauss HW, Dubinett S, Kurnick JT (1987) Tumor-derived interleukin-2-dependent lymphocytes in adoptive immunotherapy of lung cancer. *Cancer Immunol Immunother* 24: 76–85.
60. Radhakrishna Pillai M, Balaram P, Padmanabhan TK, Abraham T, Hareendran NK, Nair MK (1989) Immunocompetence in lung cancer: Relationship to extent of tumor burden and histologic type. *Cancer* 64: 1853–1858.
61. Dalbow MH, Concannon JP, Eng CP, Weil CS, Conway J, Nambison PTN (1977) Lymphocyte mitogen stimulation studies for patients with lung cancer: Evaluation of prognostic significance of preirradiation therapy studies. *J Lab Clin Med* 90: 295–302.
62. Buccheri G, Marino P, Preatoni A, Ferrigno D, Moroni GA (1991) Soluble interleukin-2 receptor in lung cancer: An indirect marker of tumor activity? *Chest* 99: 1433–1437.
63. Watanabe Y, Shimizu J, Hashizume Y, Tsunamura Y, Yamada T, Iwa T (1990) Immune reactivity in bronchogenic carcinoma and its relation to 5-year survival rate. *J Surg Oncol* 45: 103–109.
64. Ettensohn DB, Lalor PA, Roberts NJ Jr (1986) Human alveolar macrophage regulation of lymphocyte proliferation. *Am Rev Respir Dis* 133: 1091–1096.
65. Bordignon C, Villa F, Allavena P, Introna M, Biondi A, Avallone R (1982) Inhibition of natural killer activity by human bronchoalveolar macrophages. *J Immunol* 129: 587–591.
66. Lukacs K, Carroll MP, Hodson ME, Kay AB (1984) Receptor-associated defects of cultured monocytes in bronchial carcinoma. *Clin Exp Immunol* 56: 321–329.
67. Gelber C, Eisenbach L, Feldman M, Goodenow RS (1992) T-cell subset analysis of Lewis lung carcinoma tumor rejection: Heterogeneity of effectors and evidence for negative regulatory lymphocytes correlating with metastasis. *Cancer Res* 52: 6507–6515.
68. Romano PJ, Bartholomew M, Smith PJ, Kloszewski F, Stryker J, Houck J, Vesell ES (1991) HLA antigens influence resistance to lung carcinoma. *Hum Immunol* 31: 236–240.
69. Mentzer SJ, Barbosa JA, Burakoff SJ (1990) Induction of HLA class I surface expression recruits low-affinity cytolytic T lymphocytes. *Int Arch Allergy Appl Immunol* 91: 437–440.
70. Abe J, Wakimoto H, Tsunoda R, Okabe S, Yoshida Y, Aoyagi M, Hirakawa K, Hamada H (1996) *In vivo* antitumor effect of cytotoxic T lymphocytes engineered to produce interferon-gamma by adenovirus-mediated genetic transduction. *Biochem Biophys Res Comm* 218: 164–170.
71. Mentzer SJ, Rothlein R, Springer TA, Faller D (1988) Intercellular adhesion molecule-1 (ICAM-1) is involved in the cytolytic T lymphocyte interaction with a human synovial cell line. *J Cell Physiol* 137: 173–178.
72. Barbosa JA, Mentzer SJ, Kamarck ME, Hart J, Biro PA, Strominger J et al. (1986) Gene mapping and somatic cell hybrid analysis of the role of human lymphocyte function-associated antigen-3 (LFA-3) in CTL-target cell interactions. *J Immunol* 136: 3085–3091.

73. Kawamoto S, Inoue Y, Shinozaki Y, Katakura Y, Tachibana H, Shirahata S, Murakami H (1995) Impaired tumor phenotypes in class II major histocompatibility complex antigen-inducible cells originated from human lung adenocarcinoma. *Biochem Biophys Res Commun* 215: 280–285.
74. Barbosa JA, Mentzer SJ, Minowada G, Strominger JL, Burakoff SJ, Biro PA (1984) Recognition of HLA-A2 and -B7 antigens by cloned cytotoxic T lymphocytes after gene transfer into human and monkey, but not mouse, cells. *Proc Natl Acad Sci USA* 81: 7549–7553.
75. Barbosa JA, Santos-Aguado J, Mentzer SJ, Strominger JL, Burakoff SJ, Biro PA (1987) Site-directed mutagenesis of class I HLA genes: Role of glycosylation in surface expression and functional recognition. *J Exp Med* 166: 1329–1350.
76. Garrett TP, Saper MA, Bjorkman PJ, Strominger JL, Wiley DC (1989) Specificity pockets for the side chains of peptide antigens in HLA-Aw68. *Nature* 342: 692–696.
77. Tjoa BA, Kranz DM (1994) Generation of cytotoxic T-lymphocytes to a self-peptide/class I complex: A model for peptide-mediated tumor rejection. *Cancer Res* 54: 204–208.
78. Sherman LA, Hesse SV, Irwin MJ, La Face D, Peterson P (1992) Selecting T cell receptors with high affinity for self-MHC by decreasing the contribution of CD8. *Science* 258: 815–818.
79. Santos-Aguado J, Crimmins MA, Mentzer SJ, Burakoff SJ, Strominger JL (1989) Alloreactivity studies with mutants of HLA-A2. *Proc Natl Acad Sci USA* 86: 8936–8940.
80. Schulof RS, Mai D, Nelson MA, Paxton HM, Cox JW Jr, Turner ML, Mills M, Hix WR, Nochomovitz LE, Peters LC, et al. (1988) Active specific immunotherapy with an autologous tumor cell vaccine in patients with resected non-small cell lung cancer. *Mol Biother* 1: 30–36.
81. Takita H, Hollinshead AC, Adler RH, Bhayana J, Ramundo M, Moskowitz R, Rao UN, Raman S (1991) Adjuvant, specific, active immunotherapy for resectable squamous cell lung carcinoma: A 5-year survival analysis. *J Surg Oncol* 46: 9–14.
82. Alino SF, Lejarreta M, Alfaro J, Iruarrizaga A, Bobadilla M, Blaya C, Crespo J (1995) Antimetastatic effect of immunization with liposome-encapsulated tumor cell-membrane proteins obtained from experimental tumors. *Immunopharmacol Immunotoxicol* 17: 419–436.
83. Mandelboim O, Vadai E, Fridkin M, Katz-Hillel A, Feldman M, Berke G, Eisenbach L (1995) Regression of established murine carcinoma metastases following vaccination with tumour-associated antigen peptides. *Nature Medicine* 1: 1179–1183.
84. Reisfeld RA, Gillies SD, Mendelsohn J, Varki NM, Becker JC (1996) Involvement of B lymphocytes in the growth of inhibition of human pulmonary melanoma metastases in athymic nu/nu mice by an antibody-lymphotoxin fusion protein. *Cancer Res* 56: 1707–1712.
85. Lee CT, Chen HL, Carbone DP (1995) Gene therapy for lung cancer. *Ann Oncol* 3: S61–S63.

Autoimmune Aspects of Lung Disease
ed. by D.A. Isenberg and S.G. Spiro
© 1998 Birkhäuser Verlag Basel/Switzerland

CHAPTER 8
Asthma

Douglas S. Robinson

Allergy and Clinical Immunology, Imperial College School of Medicine at the National Heart and Lung Institute, London, UK

1. Introduction

Asthma is a common disease with increasing prevalence. There are roughly 3 million asthmatics in the UK (1.2 million children and 1.8 million adults), and direct costs to the National Health Service in 1994 were estimated at £4.5 billion [1]. In recent years perceptions of asthma have changed, and it is now seen as a chronic inflammatory disorder, akin to rheumatoid arthritis or psoriasis, likely to require lifelong therapy in most asthmatic subjects whose disease persists into adulthood. Asthma definitions now include the presence of an eosinophilic bronchial infiltrate [2], and although it is not an autoimmune disease *per se*, it has become clear that a form of cell-mediated immune response is as important as the immunoglobulin (Ig)E-dependent pathology in most cases. Thus the mast cell hypothesis has moved on to the eosinophil and Th2 hypothesis of asthma.

Unlike those studying other immune-mediated pathologies, researchers in asthma have the advantage that in most cases the likely inciting antigen is known, since most asthma has an allergic (atopic) basis, and many occupational triggers are well characterised. However, in a subset of cases asthma has no clear environmental trigger, and this has been termed "intrinsic asthma" [3]. This chapter will review current evidence on the immunological basis of the pathology of asthma, effector cells contributing to airway hyper-responsiveness and recent advances in understanding the genetic basis predisposing to atopy and asthma. Human and animal models of asthma will be reviewed, and current and possible future treatments will be considered in the context of the immunopathology of asthma.

2. Immunological Mechanisms in Asthma

2.1. Cellular Pathology of Asthma

Initial information on cells involved in asthma came from post-mortem studies and analysis of peripheral blood. The pathology of subjects dying of asthma showed desquamative bronchitis with marked eosinophil and mononuclear cell infiltrate, epithelial shedding and mucous hypersecretion leading to plugging of airways [4]. Eosinophils were also prominent in the airways of subjects with asthma dying from other causes [5], suggesting a role in less severe disease, and immunofluorescent staining showed marked deposition of the eosinophil granule protein, major basic protein (MBP), in the bronchial mucosa [6]. Peripheral blood eosinophilia has long been associated with asthma, and the eosinophil count and serum concentrations of eosinophil granule proteins have been correlated with the degree of airway obstruction, and with bronchial responsiveness to methacholine [7–9]. Similar findings are described for sputum eosinophilia in asthma [10]. Investigation of allergic skin disease led to the discovery of IgE [11], and the demonstration of IgE-dependent triggering of mediator release from mast cells and basophils led to the association of these mechanisms in allergen-induced symptoms in asthma. The application of fibreoptic bronchoscopy to the study of asthma has allowed sampling of airway cells in patients with mild to moderate disease by bronchial biopsy and broncho-alveolar lavage (BAL). These studies confirmed the presence of eosinophils and mast cells in the bronchial mucosa in asthma, and suggested eosinophil activation through immunohistochemical staining for eosinophil granule proteins in biopsies and increased concentrations of granule proteins in lavage fluids when compared with non-asthmatic controls [12–18]. Eosinophil numbers, and eosinophil cationic protein concentrations in both BAL and bronchial biopsies from asthmatic subjects were shown to be related to symptom scores, airway reactivity and airflow obstruction [9, 14, 17]. Mast cell histamine releasability was increased in atopic asthmatics, supporting the concept of IgE-mediated mechanisms contributing to symptoms [17].

Appreciation of the central role of the CD4+ T-helper lymphocyte in both IgE synthesis and eosinophil and mast cell development allowed the hypothesis that activated CD4 T cells might drive the inflammatory process in the airway in asthma [19]. Evidence for activation of CD4 T-cells in asthma came initially from the demonstration of increased surface expression of the activation markers CD25 [interleukin (IL)-2 receptor α], HLA DR and VLA-1 by blood CD4 T-cells (but not CD8 cells) in patients with exacerbations of asthma, but not control subjects with chronic obstructive airways disease, asymptomatic asthmatics or healthy controls [20]. Bronchoscopic biopsies from asthmatic subjects showed lymphocytes with electron microscopic features of activation, and immunohistochemistry confirmed increased numbers of CD25-positive cells in the bronchial mucosa of asthmatics compared with non-asthmatic control subjects [12, 13, 16]. BAL CD4 T-cells showed increased expression of activation markers in asthma when compared with controls, and the degree of activation was related to both eosinophil infiltration and disease severity as measured by symptom scores, airflow obstruction and bronchial responsiveness [21–23].

2.2. Type-2 T-Cell Activation in Asthma

2.2.1. Type-1 and type-2 T-cells: A major advance in immunology over the last 10 years has been the discovery that the pattern of cytokines produced by T lymphocytes determines the outcome of T-cell activation, both in terms of directing antibody synthesis and through cell-mediated responses, and that this has a pivotal role in response to infection and in immunopathology. A dichotomy of CD4 Th responses was first described by Mosmann and Coffman, who described Th1 mouse T-cell clones producing interferon γ and IL-2, but not IL-4 and IL-5, and Th2 clones which made IL-4 and IL-5 but not IFNγ and IL-2 [24]. Th1 cytokines activate macrophages and T-cells, and these clones were shown to induce a delayed-type cellular response on injection into the footpad of syngeneic recipients [25]. Conversely, Th2 clones were not able to induce a delayed-type hypersensitivity (DTH) cellular response on injection, but were good providers of B-cell help for antibody synthesis. Analysis of the T-cell response to infection showed a predominant Th1 response to the intracellular pathogen *Brucella abortus*, whereas the helminth *Nippostrongylus brasiliensis*, which evokes an IgE and eosinophil response to infection, was associated with increased cloning frequency of Th2 clones [26]. Since IL-4, unopposed by

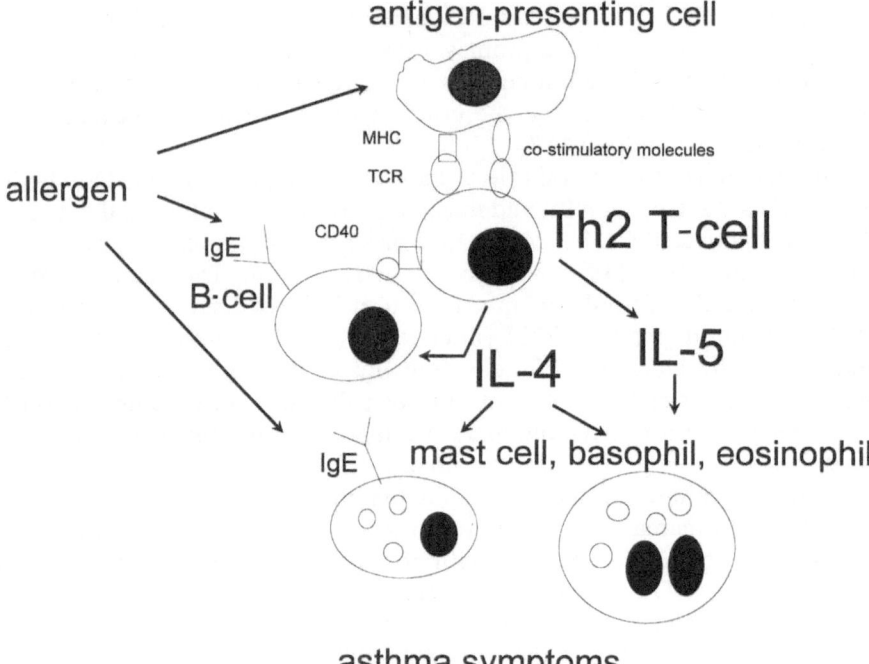

Figure 1. Proposed cellular interactions in asthma. Allergen is processed by antigen-presenting cells, and presented to CD4 T-cells. Th2 T-cells produce IL-4 and help B-cells in IgE synthesis, and IL-5, which with IL-3 and GM-CSF, acts in eosinophil recruitment.

IFNγ, was shown to be essential for IgE synthesis by B-cells [27], and IL-5 is a key cytokine in eosinophil maturation and tissue survival [28], it was clear that the Th2 pattern of cytokines might be important in human allergic disease. The importance of the cytokine profile in determining disease outcome was shown in murine *Leishmania major* infection, where the Th2 response mounted by the BALB/c strain resulted in disease progression and death after inoculation of the organism, whereas the C57/BL6 strain mounted a Th1 T-cell response leading to a self-limiting healing reaction [29, 30]. Furthermore, the cytokine dependence of these differences was seen by the conversion of the Balb/c response to healing Th1 pattern following either blocking antibody to IL-4 [31].

More recently, the concept of the dichotomy of cytokine pattern has been extended to CD8 cells, termed Tc1 and Tc2 [32], and the cytokine patterns are now referred to more broadly as type 1 (IFNγ and IL-2) and type 2 (IL-4 and IL-5).

2.2.2. Th1 and Th2 cells in humans: Initial analysis showed a diverse cytokine pattern in human T-cell clones, and the Th1/Th2 dichotomy seems to represent only two of many possible T-cell cytokine responses in humans [33, 34]. However, allergen-specific CD4+ T-cell clones from atopic donors were shown to be Th2-like by Wierenga et al., and the group of Romagnani has shown that both Th1 and Th2 clones can indeed be derived from human T-cells [35–37]. In particular these investigators have shown that the majority of allergen-specific T-cell clones both from the blood and tissues of atopic donors are of a Th2-like phenotype [38, 39]. However, there are important differences between murine and human Th1 and Th2 cells, which might have an important bearing on future treatment strategies based on this dichotomy. Human Th2 cells produce variable amounts of what are Th1 cytokines in the mouse, particularly IL-2, whilst human Th1 cells produce IL-6 and IL-10. Although the murine system has proven very useful in dissecting out the basis of the Th1/Th2 dichotomy, the results cannot always be directly applied to human T cells. Nonetheless, the isolation of allergen-specific Th2 clones from skin in atopic dermatitis, conjunctiva in vernal conjunctivitis (a form of allergic eye disease), in addition to blood from atopic subjects, strongly supports the concept that a Th2 T-cell response to allergen is a major determinant of the IgE and eosinophilic pathology in atopic disease [35, 38, 39]. Analysis of cytokine mRNA expression in the allergen-induced late cutaneous response, which is characterised by eosinophil infiltration and T-cell activation [40], showed increased numbers of infiltrating cells encoding IL-3, IL-4, IL-5 and granulocyte-macrophage colony-stimulating factor (GM-CSF), but not IL-2 or IFNγ when compared with diluent control-injected sites [41]. On this background, the hypothesis that a Th2-like CD4 T-cell response drives the pathology of airway disease in asthma is attractive.

2.2.3. Evidence for type-2 T-cell activation in asthma: Initial evidence for a Th2 pattern of cytokine expression in atopic asthma came from detection of increased numbers of cells with positive signals for mRNA encoding IL-2, IL-3, IL-4, IL-5 and GM-CSF, but not IFNγ in BAL fluid from asthmatic subjects when compared with non-atopic, non-asthmatic control subjects [42]. The majority of cells expressing IL-4 and IL-5 mRNA were shown to be BAL T-cells in asthmatic subjects. This pattern of cytokine mRNA expression has been confirmed in a number of separate studies [43], and other studies have confirmed increased expression of IL-4 and IL-5 mRNA in atopic asthma both by *in situ* hybridisation and polymerase chain reaction (PCR) of bronchial biopsies [44, 45]. Although one report did not find differences in the pattern of cytokine mRNA detected by PCR in BAL cells from atopic asthmatics compared with control subjects, they did show upregulation of IL-5 mRNA by a competitive PCR assay after allergen challenge compared with diluent inhalation, and localised this signal to the mononuclear cells within BAL [46]. The lack of difference between asthmatics and controls at baseline by PCR is compatible with other data, since mRNA-positive cells were detected in control subjects in addition to asthmatics by *in situ* hybridisation [42]. In recent studies we have localised IL-4 and IL-5 mRNA to both CD4+ and CD8+ T-cells, suggesting a possible contribution from type-2 CD8+ T cells in addition to CD4+ T-cells in asthma [47]. Measurement of cytokines in concentrated BAL fluid from atopic asthmatic subjects compared with non-asthmatic controls also showed detectable IL-4 and IL-5 in asthmatic subjects, but not controls, with IFNγ undetectable in both groups [48].

BAL T-cell lines from atopic asthmatic subjects produced IL-3, GM-CSF and IL-5 [49], and supernatants from such T-cell lines were shown to support eosinophil colony-forming activity *in vitro* [50]. Although cloning of Th2-like allergen-specific CD4+ cells has been described from one bronchial biopsy from an atopic asthmatic subject [51], there is very little evidence on Th2 clones or the frequency of allergen-specific T-cells in airway samples from asthmatic subjects compared with controls without asthma.

Recently, a technique for intracellular immunostaining of cytokines has been applied to BAL cells from asthmatic and control subjects, and flow cytometric analysis of such staining showed increased IFNγ staining in cells from asthmatic subjects with a non-significant and much lower signal for IL-4 when compared with controls [52]. However, this technique relies on *in vitro* activation with non-specific mitogens to achieve sufficient cytokine detection, and may have produced a skewed result. Further data, preferably analysing both mRNA and protein expression in the same subjects, and on allergen-induced T-cell cytokine production is needed. The balance of evidence at present suggests increased expression if IL-4 and IL-5 in the airway in atopic asthma.

2.3. Effector Cells in Asthma

2.3.1. Eosinophils: Eosinophils are characterised by granules containing proteins rich in arginine residues, giving a basic pI, and which stain with acidic dyes: hence "eosinophil". The granules have a crystalline core of major basic protein (MBP), and also contain eosinophil cationic protein (ECP), eosinophil peroxidase (EPO) and eosinophil-derived neurotoxin (EDN) [53, 54]. MBP is also found in basophils, but the other proteins are unique to eosinophils. ECP and EDN are shown to have ribonuclease activity [55]. *In vitro* studies show that MBP, ECP and EPO are toxic to respiratory epithelium, and MBP increases ion efflux [56]. Increased concentrations of ECP and MBP have been detected in serum, sputum and BAL from asthmatic subjects when compared with controls, and epithelial damage by these cationic proteins is thought to contribute to bronchial hyper-responsiveness in asthma.

Eosinophils are also a potent source of leukotriene C_4 and platelet-activating factor, and both of these mediators may contribute to bronchoconstriction, increased vascular permeability and mucus secretion in asthma [57].

Eosinophil development from bone marrow precursor cells is dependent on the actions of IL-3 and GM-CSF, and the eosinophil-specific cytokine IL-5 acts later in maturation of eosinophil precursors [58]. IL-3, IL-5 and GM-CSF also prime for degranulation of eosinophils, increase adhesion to vascular endothelium and prolong eosinophil survival by inhibiting apoptosis [59–63]. These cytokines have heterodimeric receptors, sharing a common β chain which is active in signal transduction and associates with a cytokine-specific α chain (IL-3Rα, IL-5Rα or GM-CSFRα) for high-affinity ligand binding [64, 65]. Eosinophils express all three receptor α chains, whereas neutrophils have only IL-3Rα, and monocytes have IL-3Rα and GM-CSFRα, so these cells are not IL-5-responsive [66]. Further analysis of IL-5Rα mRNA has revealed that, in common with some other cytokine receptors, membrane-associated and soluble isoforms of the IL-5Rα are produced, and the soluble IL-5Rα chain may inhibit binding of IL-5 to the high-affinity receptor [67]. The function of this mechanism in regulating IL-5 responsiveness *in vivo* is not yet clear, although recent *in situ* hybridisation studies showed preferential expression of the membrane-associated IL-5Rα isoform mRNA in bronchial biopsies from asthmatic subjects, as opposed to a preponderance of the soluble form in non-asthmatic controls [68].

Eosinophil adhesion to vascular endothelium is dependent on p-selectin [69], E-selectin, and β_2-integrin (LFA1-ICAM1) pathways [70, 71], but selective recruitement of eosinophil (as opposed to neutrophils) may partly depend on adhesion via $\alpha_4\beta_1$ (VLA$_4$)/VCAM1 interaction, since VLA$_4$ is expressed on eosinophils but not neutrophils, and VCAM-1 is upregulated on endothelial cells by IL-4. Bentley et al. showed increased intensity of immunostaining for E-selectin at baseline and VCAM1 after allergen challenge in the bronchial mucosa from asthmatic subjects when compared with control individuals [72].

Eosinophils were shown to be capable of production of IL-3 and GM-CSF *in vitro* in 1991 [73, 74], and have now been shown to produce a wide array of cytokines [75], including IL-5 [76] and the chemoattractant chemokine RANTES [77], both *in vitro* and *in vivo* in bronchial biopsies and BAL from asthmatic subjects. Thus, eosinophils may contribute to further recruitment and activation of eosinophils at sites of allergic inflammation in a positive-feedback amplification loop [75–78].

Eosinophils can also produce IL-4 [78], and express both CD40 and CD40 ligand (CD40L) [79, 80]. CD40L and IL-4 are critical for IgE switching by B cells (see Section 2.3.7). However, although they were able to support B-cell proliferation, eosinophils did not support B-cell IgE synthesis *in vitro*. It is of note that eosinophils also respond to IFNγ with increased cytotoxicity [81]. This may be relevant to eosinophil involvement in pulmonary fibrosis.

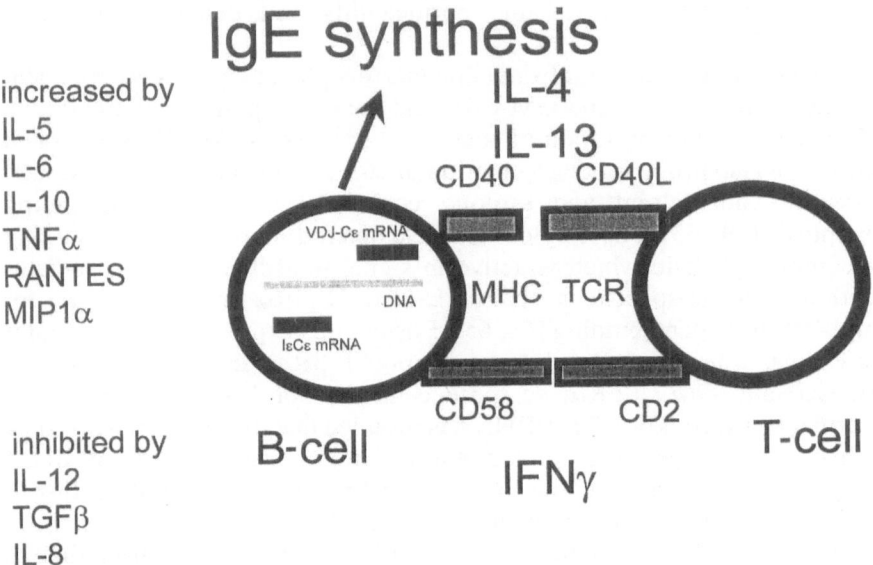

Figure 2. Regulation of IgE synthesis. B lymphocyte genes are switched to Iε and Cε RNA production by IL-4 and a cell surface interaction which may involve CD40, CD58 or interaction between MHC on the B-cell and antigenic peptide in the T-cell receptor (TCR). Interferon γ inhibits this process. Other cytokines and chemokines effecting IgE synthesis are shown.

For some years there has been debate about the precise mechanisms leading to eosinophil degranulation in asthma. Opsonised particles and particulate parasite antigens such as schistosomula larval forms [82] were shown to be potent inducers of eosinophil degranulation, and the potential mechanisms in parasitic disease are well defined. But what causes degranulation in allergic disease? Eosinophils have surface receptors for complement components (C3a, C5a) and Fc portions of immunoglobulin G and A, and these can stimulate leukotriene synthesis [57]. Serum-coated beads, and beads coated with IgG or secretory IgA lead to both ECP and EPO release, whilst interaction with IgG-coated surfaces leads to release of ECP, but not EPO [83]. This process is enhanced by cytokines, particularly IL-3, IL-5 and GM-CSF, and chemokines such as RANTES, which act to prime for degranulation. The role of IgE in triggering eosinophil degranulation remains to be fully clarified, but IgE-dependent stimulation was shown to release MBP and EPO, but not ECP. Presumably, allergen interaction with immunoglobulin at the epithelial surface may create conditions for eosinophil degranulation.

Recently, eosinophils have been shown to have express high-affinity surface IgE receptors (FcεR1) [84]. This observation may have functional significance, since EPO release on FcεR1 cross-linking was reported (although others could not detect IgE-mediated release of granule proteins). We have recently studied FcεR1 expression on blood eosinophils from atopic and non-atopic donors and compared intensity of expression with that seen on basophils and monocytes [85]. Eosinophil FcεR1 expression was several orders of magnitude less than other cell types. However, immunohistochemistry did suggest FcεR1 in up to 30% of tissue eosinophils at sites of allergic inflammation [86]. It remains to be seen whether allergen cross-linking of FcεR1 has a role in either eosinophil degranulation, lipid mediator synthesis or cytokine release.

2.3.2. Mast cells: Cross-linking of high-affinity IgE receptors on mast cells by allergens is believed to be the major factor initiating the immediate response to allergen challenge in the airway. Increasingly, these cells are seen as contributing to allergic airway inflammation through many additional pathways.

The ontogeny of the mast cell has been something of a puzzle, since this is a tissue-dwelling cell, but recent data suggest a specific precursor [87]. The major factor leading to human mast cell development is stem cell factor (SCF) which is derived from bone marrow stromal cells. This interacts with the *c-kit* (protooncogene) receptor, and circulating mast cell progenitors may be *c-kit*$^+$, although they may be deficient in FcεR1 [88]. Mast cell degranulation leads to release of a variety of preformed enzymes and mediators, including histamine, heparin, tryptase, chymase, carboxypeptidase and cathepsin G [89, 90]. Histamine release leads to rapid bronchospasm, vasodilatation and airway oedema, though histamine is rapidly broken down [91]. Heparin probably functions in storage of both histamine and tryptase, which functions as a tetramer. Tryptase is present in all mast cells, and may contribute to airway symptoms in asthma through cleavage of bronchodilator neuropeptides such as vasoactive peptide (VIP), but not bronchoconstrictor peptides such as substance P [92]. Tryptase sensitises bronchial smooth muscle in experimental animals [93]. Chymase is only present in a subset of mast cells (thus termed MC_{TC}, which are a minority in the bronchus, where most mast cells are MC_T, i.e. tryptase-only mast cells) [94]. It cleaves angiotensin I to angiotensin II, and more relevant to asthma may convert IL-1 to its active form, and can degrade IL-4. It may also act in airway remodelling, since it cleaves type IV collagen.

Mast cells also synthesise lipid mediators, prostaglandin D_2 and leukotriene C_4. These are both potent bronchoconstrictors [95].

Production of cytokines by mast cell lines was first described in 1989 [96, 97], and it is now established that human mast cells have the capacity to make a wide variety of cytokines upon FcεR1 cross-linking. In particular, mast cells appear to store preformed tumour necrosis factor (TNFα) and probably IL-4, and these may be release very rapidly after allergen challenge [98]. Anti-IgE stimulation of dispersed human dermal mast cells lead to rapid release of TNFα [99], and mRNA and protein were detected within 2 h of stimulation of human lung mast cells [100]. Although IL-4 has been localised to mast cells in nasal [101] and bronchial biopsies [102] from subjects with rhinitis and asthma, the importance of mast cells as a source of IL-4 is uncertain. Anti-IgE stimulation of human lung mast cells did not lead to detectable protein release, although mRNA was detected in some experiments [103]. We have shown that 10–15% of IL-4 mRNA-positive cells in the bronchial mucosa of atopic asthmatic subjects were mast cells (by tryptase immunohistochemistry), whereas a majority of IL-4 mRNA-positive cells were T lymphocytes [45]. However, immuno-histochemical studies co-localising cytokine protein (IL-4) with cell phenotype markers appear to give contradictory results. Bradding et al. found that the majority of IL-4+ cells in bronchial biopsies from atopic asthmatics were mast cells, and could not localise IL-4 protein to T-cells [104]. Our findings are similar, although it is of note that the numbers of IL-4 protein-positive cells were considerably less (around 30%) than numbers expressing mRNA [105]. Since T-cell IL-4 secretion appears to be directed at areas of cell-cell contact [106], it is likely that T-cells that are secreting IL-4 are not detected by immunohistochemical methods, since these rely on accumulation of the cytokine within the cell being stained. In support of this possibility, we have recently shown that blocking secretion of IL-4 by the agent monensin (which disrupts the Golgi apparatus), considerably enhanced immunocytochemical staining of IL-4 in a T-cell line.

Mast cells also have the capacity for IL-13 production [107], and with IL-4 this may be important in amplifying IgE synthesis in allergic inflammation, since mast cells express CD40L and can induce IgE synthesis by human B-cells *in vitro* [108]. Both IL-4 and IL-13 act to upregulate endothelial cell expression of the adhesion molecule VCAM1, and this may act in specific recruitment of eosinophils and T-cells through interaction with VLA-4 [109]. TNFα activates macrophages, and will also enhance endothelial cell adhesion through upregulation and activation of both E-selectin and ICAM, and there is evidence that this occurs during the early phase of allergen challenge in the skin [110, 111].

Increased mast cell numbers and concentrations of mast cell mediators such as histamine, tryptase and LTE$_4$ have been detected in BAL from atopic asthmatics compared with control subjects in a number of studies, although bronchial biopsies do not show increased mast cell numbers [14–16].

2.3.3. Basophils: Basophils originate from a separate haematopoietic lineage to mast cells, and are more closely "related" to eosinophils. Indeed, basophils develop from bone marrow progenitors in response to IL-3 and GM-CSF and differentiate in response to IL-5, and mixed eosinophil/basophil colonies are described in such cultures [112]. What determines the differentiation of these common precursors into either eosinophils or basophils is unknown.

Like mast cells, basophils express FcεR1 and will release histamine on IgE cross-linking by allergen. They also produce LTC$_4$ but do not synthesise PGD$_2$ [113]. These cells may also be triggered by IgG via CD16 (FcγRIII), CD32 (FcγRII), and via complement receptors by C3a and C5a. Numerous histamine releasing factors have been described in *in vitro* assays, and it is suggested that such agents are produced by mononuclear cells in response to allergen, and enhance or themselves trigger basophil histamine release [114]. This activity is increased by IL-3 [115]. Recently, many of these factors have been shown to be chemokines, and they include MCP-1, MCP-3, MIPα, RANTES and MCP2 [114, 116]. In addition, an IgE-independent factor has been recently cloned [117].

Basophils are also shown to be capable of cytokine synthesis, and may be an important source of IL-4 [118]. IL-3 enhances basophil IL-4 production in response to IgE cross-linking, and the amount of IL-4 produced can be comparable to that from T-cells on a cell-per-cell basis [119, 120]. Since basophils also express CD40L, these cells too can support B-cell IgE synthesis. Non-B- non-T-cell IL-4 production by spleen cells has been shown to be a potentially important factor in priming for a Th2 response in animal infection models, and basophil cytokine production is proably the most relevant non-T-cell source to allergic disease, at least for IL-4.

Because there is no specific marker for basophils, it has proved difficult to demonstrate these cells at sites of allergic inflammation. Increased basophil numbers are reported in nasal washings [121] and BAL after allergen challenge [122], although cell numbers are still small. Indirect evidence for a role for basophils came from the demonstration of histamine and LTC$_4$, but not PGD$_2$, in the late response to allergen challenge in the skin, nose and airway.

2.3.4. Macrophages and monocytes: Increased numbers of macrophages are reported in bronchial biopsies from atopic asthmatics, and particularly from subjects with intrinsic (non-atopic) asthma, when compared with control subjects [123, 124]. Immunohistochemical analysis suggests infiltration of relatively immature monocyte-like macrophages into the airway mucosa in asthma [123]. These cells have a wide variety of functions, in addition to their phagocytic capacity. Macrophages can produce lipid mediators, including PGD$_2$, and may do so in response to allergen stimulation via low-affinity IgE receptors (CD23) [125]. These cells are a source of a number of cytokines important in upregulation of adhesion molecules, such as TNFα, IL-1 and IL-6; GM-CSF, which may act in eosinophil recruitment and activation; and IL-1, which may act as a co-stimulator of T lymphocytes (particularly Th2 cells) [126, 127]. Macrophage recruitment and differentiation from monocytes results, in part, from the actions of GM-CSF, and since macrophage production of GM-CSF has been demonstrated in the asthmatic airway, this cytokine may be important in regulation of macrophage numbers and function in asthma [128]. However, macrophages are also potent sources of IL-10 and IL-12, which act to inhibit T-cell activation or skew towards expansion of a Th1 phenotype, respectively [129, 130]. Alveolar macrophages from normal donors show poor antigen-presenting cell activity to autologous T cells, possibly because of low expression of the B7 co-stimulator molecules [131]. However, some reports suggest that BAL macrophages from atopic asthmatic subjects may act in T-cell activation [132], and enhance T-cell activation *in vitro* [133]. We have recently shown an increase in numbers of BAL cells expressing IL-10 mRNA in asthmatic subjects when compared with controls [129]. Both macrophages and T-cells encoded IL-10 mRNA in both groups of subjects, although the T-cell contribution was increased in the asthmatic. IL-10 expression was further increased after allergen inhalation challenge, when compared with diluent control challenge in the same mild asthmatic subjects, and this may be a regulatory pathway tending to turn off allergen-induced inflammation in the airway, although this remains to be confirmed.

Monocytes have recently been shown to have high-affinity IgE receptors, and we have shown that these are increased in atopic subjects. This may be relevant to T-cell activation, since *in vitro* interaction with surface IgE on monocytes was shown to lead to processing and antigen presentation, and allergens might be presented preferentially to T-cells by this route [134]. Whether this occurs in the airway is unknown.

2.3.5. Dendritic cells: The presence of a dense network of interdigitating dendritic cells has been demonstrated in human bronchial mucosa [135]. These cells are important in antigen processing and presentation, and have also been shown to express FcεR1, at least in the skin. Isolation of sufficient dendritic cells for functional studies from human airways has so far proved difficult. It is thus not known whether allergen can be presented at the mucosal surface to resident memory T-cells, or whether this occurs at regional lymph nodes. Murine dendritic cells have been shown to be capable of producing IL-12, and can induce a Th1 phenotype during primary T-cell activation [136]. Whether dendritic cells produce IL-12 or other cytokines in the human airway is unknown.

2.3.6. Epithelial cells: Epithelial damage with loss of epithelial-derived relaxing factors and increased access of allergens is thought to be an important contributor to bronchial hyper-responsiveness in asthma. However, epithelial cells may also contribute to airway inflammation through production of cytokines, including GM-CSF and IL-3, and chemokines such as IL-8 and possibly eotaxin [137, 138]. These cells can also be induced to present antigen to T-cells *in vitro*, since they express HLA class II molecules at the site of inflammation [139].

Epithelial cells, with macrophages, are also an important potential source of nitric oxide, which may be a proinflammatory mediator in asthma. Although low doses of nitric oxide have a bronchodilator effect, higher doses activate inflammatory cells and may contribute to tissue damage. One such pathway is through skewing T-cell responses towards the Th2 subtype. Elevated concentrations of exhaled nitric oxide have been detected in asthmatics when compared with control subjects [140–142].

2.3.7. B lymphocytes: The major contribution of B-cells to atopic allergic inflammation is clearly through IgE synthesis, although these cells also have an important potential as antigen-presenting cells and may preferentially activate a Th2 phenotype.

In recent years the factors involved in switching B-cells to produce IgE have been determined in some detail [143]. Isotype switching in B-cells results from DNA recombination, leading to juxtaposition of different heavy chain genes (C_H) to the expressed variable, diversity and junctional (VDJ) gene regions which determine antigen specificity. This proceeds through a step of transcriptional activation of the same gene in its germline configuration so that exons (I regions) just upstream of the switch region (this part of the Ig gene sequences switches to different isotypes) join to the C_H. This I-C_H mRNA is slightly shorter than the fully rearranged coding mRNA, and contains multiple stop codons, so that it is not translated: this is termed a "sterile germline transcript". It appears that this step is necessary before further rearrangement and editing lead to combination of VDJ regions encoding the antigen-binding portion of Ig, and $C\varepsilon$ leading to productive IgE mRNA. In both murine and human *in vitro* studies, IL-4 was defined was the obligatory first signal leading to germline mRNA switching [144, 145]. More recently, IL-13 has been shown to act in IgE switching, and can substitute for IL-4 [146]. This cytokine probably represents a gene duplication of IL-4, and binds to a shared receptor [147]. A number of other cytokines have a role, or can potentiate IgE synthesis. IL-6 is required for human IgE production, whilst IL-5 can potentiate IgE production [148, 149]. INFα inhibits IgE synthesis, and this is also true of IL-12 [150] and IL-8 [151]. Recently, the chemokines RANTES and MIP1α were shown to upregulate human IgE synthesis *in vitro* [152].

For productive IgE switching a second signal is required, in addition to IL-4 or IL-13. The best characterised is via CD40L, which interacts with CD40 on the B-cell [153]. This function can also be subsumed by CD2 (T-cell) and CD58 (B-cell) [154], and by soluble factors such as hydrocortisone, at least *in vitro*.

B-cells express surface HLA DR, and interaction with the T-cell receptor leading to T-cell activation via B-cell antigen presentation and T-cell IL-4 production and interaction at the level of CD2, CD58, CD40 and CD40L leads to production of IgE directed against the specific antigen leading to B- and T-cell activation. This is termed "cognate" B-cell IgE switching. Since other cell types, including mast cells and basophils, both produce IL-4 and express CD40L, these cells can switch to IgE production but will not do so in an antigen-specific manner: this is non-cognate B-cell activation (which T-cells can also do). Thus, both specific and polyclonal IgE production will occur at sites of allergic inflammation.

B-cell antigen presentation appears to favour Th2 cell activation in both murine and human systems *in vitro* [155–157]. The mechanism is uncertain, although recent data suggest that CD40-CD40L interaction may favour Th2 expansion [158].

The site of IgE synthesis in allergic asthma is presumed to be in local lymph nodes in specialised germinal centres. However, recent data suggest that local mucosal IgE synthesis may occur in the nasal mucosa of atopic subjects after allergen challenge, since upregulation of mRNA containing both Iε and Cε suggests that switching to IgE synthesis may be a mucosal event. This has important implications for directing therapy at IgE synthesis, and Durham et al. were able to show that topical nasal steroid treatment reduced Iε expression [159].

CD23 is the low-affinity IgE receptor, but is also present in soluble form. This molecule has been rather enigmatic in that the appears to both enhance and inhibit IgE synthesis. The basis of these findings has recently been elucidated in elegant experiments by the group of Hannah Gould [160, 161]. Unlike other Fc receptors, FcεRII (CD23) is a lectin-like molecule with a trimeric helical structure. It is cleaved into three subfragments by endogenous proteases, and all of these bind both IgE and, like the intact receptor, the complement 2 receptor (CR2 or CD21). Downregulation of IgE production occurs through interaction of membrane bound-CD23 and IgE in antigen-antibody complexes. However, upregulation of IgE synthesis is induced by interaction of soluble fragments of CD23 with CD21 on the B-cell surface. Gould et al. suggest that these findings provide a regulatory mechanism for IgE synthesis, so that if serum IgE is high, this binds to surface CD23, leading to inhibition of IgE synthesis and preventing proteolysis so that soluble CD23 fragments are not released and cannot therefore interact with CD21 to increase IgE synthesis. Conversely, if serum IgE is low, CD23 is "exposed" to proteases, and CD21 is activated by sCD23, leading to increased IgE synthesis [162]. Whether this system can be exploited for therapy remains to be seen.

2.3.8. Other cell types: Neutrophils, platelets, airway nerves and myofibroblasts: Although neutrophils are prominent in experimental allergen challenge [163], and neutrophil chemoattractants [164, 165] have been described in serum and airway samples from asthmatic subjects, neutrophil numbers and elastase staining are not increased in either bronchial biopsies or BAL samples from asthmatics when compared with control subjects. Neutrophils are a potential source of inflammatory cytokines (TNFα, RANTES) and cytotoxic enzymes, and it is possible that neutrophil recruitment plays a role in asthma exacerbations due to allergen challenge or infection [166]. It is of note that a subgroup of subjects who died of asthma showed neutrophil, and not eosinophil, infiltration into the airway, although this is an unusual finding [167].

Platelets are a potential source of proinflammatory lipid mediators which might contribute to airway changes in asthma, and these cells can also produce chemokines which may amplify inflammatory cell infiltration [168].

Numerous vasoactive neuropeptides, including endothelin, vasoactive intestinal peptide and substance P may lead to mucosal oedema and vascular leak. Nitric oxide also functions as a neurotransmitter. The role of these factors in airway inflammation in asthma remains to be defined [169].

A characteristic appearance in bronchial biopsies from asthmatic subjects is apparent basement membrane thickening. This is shown to result from sub-basement deposition of collagen from myofibroblasts [170]. Whether this airway remodelling leads to irreversible airway obstruction is not known. In most studies, this sub-basement membrane thickening persists after treatment [171], although two reports suggest partial resolution after inhaled corticosteroid treatment [172, 173]. The signals that turn on collagen synthesis in the asthmatic airway are unknown, although platelet-derived growth factor (PDGF) and insulin-like growth factor (IGF) are candidates.

3. Chemokines

The chemokines are a family of structurally related peptides of 8- to 10-kDa molecular weight which were defined based on their property of attracting various leucocytes to the site of inflammation [174]. Chemokines are produced by a wide variety of inflammatory cell types, so they contribute to amplification of the inflammatory response. The recent demonstration that they are also produced by a number of resident tissue cells give them particular importance, with potential as initiators of inflammatory cell infiltration to sites of allergic reactions. There is a common structural motif of four cysteine residues with a short amino-terminal and longer carboxy-terminal sequence. The cysteine residues form disulphide bonds that give a shared secondary and tertiary structure seen on X-ray crystallography. The presence or absence or an amino acid residue separating the first two cysteine groups is used to define C-X-C chemokines and C-C chemokines, and this subdivision also holds on a functional basis, since the C-X-C chemokines are encoded on chromosome 4 and act principally on neutrophils, whereas the C-C chemokine genes are on chromosome 17, and these agents act principally on eosinophils, basophils and mononuclear cells. The C-C chemokines are thus clear candidates for a role in allergic inflammation in asthma.

The C-C chemokines RANTES [175], monocyte chemotactic peptide-3 (MCP-3), MCP-2, and MIP-1α are chemoattractants for both eosinophils and basophils [176], and MCP-1 acts on basophils but not eosinophils. The chemokines are also chemoattractants for monocytes and lymphocytes [177, 178], and thus may have roles in accumulation of the major cellular players in allergic inflammation. The number of chemokines described is increasing rapidly, and of great interest are eotaxin [179, 180] and MCP-4 [181], which seem to be selective eosinophil chemoattractants. Many other agents are likely to be identified. The bewildering array of C-C chemokines can be grouped functionally on the basis of receptor binding and activation: of relevance to selective accumulation of eosinophils is the C-C-chemokine receptor 3, which binds eotaxin, RANTES and MCP-3 [182]. Selective blockade of this receptor might have therapeutic potential in asthma.

In addition to their chemoattractant properties, C-C chemokines also act in both eosinophil and basophil degranulation and stimulating leukotriene synthesis, particularly after priming by IL-3 and IL-5. As described above, RANTES and MIP-1α may also have a role in IgE regulation [174].

Although IL-8 has been reported to be a weak eosinophil chemoattractant, and it acts in basophil chemotaxis and activation, it is uncertain what role, if any, the C-X-C chemokines play in orchestrating airway inflammation in asthma.

RANTES, MCP-3 and MIP-1α have been detected at both mRNA and protein level in airway tissue and in BAL fluid from asthmatic subjects, as well as in skin, nasal samples and BAL after allergen challenge [183–185]. The source of these cytokines in asthma is uncertain, although many cell types have the capacity to synthesise them *in vitro*, and production from both epithelial cells and eosinophils has been demonstrated in bronchial biopsies.

4. Non-atopic Asthma

4.1. Clinical Variants of Asthma

Although most asthma occurs in atopic individuals, and allergic triggers can be recognised, there exist other clinical patterns of disease. Occupational triggers to asthma vary from low molecular weight chemicals, such as isocyanates, to protein antigens such as flour and laboratory animal proteins, which may act as allergens and evoke specific IgE responses [186]. Although IgE responses to some low molecular weight compounds have been reported, and this may result from chemical association with host proteins (haptens) leading to allergic response to the altered self peptide, it is not certain that all these agents produce such an immune response. Clinically, development of occupational asthma is not necessarily associated with previous atopic disease. Avoidance of the inciting agent may lead to resolution of symptoms, but asthma may also persist. Thus, study of occupational asthma may provide information on initiation of asthmatic airway inflammation which is difficult to gain in atopic disease.

The other major clinical variant of asthma is non-atopic asthma, where there is no history to suggest an environmental trigger and no evidence of specific IgE. This has been termed "intrinsic" asthma, and onset is generally around the age of 30–40; it is more prevalent in women. It is unknown whether this variant represents sensitivity to unidentified "allergen" or whether it is possibly a form of autoimmune disease which might be triggered by viral exposure. Despite the lack of specific IgE, it is of note that in asthma generally there is a correlation between total serum IgE and both bronchial responsiveness and the presence of asthma symptoms [187], whether the subject is atopic or not.

These forms of asthma respond to treatment similar to that for atopic asthma.

4.2. Immunopathology of Non-atopic Asthma

The pathology of subjects dying of occupational or intrinsic asthma shows features similar to atopic asthma, with a prominent infiltrate of eosinophils and mononuclear cells and epithelial desquamation [188]. This is confirmed by immunohistological studies comparing bronchoscopic bronchial biopsies from atopic, intrinsic and occupational asthma [189]. These show increased numbers of activated eosinophils and T lymphocytes in the airway mucosa, and increased macrophages in intrinsic asthma. BAL also showed evidence of CD4$^+$ T-cell activation in intrinsic asthma, but also, in contrast to atopic disease, CD8$^+$ T-cell activation [190]. Analysis of cytokines in concentrated BAL fluid showed increased IL-4 and IL-5, but not IL-2 or IFNγ in atopic asthmatics compared with control subjects, whilst IL-5 and IL-2, but not IL-4, were present in increased concentrations in BAL fluid from intrinsic asthmatics [48]. However, more recently we have analysed cytokine expression in bronchial biopsies from atopic and intrinsic asthmatics with atopic and non-atopic control subjects by RT-PCR and in situ hybridisation for cytokine mRNA, and immunohistochemistry for cytokine protein [44]. These studies suggested increased expression of IL-4 and IL-5 in both atopic and non-atopic asthma, both at the mRNA and protein level. Furthermore, FcεR1+ cells were increased in number in bronchial biopsies from both atopic and non-atopic asthmatics, suggesting that IgE-dependent mechanisms might apply in both atopic and intrinsic asthma [191].

Recently T cells have been cloned from bronchial biopsies from subjects with occupational asthma due to toluene di-isocyanate exposure. These clones were CD8$^+$ and produced IL-5 and IFNγ [192].

Overall, it appears that both atopic and non-atopic asthma are characterised by eosinophilic airway inflammation, and this may result from a common pattern of Th2-type T-cell activation, although additional T-cell cytokine patterns may contribute.

5. Allergen Challenge

Inhalational challenge of sensitised asthmatic subjects with allergen extract leads to immediate airway narrowing with 15 min which may persist for 1–2 h and is termed the "early asthmatic response". This may be followed at 3–8 h by further airway narrowing which is accompanied by increased airway responsiveness to non-specific stimuli and may be followed by increased symptoms for several days [193, 194]. This late asthmatic response is also associated with airway hyperexpansion [195]. Allergen challenge has been used as a model for airway inflammation in asthma, and is widely used in drug testing. With the advent of bronchoscopic study of asthma, this has been complemented by direct instillation of allergen extract into the segmental airways in a local allergen challenge.

Bronchoscopic study of the airway after allergen challenge confirms the role of mast cell degranulation in the early asthmatic response, since PGD_2, histamine, tryptase and LTC_4 are all increased in BAL fluid immediately after allergen challenge [122]. In contrast, there is a second rise in histamine and LTC_4 but not PGD_2 in the late response, possibly implicating basophils. However, the main feature of the late response is infiltration of eosinophils and neutrophils with evidence of eosinophil degranulation. Examination of cytokine gene expression at 24 h after allergen challenge showed increased mRNA+ cells for IL-4, IL-5 and GM-CSF in both BAL and biopsies from atopic asthmatic subjects [196, 197]. These changes were localised predominantly to T lymphocytes, and GM-CSF mRNA was demonstrated in lymphocytes and macrophages after allergen challenge in a separate study [198]. IL-5 was measured by enzyme-linked immuno-sorbent assay (ELISA) in lavage fluid following local allergen challenge [199]. Correlations amongst IL-5 mRNA expression, T-cell activation and eosinophil numbers in BAL 24 h after challenge and the preceding fall in FEV_1 during late response supported a link between T-cell activation of eosinophils and clinical effects of allergen inhalation [197].

6. Animal Models of Asthma

Animal models of asthma are described more accurately as models of allergen challenge. Almost all rely on initial sensitisation to antigen followed by inhaled challenge, which may lead to airway eosinophil influx, hyper-responsiveness or both. Such models have allowed interventions not possible in human volunteers. Depletion of CD4+ T-cells or prior administration of monoclonal antibody to IL-5 blocked airway eosinophil infiltration in a mouse model of allergen challenge [200]. Blockade of IL-4 with monoclonal antibody abrogated bronchial hyper-responsiveness to airway challenge with ovalbumin in BALB/c mice [201]. In a similar model in a different mouse strain, the application of gene knockout technology showed that disruption of the IL-5 gene also prevented antigen-induced airway responsiveness and eosinophil infiltration [202]. These apparently contradictory results may reflect the different mouse strains used [203]. Other investigators have recently shown that CD8[+] T-cells were required for IgE synthesis and hyper-responsiveness in a similar mouse model [204], and this system has also been used to show blockade of antigen-induced hyper-responsiveness by anti-IgE antibodies [205].

A rat model showed that hyperresponsiveness was transferred on adoptive transfer of CD4[+] T-cells from allergen-sensitised animals to naive recipients and led to acquisition of hyper-responsiveness in the recipient animals [206, 207]. Guinea pig ovalbumin sensitisation was used to isolate a specific eosinophil chemoattractant, later cloned as eotaxin [138].

A monkey model has been employed to show that airway instillation of eosinophil major basic protein led to airway hyper-responsiveness [208], and eosinophil influx and hyper-responsiveness to allergen inhalation was blocked by monoclonal antibody to ICAM-1 in the same model [209]. A humanised anti-IL-5 monoclonal antibody has recently been applied to this model, and this treatment was shown to inhibit both eosinophil infiltration and hyper-responsiveness to allergen challenge; these effects persisted for up to 3 months after treatment [210].

Airway challenge of mice sensitised to ovalbumin with viral proteins led to increased airway responsiveness and eosinophil infiltration which was dependent on IL-5 from CD8[+] T-cells [211]. Certain respiratory syncytial virus (RSV) peptides will also induce a Th2-type airway response after sensitisation in mice [212]. It is possible that similar mechanisms underlie the demonstrated increased response to allergen in asthmatics with experimental rhinovirus infection.

7. Treatment of Asthma

7.1. Current Treatments

Current national and international treatment guidelines for asthma stress the combination of β_2 agonists for symptomatic relief with anti-inflammatory therapy in all but the most mild asthmatics [213]. Other bronchodilator therapy includes theophylline, and ipratropium bromide. The most effective anti-inflammatory therapy is inhaled corticosteroids, although cromoglycate or nedocromil sodium may be effective in some subjects, and a few severe asthmatics require oral corticosteroid treatment. Treatment guidelines follow a step therapy approach with grades of treatment in terms of agents an dosage.

β_2 agonists act principally as functional antagonists of smooth muscle constriction, thus reversing the acute symptoms of asthma [214]. These agents also have actions on mast cells and eosinophils, and β receptors are present on lymphocytes. The role of such effects *in vivo* is uncertain. Although β agonists will act to increase intracellular cyclic adenosine monophosphate (cAMP) at relatively high concentrations, leading to muscle relaxation, they may also interact with high-conductance potassium channels to produce these effects. It has been suggested that interaction with cAMP may explain the potential for high-dose β agonists to worsen asthma control, at least in some studies. cAMP binds to and activates a cytoplasmic transcription factor termed CREB (cAMP binding protein), and this interacts with genes at specific nuclear CREB binding regions. However, CREB can interact directly with the glucocorticoid receptor in the cytoplasm, and this may prevent translocation of the steroid-receptor complex to the nucleus, where interaction at steroid response elements has beneficial effects downregulating a number of proinflammatory gene products [215].

Corticosteroids are the mainstay of asthma treatment. These agents are potent inhibitors of T-cell activation and cytokine synthesis *in vitro*, and recent studies have demonstrated inhibition of eosinophil and T-cell infiltration and activation in the bronchial mucosa of asthmatic subjects after inhaled corticosteroid treatment [216, 217]. We examined cellular infiltration and cytokine mRNA expression in both BAL cells and bronchial biopsies from symptomatic asthmatic subjects treated for a 2-week period with either prednisolone or matched placebo in a double-blind, parallel-group study. The subjects receiving prednisolone showed an over fivefold decrease in bronchial responsiveness to methacholine, and this was accompanied by reduction in BAL eosinophils, mucosal eosinophils, T-cells and mast cells in the prednisolone group [218, 219]. Furthermore there was a reduction in numbers of BAL or biopsy cells expressing mRNA for both IL-4 and IL-5, but an increse in those expressing IFNγ. Similar findings were reported by Leung et al., and this group extended the study to show that a group of patients whose asthma did not improve with corticosteroid therapy (corticosteroid-resistant asthmatics) did not show any changes in airway mucosal cytokine mRNA for IL-4, IL-5 and IFNγ after prednisolone therapy [43].

Corticosteroids undoubtedly have many other actions relevant to their efficacy in asthma. In addition to reduction in inflammatory cell numbers and activation, which may relate to inhibitory effects on cytokines, glucocorticoids also reduce tissue oedema by effects on vascular permeability. This may result from synthesis of lipocortin, principally in monocytes and macrophages, which blocks phospholipase A_2, thus preventing mobilisation of arachidonic acid for lipid mediator synthesis. Lipocortin 1 has been cloned and shown to act *in vitro* to inhibit monocyte prostanoid synthesis [220]. It was suggested that this mechanism might underlie many of the biological actions of glucocorticoids, but most effects seem to result from direct interaction between the glucocorticoid-receptor complex binding at both negative and positive glucocorticoid-response elements in genes relevant to inflammation [221]. In this way lipid mediator synthesis is affected by downregulation of the cyclo-oxygenase 2 gene (COX2), and inducible nitric oxide synthetase (iNOS) is also switched off at the gene level by steroids [222, 223].

It has become possible to determine more accurately the role of leuko-trienes in airway inflammation in asthma with the advent of specific leuko-triene antagonists. Various drugs have been developed that either block the leukotriene D_4 receptor or interfere with synthesis via 5-lipoxygenase or membrane transport via 5-lipoxygenase-associated protein (FLAP) [224]. These agents block both the early and late response to allergen inhalation challenge in atopic subjects, and appear to have some benefit in short-term clinical studies, both reducing nocturnal asthma symptoms and producing a modest improvement in airflow obstruction [225]. There is little current information about the effect of the agents on inflammatory cell infiltration or cytokine expression in the airway in asthma.

Recent evidence suggests that theophyllines might have an anti-inflam-matory effect in addition to the well-described bronchodilator properties of these drugs. In biopsy studies, theophylline, at sub-bronchodilator doses, reduced mucosal eosinophil infiltration during late asthmatic response and inhibited the associated fall in FEV_1 [226]. In a withdrawal study, as theo-phylline treatment was discontinued, there was evidence for increased T-cell numbers and activation in the airways of asthmatic subjects [227]. Selective blockade of phosphodiesterase isoenzymes might hold the poten-tial for selection of anti-inflammatory effects on both T lymphocytes and eosinophils, which can be demonstrated *in vitro* to result from type-IV phosphodiesterase inhibition [228]. The basis for apparent anti-inflamma-tory effects of cromoglycate and nedocromil is uncertain, although these agents also inhibit both early and late asthmatic responses to allergen chal-lenge. Recent data suggests these drugs may also inhibit airway eosinophil infiltration and activation, although the mechanism remains obscure.

A subgroup of asthmatic subjects requires oral prednisolone to control their symptoms, and a much smaller subgroup of these asthmatics do not appear to respond to glucocorticoids with improvement in lung func-tion (usually defined on the basis of a less than 15% change in FEV_1 after 2 weeks of treatment with 20 mg equivalent of prednisolone), and are term-ed corticosteroid-resistant. Corrigan et al. showed defects in suppression of CD4 T-cell proliferation to mitogens by dexamethasone *in vitro* in steroid-resistant asthmatics, but could not account for resistance on the grounds of minor changes seen in steroid pharmacokinetics and binding in these subjects [229]. This suggests a T-lymphocyte defect, and Leung et al. sug-gested that in some steroid-resistant subjects this was fixed, but that in others it resulted from the effects of exposure to cytokines, particularly the combination of IL-2 and IL-4, which could induce steroid resistance *in vitro* [230, 231]. A possible molecular basis for this effect was described by Adcock et al., who showed an increase in cytoplasmic expression of the transcription factor AP-1 in steroid-resistant subjects [232]. This ubiquitous transcription factor is involved in the action of many cytokine effects, and has the capacity to bind to the glucocorticoid receptor-steroid complex in the cytoplasm, blocking nuclear translocation of both DNA binding factors. It is suggested that this usually contributes to the anti-inflammatory effects of steroids, which "mop up" AP-1 before it can exert its effects in the nucleus, but in steroid-resistant subjects an excess of AP-1 has the converse effect, preventing beneficial effects of the gluco-corticoid receptor in downregulation of inflammatory genes.

As a logical extension of the findings suggesting a dominant role for CD4+ T-cell activation in asthma, Alexander et al. studied the effect of cyclosporin A in chronic steroid-dependent asthmatics [233]. They demon-strated improvements in lung function over the 12-week duration of this placebo-controlled crossover study, and Lock et al. went on to show a sustained steroid-sparing effect over a much longer 44-week study period [234]. Cyclosporin A is widely used in transplant medicine, and as an anti-inflammatory treatment in inflammatory skin disorders, and has profound effects on T-cell proliferation and cytokine gene expression, particularly IL-2. The molecular basis of this action has been elegantly demonstrated by Crabtree and others, who show that the cyclosporin binding protein cyclophilin interferes with dissociation of a blocking factor from the T-cell-specific transcription factor NFAT, and this prevents nuclear translocation and gene activation (or repression) [235]. However, additional effects of cyclosporin on mast cell and basophil degranulation have been described, and it remained possible that some of the effects described in asthma were attributable to these actions. However, recently we have examined the effect of cyclosporin A on allergen challenge in mild atopic asthmatics. Cyclosporin inhibited late response, but not early asthmatic reaction (analagous to corticosteroids), supporting the hypothesis that the major effects in asthma result from inhibition of T-lymphocyte activation [236].

Other steroid-sparing agents have been demonstrated to have effects in asthma. In particular, methotrexate was shown to reduce steroid require-ment in a placebo-controlled study [237]. The mechanism of action is uncertain.

Allergen injection immunotherapy is not used for treatment of asthma in the UK, following recommendations from the Committee on Safety of Medicines in 1986 and, more recently, a position paper from the British Society of Allergy and Clinical Immunology [238, 239]. However, a placebo-controlled study showed that this treatment was effective in severe summer hayfever, and suggested possible modulation of T-cell cytokine production as a potential mechanism [240]. Allergen immunotherapy has been used in asthma, and double-blind placebo controlled studies have shown significant improvements in asthma due to house dust mite, cat and ragweed [241–243]. However, the improvements seen are probably achiev-able with more conventional therapy, particularly inhaled steroids, and the possible risk of anaphylaxis, in addition to the cost, makes imunotherapy for asthma difficult to justify [244]. Recent reports in abstract form raise the possibility of using peptides derived from allergens which do not bind IgE but act specifically at the T-cell to induce non-responsiveness to whole allergen [245]. However, these studies will need careful analysis.

References

1. National Asthma Campaign (1995) *Purchasing and providing asthma care*. National Asthma Campaign, London.
2. Anonymous (1992) International Consensus Report on diagnosis and management of asthma. *Clin Exp Allergy* (Suppl 1): 1–72.
3. Rackeman FM (1947) A working classification of asthma. *Am J Med* 3: 601–606.
4. Dunnill MS (1960) The pathology of asthma with special reference to changes in the bronchial mucosa. *J Clin Pathol* 13: 27–33.
5. Houston JC, de Navasquez S, Trounce JR (1953) A clinical and pathological study of fatal cases of status asthmaticus. *Thorax* 8: 207–213.
6. Filley WV, Holley HE, Kephardt GM, Gleich GJ (1982) Identification by immunofluorescence of eosinophil granule major basic protein in lung tissue of patients with bronchial asthma. *Lancet* ii: 11–16.
7. Horn BR, Robin ED, Theodore J, Van-Kessel A (1975) Total eosinophil counts in the management of bronchial asthma. *N Engl J Med* 292: 1152–1155.
8. Durham-SR, Loegering DA, Dunnette S, Gleich GJ, Kay AB (1989) Blood eosinophils and eosinophil-derived proteins in allergic asthma. *J Allergy Clin Immunol* 84: 931–936.
9. Bousquet J, Chanez P, Lacoste JY, Barneon G, Ghavanian N, Enander I, Venge P, Ahlstedt S, Simony-Lafontaine J, Godard P et al. (1990) Eosinophilic inflammation in asthma. *N Engl J Med* 323: 1033–1039.
10. Hansel TT (1994) The cardinal importance of sputum microscopy. *Clin Exp Allergy* 24: 695–697.
11. Ishizaka K, Ishizaka T (1967) Identification of γE-antibodies as a carrier of reaginic activity. *J Immunol* 99: 1187–1198.
12. Azzawi M, Bradley B, Jeffery PK, Frew AJ, Wardlaw AJ, Knowles GK, Assoufi B, Collins JV, Durham SR, Kay AB (1990) Identification of activated T lymphocytes and eosinophils in bronchial biopsies in stable atopic asthma. *Am Rev Respir Dis* 142: 1407–1413.
13. Jeffery PK, Wardlaw AJ, Nelson FC, Collins JV, Kay AB (1989) Bronchial biopsies in asthma: An ultrastructural, quantitative study and correlation with hyperreactivity. *Am Rev Respir Dis* 140: 1745–1753.
14. Beasley R, Roche WR, Roberts JA, Holgate ST (1989) Cellular events in the bronchi before and after bronchial provocation. *Am Rev Respir Dis* 139: 806–817.
15. Djukanovic R, Wilson JW, Britten KM, Wilson SJ, Walls AF, Roche WR, Howarth PH, Holgate ST (1990) Quantitation of mast cells and eosinophils in the bronchial mucosa of symptomatic atopic asthmatics and healthy control subjects using immunohistochemistry. *Am Rev Respir Dis* 142: 863–871.
16. Bradley BL, Azzawi M, Jacobson M, Assoufi B, Collins JV, Irani A-M, Schwartz LB, Durham SR, Jeffery PK, Kay AB (1991) Eosinophils, T-lymphocytes, mast cells, neutrophils and macrophages in bronchial biopsy specimens from atopic subjects with asthma: Comparison with biopsy specimens from atopic subjects without asthma and normal control subjects and relationship to bronchial hyperresponsiveness. *J Allergy Clin Immunol* 88: 661–674.
17. Wardlaw AJ, Dunnette S, Gleich GJ, Collins JV, Kay AB (1988) Eosinophils and mast cells in bronchoalveolar lavage in mild asthma: Relationship to bronchial reactivity. *Am Rev Respir Dis* 137: 62–69.
18. Godard P, Chaintreuil J, Damon M, Michel FB (1982) Functional characterisation of alveolar macrophages: Comparison of cells from asthmatics and normal subjects. *J Allergy Clin Immunol* 70: 88–93.
19. Corrigan CJ, Kay AB (1992) T-cells and eosinophils in the pathogenesis of asthma. *Immunol Today* 13: 501–506.

20. Corrigan CJ, Hartnell AH, Kay AB (1988) CD4 T lymphocyte activation in acute severe asthma. *Lancet* 1: 1129–1132.
21. Wilson JW, Djukanovic R, Howarth PH, Holgate ST (1992) Lymphocyte activation in bronchoalveolar lavage and peripheral blood in atopic asthma. *Am Rev Respir Dis* 145: 958–960.
22. Robinson DS, Bentley AM, Hartnell AH, Kay AB, Durham SR (1993) Activated memory T helper cells in bronchoalveolar lavage fluid from patients with atopic asthma: Relation to asthma symptoms, lung function and bronchial responsiveness. *Thorax* 48: 26–32.
23. Walker C, Kaegi MK, Braun P, Blaser K (1991) Activated T-cells and eosinophilia in bronchoalveolar lavages from subjects with asthma correlated with disease severity. *J Allergy Clin Immunol* 88: 935–942.
24. Mosmann TR, Cherwinski H, Bond MW, Gieldin MA, Coffman RL (1986) Two types of murine helper T-cell clones. *J Immunol* 136: 2348–2357.
25. Fong TAT, Mosmann TR (1989) The role of IFNγ in delayed-type hypersensitivity mediated by Th1 clones. *J Immunol* 143: 2887–2893.
26. Street NE, Schumacher JH, Fong TAT, Bass H, Fiorentino DF, Leverah JA, Mosmann TR (1990) Heterogeneity of mouse helper T-cells: Evidence from bulk cultures and limiting dilution cloning for precursors of Th1 and Th2 cells. *J Immunol* 144: 1629–1639.
27. Del Prete GF, Maggi E, Parronchi P, Chretien I, Tiri A, Macchia D, Rici M, Banchereau J, de Vries J, Romagnani S (1988) IL-4 is an essential factor for the IgE synthesis induced *in vitro* by human T-cell clones and their supernatants. *J Immunol* 140: 4193–4198.
28. Sanderson CJ (1992) Interleukin 5, eosinophils and disease. *Blood* 79: 3101–3109.
29. Heinzel FP, Sadick MD, Holaday BJ, Coffman RL, Locksley RM (1989) Reciprocal expression of interferon γ or IL-4 during the resolution or progression of murine leishmaniasis: Evidence for expansion of distinct helper T-cell subsets. *J Exp Med* 169: 59–72.
30. Sadick MD, Heinzel FP, Holaday BJ, Pu RT, Dawkins RS, Locksley RM (1990) Cure of murine leishmaniasis with anti-interleukin-4 monoclonal antibody: Evidence for a T-cell-dependent, interferon γ-independent mechanism. *J Exp Med* 171: 115–127.
31. Scott P, Natovitz P, Coffman RL, Pearce E, Sher A (1988) Immunoregulation of cutaneous leishmaniasis: T-cell lines that transfer protective immunity or exacerbation belong to different T helper subsets and respond to distinct parasite antigens. *J Exp Med* 168: 1675–1694.
32. Mosmann TR, Sad S (1996) The expanding universe of T-cell subsets: Th1, Th2 and more. *Immunol Today* 17: 139–146.
33. Paliard X, de Waal Malefijt R, Yssel H, Blanchard D, Chretien I, Abrams J, de Vries J, Spits H (1988) Simultaneous production of IL-2, IL-4 and IFNγ by activated human CD4+ and CD8+ T-cell clones. *J Immunol* 414: 849–855.
34. Umetsu DT, Jabara HH, DeKruyff RH, Abbas AK, Abrams JS, Geha RS (1988) Functional heterogeneity among human inducer T-cell clones. *J Immunol* 140: 4211–4216.
35. Wierenga EA, Snoek M, deGroot C, Chretien I, de Bos J, Jansen HM, Kapsenberg ML (1990) Evidence for compartmentalization of functional subsets of CD4+ T lymphocytes in atopic patients. *J Immunol* 44: 4651–4656.
36. Del Prete GF, De Carli M, Mastromauro C, Macchia D, Biagiotti R, Ricci M, Romagnani S (1991) Purified protein derivative of *Mycobacterium tuberculosis* and excretory antigens of *Toxocara canis* expand *in vitro* human T-cells with stable and opposite (type 1 T helper or type 2 T helper) profile of cytokine production. *J Clin Invest* 88: 346–350.
37. Romagnani S (1991) Human Th1 and Th2: Doubt no more. *Immunol Today* 12: 256–257.
38. Maggi E, Biswas P, Del Prete G, Parronchi P, Macchia D, Simonelli C, Emmi L, De Carli M, Tiri A, Ricci M et al. (1991) Accumulation of Th2-like helper T-cell in the conjunctiva of patients with vernal conjunctivitis. *J Immunol* 146: 1169–1174.
39. van Reijsen FC, Brujnzeel-Koomen CAFM, Kalthoff FS, Maggi E, Romagnani S, Westland JKT, Mudde GC (1992) Skin-derived aeroallergen-specific T-cell clones of Th2 phenotype in patients with atopic dermatitis. *J Allergy Clin Immunol* 90: 184–192.
40. Frew AJ, Kay AB (1988) The relationship between infiltrating CD4+ lymphocytes, activated eosinophils and the magnitude of the allergen-induced late-cutaneous reaction in man. *J Immunol* 141: 4158–4162.

41. Kay AB, Ying S, Varney V, Gaga M, Durham SR, Moqbel R, Wardlaw AJ, Hamid Q (1991) Messenger RNA expression of the cytokine gene cluster interleukin 3 (IL-3), IL-4, IL-5 and granulocyte/macrophage colony-stimulating factor, in allergen-induced late-phase cutaneous reactions in atopic subjects. *J Exp Med* 173: 775–778.
42. Robinson DS, Hamid Q, Ying S, Tsicopoulos A, Brkans J, Bentley AM, Corrigan CJ, Durham SR, Kay AB (1992) Predominant Th2-like bronchoalveolar T lymphocyte population in atopic asthma. *N Engl J Med* 326: 298–304.
43. Leung DY, Martin RJ, Szefler SJ, Sher ER, Ying S, Kay AB, Hamid Q (1995) Dysregulation of interleukin 4, interleukin 5 and interferon gamma gene expression in steroid-resistant asthma. *J Exp Med* 181: 33–44.
44. Humbert M, Durham SR, Ying S, Kimmitt P, Barkans J, Assoufi B, Pfister R, Menz G, Robinson DS, Kay AB et al. (1996) Bronchial mucosal interleukin-4 (IL-4) and IL-5 expression is a feature of both atopic and non-atopic asthma. *Am J Respir Crit Care Med.* 154: 149.
45. Ying S, Durham SR, Corrigan CJ, Hamid Q, Kay AB (1995) Phenotype of cells expressing mRNA for Th2-type (interleukin 4 and interleukin 5) and Th10-type (interleukin 2 and interferon γ) cytokines in bronchoalveolar lavage and bronchial biopsies from atopic asthmatic and normal control subjects. *Am J Respir Cell Mol Biol* 12: 477–487.
46. Krishnaswamy G, Liu MC, Su SN, Kumai M, Xiao HQ, Marsh DG, Huang SK (1993) Analysis of cytokine transcripts in the bronchoalveolar lavage cells of patients with asthma. *Am J Respir Cell Mol Biol* 9: 279–286.
47. Ying S, Humbert M, Barkans J, Corrigan CJ, Pfister R, Menz G, Robinson DS, Larche M, Durham SR, Kay AB (1997). Expression of IL-4 and IL-5 mRNA and protein product by CD4+ and CD8+ T-cells, eosinophils and mast cells in bronchial biopsies obtained from atopic and non-atopic (intrinsic) asthmatics. *J Immunol* 158: 355.
48. Walker C, Bode E, Boer L, Hansel TT, Blaser K, Virchow J-C Jr (1992) Allergic and non-allergic asthmatics have distinct patterns of T-cell activation and cytokine production in peripheral blood and bronchoalveolar lavage. *Am Rev Respir Dis* 146: 109–115.
49. Till S, Li B, Durham SR, Humbert M, Assoufi B, Huston D, Dickason R, Jeannin P, Kay AB, Corrigan CJ (1995) Secretion of the eosinophil-active cytokines interleukin 5, granulocyte macrophage colony stimulating factor and interleukin 3 by bronchoalveolar lavage CD4+ and CD8+ T-cell lines in atopic asthmatics. *Eur J Immunol* 25: 2727–2731.
50. Kamei T, Ozaki T, Kawaji K, Banno K, Sano T, Azuma M, Ogura T (1993) Production of interleukin-5 and granulocyte/macrophage colony-stimulating factor by T-cells of patients with bronchial asthma in response to *Dermatophagoides farinae* and its relation to eosinophil colony-stimulating factor. *Am J Respir Cell Mol Biol* 9: 378–385.
51. Del-Prete GF, De Carli M, D'Elios MM, Maestrelli P, Ricci M, Fabbri L, Romagnani S (1993) Allergen exposure induces the activation of allergen-specific Th2 cells in the airway mucosa of patients with allergic respiratory disorders. *Eur J Immunol* 23: 1445–1449.
52. Krug N, Madden J, Redington AE, Lackie P, Djukanovic R, Schauer U, Holgate ST, Frew AJ, Howarth PH (1996) T-cell cytokine profile evaluated at the single cell level in BAL and blood in allergic asthma. *Am J Respir Cell Mol Biol* 14: 319–326.
53. Gleich GJ (1990) The eosinophil and bronchial asthma: Current understanding. *J Allergy Clin Immunol* 85: 422–436.
54. Weller PF (1991) The immunobiology of eosinophils. *N Engl J Med* 324: 1110–1118.
55. Gleich GJ, Loegering DA, Bell MP, Checkel JL, Ackerman SJ, McKean DJ (1986) Biochemical and functional similarities between eosinophil derived neurotoxin and eosinophil cationic protein: homology with ribonuclease. *Proc Natl Acad Sci USA* 83: 3146–3150.
56. Frigas E, Loergering DA, Solley G, Farrow G, Gleich GJ (1981) Elevated levels of the eosinophil major basic protein in the sputum of patients with bronchial asthma. *Mayo Clin Proc* 56: 345–353.
57. Shaw RJ, Walsh GM, Cromwell O, Moqbel R, Spry CJF, Kay AB (1985) Activated human eosinophils generate SRS-A leukotrienes following physiological (IgG-dependent) stimulation. *Nature* 316: 150–152.
58. Clutterbuck EJ, Hirst EM, Sanderson CJ (1989) Human interleukin 5 (IL-5) regulates the production of eosinophils in human bone marrow cultures: Comparison and interaction with IL-1, IL-3, IL-6 and GM-CSF. *Blood* 73: 1504–1512.

59. Rothenberg ME, Owen WF Jr, Silberstein DS, Woods J, Soberman RJ, Austen KF, Stevens RL (1988) Human eosinophils have prolonged survival, enhanced functional properties and become hypodense when exposed to interleukin 3. *J Clin Invest* 81: 1986–1992.

60. Owen WF Jr, Rothenberg ME, Silberstein DS, Gasson J, Stevens RL, Austen KF, Soberman RJ (1987) Regulation of human eosinophil viability, density and function by granulocyte/macrophage colony stimulating factor in the presence of 3T3 fibroblasts. *J Exp Med* 166: 129–141.

61. Fujisawa T, Abu-Ghazaleh R, Kita H, Sanderson CJ, Gleich GJ (1990) Regulatory effect of cytokines on eosinophil degranulation. *J Immunol* 144: 642–646.

62. Walsh GM, Hartnell A, Wardlaw AJ, Kurihara K, Sanderson CJ, Kay AB (1990) IL-5 enhances the *in vitro* adhesion of human eosinophils, but not neutrophils in a leucocyte integrin (CD11/CD18)-dependent manner. *Immunology* 71: 258–265.

63. Her E, Frazer J, Austen KF, Owen WF Jr (1991) Eosinophil haematopoietins antagonise the programmed cell death of eosinophils. *J Clin Invest* 88: 1982–1987.

64. Tavernier J, Devos R, Cornelis S, Tuypens T, van der Heyden J, Fiers W, Plaetinck G (1991) A human high affinity interleukin-5 receptor (IL5R) is composed of an IL-5 specific α chain and a β chain shared with the receptor for GM-CSF. *Cell* 66: 1175–1184.

65. Kitamura T, Sato N, Arai K, Miyajima A (1991) Expression cloning of the human IL-3 receptor cDNA reveals a shared β subunit for the human IL-3 and GM-CSF receptors. *Cell* 66: 1165–1174.

66. Lopez AF, Elliott MJ, Woodcock J, Vadas MA (1992) GM-CSF, IL-3 and IL-5: Cross-competition on human haemopoietic cells. *Immunol Today* 13: 495–500.

67. Tavernier J, Tuypens T, Plaetinck G, Verhee A, Fiers W, Devos R (1992) Molecular basis of the membrane-anchored and two soluble isoforms of the human interleukin-5 receptor α subunit. *Proc Natl Acad Sci USA* 89: 7041–7045.

68. Yasruel Z, Humbert M, Kotsimbos ATC, Ploysongsang Y, Minshall E, Durham SR, Pfister R, Menz G, Tavernier J, Kay AB et al. (1997) Expression of the membrane-bound and soluble interleukin-5 α receptor mRNA in the bronchial mucosa of atopic and non-atopic asthmatics. *Am J Respir Crit Care Med.* 155: 1413–1418.

69. Symon FA, Walsh GM, Watson SR, Wardlaw AJ (1994) Eosinophil adhesion to nasal polyp endothelium is P-selectin-dependent. *J Exp Med* 180: 371–376.

70. Walsh GM, Hartnell AH, Mermod JJ, Kay AB, Wardlaw AJ (1991) Human eosinophil, but not neutrophil, adherence to IL-1 stimulated HUVEC is $\alpha4\beta1$ (VLA-4) dependent. *J Immunol* 146: 3419–3123.

71. Schleimer RP, Sterbinsky SA, Kaiser J, Bickel CA, Klunk DA, Tomioka K, Newman W, Luscinskas FW, Gimbrone MA, McIntyre BW et al. (1992) IL-4 induces adherence of human eosinophils and basophils, but not neutrophils, to endothelium. *J Immunol* 148: 1086–1089.

72. Bentley AM, Robinson DS, Durham SR, Cromwell O, Kay AB, Wardlaw AJ (1993) Expression of the endothelial and leukocyte adhesion molecules ICAM-1, E-selectin and VCAM-1 in the bronchial mucosa in steady state and allergen-induced asthma. *J Allergy Clin Immunol* 92: 857–868.

73. Kita H, Ohnishi T, Okubo Y, Weiler D, Abrams JS, Gleich GJ (1991) GM-CSF and interleukin-3 release from human peripheral blood eosinophils and neutrophils. *J Exp Med* 174: 745–748.

74. Moqbel R, Hamid Q, Ying S, Barkans J, Hartnell A, Tsicopoulos A, Wardlaw AJ, Kay AB (1991) Expression of mRNA for the granulocyte macrophage colony-stimulating factor by activated human eosinophils. *J Exp Med* 174: 749–751.

75. Moqbel R, Levi-Schaffer F, Kay AB (1994) Cytokine generation by eosinophils. *J Allergy Clin Immunol* 94: 1183–1188.

76. Desreumaux P, Janin A, Colombel JF, Prin L, Plumas J, Emilie D, Torpier G, Capron A, Capron M (1992) Interleukin-5 messenger RNA expression by eosinophils in the intestinal mucosa of patients with coeliac disease. *J Exp Med* 175: 293–296.

77. Ying S, Meng Q, Taborda-Barata L, Corrigan CJ, Barkans J, Assoufi B, Moqbel R, Durham SR, Kay AB (1996) Human eosinophils express messenger RNA encoding RANTES and store and release biologically active RANTES protein. *Eur J Immunol* 26: 70–76.

78. Moqbel R, Ying S, Barkans J, Newman TM, Kimmitt P, Wakelin M, Taborda-Barata L, Meng Q, Corrigan CJ, Durham SR et al. (1995) Identification of messenger RNA for IL-4 in human eosinophils with granule localization and release of the translated product. *J Immunol* 155: 4939–4947.

79. Gauchat J-F, Henchoz S, Fattah D, Mazzei G, Aubry J-P, Jomotte T, Dash L, Page K, Solari R, Aldebert D (1995) CD40 ligand is functionally expressed on human eosinophils. *Eur J Immunol* 25: 863–865.

80. Ohkawara Y, Lim KG, Xing Z, Glibetic M, Nakano K, Dolovich J, Croitoru K, Weller PF, Jordana M (1996) CD40 expression by human peripheral blood eosinophils. *J Clin Invest* 97: 1761–1766.

81. Valerius T, Repp R, Kalden JR, Platzer E (1990) Effects of IFNγ on human eosinophils in comparison with other cytokines. *J Immunol* 145: 2950–2958.

82. Silberstein DS, Desseain AJ, Elsas PP, Fontaine B, David JR (1987) Characterisation of a factor from the U937 cell line that enhances the toxicity of human eosinophils to *Schistosoma mansoni* larvae. *J Immunol* 138: 3042–3050.

83. Abu-Ghazaleh RI, Fujisawa T, Mestecky J, Kyle RA, Gleich GJ (1989) IgA-induced eosinophil degranulation. *J Immunol* 142: 2393–2400.

84. Gounni AS, Lamkhioued B, Ochiai K, Tanaka Y, Delaporte E, Capron A, Kinet JP, Capron M (1994) High-affinity IgE receptor on eosinophils is involved in defence against parasites. *Nature* 367: 183–186.

85. Kon OM, Sihra BS, Grant JA, Kay AB (1996) Expression of high-affinity IgE receptors on peripheral blood basophils, monocytes and eosinophils in atopic subjects. *J Allergy Clin Immunol* 97: 358 (abstract).

86. Taborda-Barata L, Grant JA, Humbert M, Barkans J, Ying S, Kay AB (1996) Recruitment of high-affinity IgE receptor (FcεRI) bearing cells in allergen-induced skin late phase reactions. *J Allergy Clin Immunol* 97: 425 (abstract).

87. Rodewald HR, Dessing M, Dvorak AM, Galli SJ (1996) Identification of a committed precursor for the mast cell lineage. *Science* 271: 818–822.

88. Galli SJ (1993) New concepts about the mast cell. *N Engl J Med* 328: 257–265.

89. Schlechter NM, Fraki JE, Geesin JC, Lazarus GS (1983) Human skin chymotryptic proteinase: Iolation and relation to cathepsin G and rat mast cell protease. *J Biol Chem* 258: 2973–2978.

90. Schwartz LB, Lewis RA, Austen KF (1981) Tryptase from human pulmonary mast cells: Purification and characterization. *J Biol Chem* 256: 11939–11943.

91. Liu MC, Hubbard WC, Proud D, Stealey BA, Galli SJ, Kagey-Sobotka A, Bleeker ER, Lichtenstein LM (1991) Immediate and late inflammatory responses to ragweed antigen challenge of the peripheral airways in allergic asthmatics. *Am Rev Respir Dis* 144: 51–56.

92. Tam EK, Caughey GH (1990) Degradation of airway neuropeptides by human lung tryptase. *Am J Respir Cell Mol Biol* 3: 27–32.

93. Sekizawa K, Caughey GH, Lazarus SC, Gold WM, Nadel JA (1989) Mast cell tryptase causes airway smooth muscle hyperresponsiveness in dogs. *J Clin Invest* 83: 175–179.

94. Irani AA, Schlechter NM, Craig SS, DeBlois G, Schwartz LB (1986) Two types of human mast cells that have distinct neutral protease compositions. *Proc Natl Acad Sci USA* 83: 4464–4468.

95. Robinson C, Benyon RC, Holgate ST, Church MK (1989) The IgE- and calcium-dependent release of eiconsanoids and histamine from human cutaneous mast cells. *J Invest Dermatol* 93: 397–404.

96. Plaut M, Pierce JH, Watson CJ, Haney-Hyde J, Nordan RP, Paul WE (1989) Mast cell lines produce lymphokines in response to cross-linkage of FcεRI or calcium ionophore. *Nature* 329: 64–67.

97. Wodnar-Filipowicz A, Heusser CH, Moroni C (1989) Production of the haemopoeitic growth factors GM-CSF and interleukin-3 by mast cells in response to IgE receptor-mediated activation. *Nature* 339: 150–152.

98. Gordon JR, Galli SJ (1991) Release of both preformed and newly synthesised tumour necrosis factor alpha (TNFα)/cachectin by mouse mast cells stimulated via the FCεRI: A mechanism for the sustained action of mast cell-derived TNFα during IgE-dependent biological responses. *J Exp Med* 174: 103–107.

99. Walsh LJ, Trinchieri G, Waldorf HA, Whitaker D, Murphy GF (1991) Human dermal mast cells contain and release tumour necrosis factor alpha, which induces endothelial leukocyte adhesion molecule 1. *Proc Natl Acad Sci USA* 88: 4220–4224.
100. Church MK, Hiroi J (1987) Inhibition of IgE-dependent histamine release from human dispersed lung mast cells by anti-allergic drugs and salbutamol. *Br J Pharmacol* 90: 421–429.
101. Bradding P, Feather IH, Wilson S, Bardin PG, Heusser CH, Holgate ST, Howarth PH (1993) Immunolocalization of cytokines in the nasal mucosa of normal and perennial rhinitic subjects: The mast cell as a source of IL-4, IL-5 and IL-6 in human allergic mucosal inflammation. *J Immunol* 151: 3853–3865.
102. Bradding P, Feather IH, Howarth PH, Mueller R, Roberts JA, Britten K, Bews JPA, Hunt TC, Okayama Y, Heuser CH et al. (1992) Interleukin-4 is localized to and released by human mast cells. *J Exp Med* 176: 1381–1386.
103. Okayama Y, Petit Frere C, Kassel O, Semper A, Quint D, Tunon-de-Lara MJ, Bradding P, Holgate ST, Church MK (1995) IgE-dependent expression of mRNA for IL-4 and IL-5 in human lung mast cells. *J Immunol* 155: 1796–1808.
104. Bradding P, Roberts JA, Britten KM, Montefort S, Djukanovic R, Mueller R, Heusser CH, Howarth PH, Holgate ST (1994) Interleukin-4, -5, -6 and tumor necrosis factor-alpha in normal and asthmatic airways: Evidence for the human mast cell as a source of these cytokines. *Am J Respir Cell Mol Biol* 10: 471–480.
105. Ying S, Humbet M, Barkans J, Corrigan CJ, Pfister R, Menz G, Larche M, Robinson DS, Durham SR, Kay AB (1997). Expression of IL-4 and IL-5 mRNA and protein product by CD4+ and CD8+ T-cells, eosinophils and mast cells in bronchial biopsies obtained from atopic and non-atopic (intrinsic) asthmatics. *J Immunol* 158: 3539–3544.
106. Kupfer A, Mosmann TR, Kupfer H (1991) Polarized expression of cytokines in cell conjugates of helper T-cells and splenic B-cells. *Proc Natl Acad Sci USA* 88: 775–779.
107. Burd PR, Thompson WC, Max EE, Mills FC (1996) Activated mast cells produce interleukin-13. *J Exp Med* 181: 1373–1380.
108. Gauchat J-F, Henchoz S, Mazzei G, Aubry J-P, Brunner T, Blasey H, Life P, Talabot D, Flores-Romo L, Thompson J et al. (1993) Induction of human IgE synthesis in B-cells by mast cells and basophils. *Nature* 365: 340–343.
109. Ying S, Meng Q, Barata LT, Robinson DS, Durham SR, Kay AB (1997). IL-13, but not IL-4, correlates with upregulation of VCAM-1 and infiltration of eosinophils, macrophages and T-cells in the allergen-induced late-phase cutaneous response in atopic subjects. *J Immunol* 158: 5050–5057.
110. Leung DY, Pober JS, Cotran RS (1991) Expression of endothelial-leukocyte adhesion molecule-1 in elicited late phase allergic reactions. *J Clin Invest* 87: 1805–1809.
111. Walsh LJ, Trinchieri G, Waldorf HA, Whitaker D, Murphy GF (1991) Human dermal mast cells contain and release tumor necrosis factor alpha, which induces endothelial leukocyte adhesion molecule 1. *Proc Natl Acad Sci USA* 88: 4220–4224.
112. Denburg JA (1992) Basophil and mast cell lineages *in vitro* and *in vivo*. *Blood* 79: 846–860.
113. MacGlashan DW, Peters SP, Warner J, Lichtenstein LM (1986) Characteristics of human basophil sulfidopeptide leukotriene release: Releaseability defined as the ability of basophils to respond to dimeric cross-links. *J Immunol* 136: 2231–2238.
114. Bischoff SC, Brunner T, DeWeck AL, Dahinden CA (1990) Interleukin-5 modifies histamine release and leukotriene generation by human basophils in response to diverse agonists. *J Exp Med* 172: 1577–1585.
115. Kurimoto Y, de Weck AL, Dahinden CA (1989) Interleukin-3-dependent mediator release in basophils triggered by C5a. *J Exp Med* 170: 467–479.
116. Baggiolini M, Dahinden CA (1994) CC chemokines in allergic inflammation. *Immunol Today* 15: 127–133.
117. MacDonald SM, Rafnar T, Langdon J, Lichtenstein LM (1995) Molecular identification of an IgE-dependent histamine-releasing factor. *Science* 269: 688–690.
118. Piccini MP, Macchia D, Parronchi P, Giudizi MG, Bani D, Alterini R, Grossi A, Ricci M, Maggi E, Romagnani S (1991) Human bone marrow non-B, non-T-cells produce IL-4 in response to cross linkage of Fcε and Fcγ receptors. *Proc Natl Acad Sci USA* 88: 8656–8660.

119. Brunner T, Heusser CH, Dahinden CA (1993) Human peripheral blood basophils primed by interleukin 3 (IL-3) produce IL-4 in response to immunoglobulin E receptor stimulation. *J Exp Med* 177: 605–611.

120. Ben-Sasson SZ, Le-Gros G, Conrad DH, Finkelman FD, Paul WE (1990) Cross-linking Fc receptors stimulate splenic non-B, non-T-cells to secrete interleukin-4 and other lymphokines. *Proc Natl Acad Sci USA* 87: 421–425.

121. Bascom R, Wachs M, Naclerio RM, Pipkorn U, Galli SJ, Lichtenstein LM (1988) Basophil influx occurs after nasal antigen challenge: Effects of topical corticosteroid pretreatment. *J Allergy Clin Immunol* 81: 580–589.

122. Liu MC, Hubbard WC, Proud D, Stealey BA, Galli SJ, Kagey-Sobotka A, Bleeker ER, Lichtenstein LM (1991) Immediate and late inflammatory responses to ragweed antigen challenge of peripheral airways in allergic asthmatics. *Am Rev Respir Dis* 144: 51–58.

123. Poston RN, Chanez P, Lacoste JY, Lichfield T, Lee TH, Bousquet J (1992) Immunohistochemical characterisation of the cellular infiltrate in asthmatic bronchi. *Am Rev Respir Dis* 145: 918–921.

124. Bentley AM, Menz G, Storz C, Robinson DS, Bradley BL, Jeffery PK, Durham SR, Kay AB (1992) Identification of T lymphocytes, macrophages and activated eosinophils in the bronchial mucosa in intrinsic asthma. *Am Rev Respir Dis* 146: 500–506.

125. Joseph M, Tonnel AB, Torpier G, Capron A, Arnoux B, Benveniste J (1983) Involvement of immunoglobulin E in the secretory processes of alveolar macrophages from asthmatic patients. *J Clin Invest* 71: 221–230.

126. Tonnel AB, Gossett P, Joseph M, Lassalle P, Dessant JP, Capron A (1986) Alveolar macrophage and its participation in the inflammatory processes of allergic asthma. *Bull Eur Physiopathol Respir* 22: 70–77.

127. Greenbaum LA, Horowitz JB, Woods A, Pasqualinin T, Reich EP, Bottomly K (1988) Autocrine growth of CD4 T-cells: Differential effects of IL-1 on helper and inflammatory T-cells. *J Immunol* 140: 1555–1560.

128. Howell CJ, Pujol JL, Crea AEG, Davidson R, Gearing AJH, Godrard PH, Lee TH (1989) Identification of an alveolar macrophage-derived activity in bronchial asthma that enhances leukotriene C4 generation by human eosinophils stimulated by ionophore A23187 as a granulocyte macrophage colony stimulating factor. *Am Rev Respir Dis* 140: 1340–1347.

129. Robinson DS, Tsicopoulos A, Meng Q, Durham SR, Kay AB, Hamid Q (1996) Increased interleukin-10 messenger RNA expression in atopic allergy and asthma. *Am J Respir Cell Mol Biol* 14: 113–117.

130. D'Andrea A, Ma X, Aste Amezaga M, Paganin C, Trinchieri G (1995) Stimulatory and inhibitory effects of interleukin (IL)-4 and IL-13 on the production of cytokines by human peripheral blood mononuclear cells: Priming for IL-12 and tumor necrosis factor alpha production. *J Exp Med* 181: 537–546.

131. Chelen CJ, Fang Y, Freeman GJ, Secrist H, Marshall JD, Hwang PT, Frankel LR, DeKruyff RH, Umetsu DT (1995) Human alveolar macrophages present antigen ineffectively due to defective expression of B7 costimulatory cell surface molecules. *J Clin Invest* 95: 1415–1421.

132. Gant V, Cluzel M, Shakoor Z, Rees JP, Lee TH, Hamblin AS (1992) Alveolar macrophage accessory cell function in bronchial asthma. *Am Rev Respir Dis* 146: 900–904.

133. Spiteri MA, Knight RJ, Jeremy JY, Barnes PJ, Chung KF (1994) Alveolar macrophage-induced suppression of peripheral blood mononuclear cell responsiveness is reversed by *in vitro* allergen exposure in bronchial asthma. *Eur Respir J* 7: 1431–1438.

134. Maurer D, Ebner C, Reininger B, Fiebiger E, Kraft D, Kinet JP, Stingl G (1995) The high-affinity IgE receptor mediated IgE-dependent allergen presentation. *J Immunol* 154: 6285–6290.

135. Holt PG, Schon-Hegrad MA, Phillips MJ, McMenamin PG (1989) Ia-positive dendritic cells form a tightly meshed network within the human airway epithelium. *Clin Exp Allergy* 19: 597–601.

136. Macatonia SE, Hosken NA, Litton M, Vieira P, Hsieh CS, Culpepper JA, Wysocka M, Trinchieri G, Murphy KM, O'Garra A (1995) Dendritic cells produce IL-12 and direct the development of Th1 cells from naive CD4[+] T-cells. *J Immunol* 154: 5071–5079.

137. Davies RJ, Wang JH, Trigg CJ, Devalia JL (1995) Expression of granulocyte/macrophage-colony-stimulating factor, interleukin-8 and RANTES in the bronchial epithelium of mild asthmatics is down-regulated by inhaled beclomethasone dipropionate. *Int Arch Allergy Immunol* 107: 428–429.

138. Garcia-Zepeda EA, Rothenberg ME, Ownbey RT, Celestin J, Leder P, Luster AD (1996) Human eotaxin is a specific chemoattractant for eosinophil cells and provides a new mechanism to explain tissue eosinophilia. *Nat Med* 2: 449–456.

139. Kalb TH, Chuang MT, Marom Z, Mayer L (1991) Evidence for accessory cell function by class II MHC antigen-expressing airway epithelial cells. *Am J Respir Cell Mol Biol* 4: 320–329.

140. Asano K, Chee CB, Gaston B, Lilly CM, Gerard C, Drazen JM, Stamler JS (1994) Constitutive and inducible nitric oxide synthase gene expression, regulation and activity in human lung epithelial cells. *Proc Natl Acad Sci USA* 91: 10089–10093.

141. Kharitonov SA, Yates D, Robbins RA, Logan-Sinclair R, Shinebourne EA, Barnes PJ (1994) Increased nitric oxide in exhaled air of asthmatic patients. *Lancet* 343: 133–135.

142. Barnes PJ, Liew FY (1995) Nitric oxide and asthmatic inflammation. *Immunol Today* 16: 128–130.

143. Geha RS (1992) Regulation of IgE synthesis in humans. *J Allergy Clin Immunol* 90: 143–150.

144. Gauchat J-F, Lebman DA, Coffman RL, Gascan H, de Vries JE (1990) Structure and expression of germline ε transcripts in human B-cells induced by interleukin-4 to switch to IgE production. *J Exp Med* 172: 463–468.

145. Del Prete GF, Maggi E, Parronchi P, Chretien I, Tiri A, Macchia D, Ricci M, Banchereau J, de Vries J, Romagnani S (1988) IL-4 as an essential factor for the IgE synthesis induced *in vitro* by human T-cell clones and their supernatants. *J Immunol* 140: 4193–4198.

146. McKenzie ANJ, Culpepper JA, de Waal Malefyt R, Briere F, Punnonen J, Aversa G, Sato A, Dang W, Cocks BG, Menon S et al. (1993) Interleukin 13, a T-cell derived cytokine that regulates human monocyte and B-cell function. *Proc Natl Acad Sci USA* 90: 3735–3739.

147. Zurawski G, de Vries JE (1994) Interleukin-13, an interleukin-4-like cytokine that acts on monocytes and B-cells but not on T-cells. *Immunol Today* 15: 19–26.

148. Pene J, Rousset F, Briere F, Chretien I, Wideman J, Bonnefoy JY, de Vries JE (1988) Interleukin-5 enhances interleukin-4-indced IgE production by normal human B-cells: The role of soluble CD23 antigen. *Eur J Immunol* 18: 929–935.

149. Vercelli D, Jabara HH, Arai K, Yokota T, Geha RS (1989) Endogenous IL-6 plays an obligatory role in IL-4-induced human IgE synthesis. *Eur J Immunol* 19: 1419–1422.

150. Kinawa M, Gateley M, Gubler R, Chizzonite R, Fargas C, Delespesse G (1992) Recombinant interleukin-12 suppresses the synthesis of immunoglobulin E by interleukin-4-stimulated human lymphocytes. *J Clin Invest* 90: 262–266.

151. Kimata H, Yoshida A, Ishioka C, Lindley I, Mikawa H (1992) Interleukin-8 (IL-8) selectively inhibits immunoglobulin E production induced by IL-4 in human B-cells. *J Exp Med* 176: 1227–1231.

152. Kimata H (1996) RANTES and macrophage inflammatory protein 1α selectively enhance immunoglobulin (IgE) and IgG4 production by human B-cells. *J Exp Med* 183: 2397–2402.

153. Zhang K, Clark EA, Saxon A (1991) CD40 stimulation provides an IFNγ-independent signal directly to human B-cells for IgE production. *J Immunol* 146: 1836–1842.

154. Diaz-Sanchez D, Chegini DS, Chang K, Saxon A (1994) CD58 (LFA3) stimulation provides a signal for human isotype switching and IgE production distinct from CD40. *J Immunol* 153: 10–19.

155. Rock KL, Benacerraf B, Abbas AK (1984) Antigen presentation by hapten-specific B lymphocytes. I. Role of surface immunoglobulin receptors. *J Exp Med* 160: 1102–1113.

156. Gajewski TF, Pinnas M, Wong T, Fitch FW (1991) Murine Th1 and Th2 clones proliferate optimally in response to distinct antigen-presenting cell populations. *J Immunol* 146: 1750–1758.

157. Secrist H, DeKruyff RH, Umetsu DT (1995) Interleukin-4 production by CD4+ T-cells from allergic individuals is modulated by antigen concentration and antigen-presenting cell type. *J Exp Med* 181: 1081–1089.

158. Blotta MH, Marshall JD, DeKruyff RH, Umetsu DT (1996) Cross-linking of the CD40 ligand on human CD4⁺ T lymphocytes generates a costimulatory signal that up-regulates IL-4 synthesis. *J Immunol* 156: 3133–3140.
159. Durham SR, Gould HJ, Thiennes CP, Jacobson MR, Masuyama K, Rak S, Lowhagen O, Schotman E, Hamid Q (1996) Local control of ε-gene expression in B-cells of the nasal mucosa in hay fever patients following allergen challenge. *J Allergy Clin Immunol* 97: 297 (abstract 460).
160. Sutton BJ, Gould HJ (1993) The human IgE network. *Nature* 366: 421–428.
161. Beavil RL, Graber P, Aubonney N, Bonnefoy JY, Gould HJ (1995) CD23/Fc epsilon RII and its soluble fragments can form oligomers on the cell surface and in solution. *Immunology* 84: 202–206.
162. Bonnefoy JY, Gauchat JF, Life P, Graber P, Aubry JP, Lecoanet-Henchoz S (1995) Regulation of IgE synthesis by CD23/CD21 interaction. *Int Arch Allergy Immunol* 107: 40–42.
163. Metzger WJ, Zavala D, Richerson HB, Moseley P, Iwamota P, Monick M, Sjoerdsma K, Hunnighake GW (1987) Local allergen challenge and bronchoalveolar lavage of allergic asthmatic lungs: Description of the model and local airway inflammation. *Am Rev Respir Dis* 135: 433–440.
164. Corrigan CJ, Collard P, Nagy L, Kay AB (1991) Cultured peripheral blood mononuclear cells derived from patients with acute severe asthma ("status asthmaticus") spontaneously elaborate a neutrophil chemotactic activity distinct from interleukin-8. *Am Rev Respir Dis* 143: 538–544.
165. Hallsworth MP, Soh CP, Lane SJ, Arm JP, Lee TH (1994) Selective enhancement of GM-CSF, TNF-alpha, IL-1 beta and IL-8 production by monocytes and macrophages of asthmatic subjects. *Eur Respir J* 7: 1096–1102.
166. Baggiolini M, Loetscher P, Moser B (1995) Interleukin-8 and the chemokine family. *Int J Immunopharmacol* 17: 103–108.
167. Sur S, Crotty TB, Kephart GM, Hyman BA, Colby TV, Reed CE, Hunt LW, Gleich GJ (1993) Sudden-onset fatal asthma: A distinct entity with few eosinophils and relatively more neutrophils in the airway submucosa? *Am Rev Respir Dis* 148: 713–719.
168. Page CP (1989) Platelets and asthma. *Agents Actions Suppl* 28: 75–84.
169. Barnes PJ (1991) Neuropeptides and asthma. *Am Rev Respir Dis* 143: S28–32.
170. Roche WR, Beasley R, Williams JH, Holgate ST (1989) Subepithelial fibrosis in the bronchi of asthmatics. *Lancet* I: 520–524.
171. Jeffery PK, Godfrey RW, Adelroth E, Nelson F, Rogers A, Johansson SA (1992) Effects of treatment on airway inflammation and thickening of basement reticular collagen in asthma. *Am Rev Respir Dis* 145: 890–899.
172. Trigg CJ, Manolitsas ND, Wang J, Calderon MA, McAulay A, Jordan SE, Herdman MJ, Jhalli N, Duddle JM, Hamilton SA et al. (1994) Placebo-controlled immunopathologic study of four months of inhaled corticosteroids in asthma. *Am J Respir Crit Care Med* 150: 17–22.
173. Maestrelli P, De Marzo N, Saetta M, Boscaro M, Fabbri LM, Mapp CE (1993) Effects of inhaled beclomethasone on airway responsiveness in occupational asthma: Placebo-controlled study of subjects sensitized to toluene diisocyanate. *Am Rev Respir Dis* 148: 407–412.
174. Baggiolini M, Dahinden CA (1994) CC chemokines in allergic inflammation. *Immunol Today* 15: 127–133.
175. Kameyoshi Y, Dorschner A, Mallet AI, Christophers E, Schroder J-M (1992) Cytokine RANTES relesed by thrombin stimulated platelets is a potent attractant for human eosinophils. *J Exp Med* 176. 587–592.
176. Bischoff SC, Krieger M, Brunner T, Rot A, von Tscharner V, Baggiolini M, Dahinden CA (1993) RANTES and related chemokines activate human basophil granulocytes through different G protein-coupled receptors. *Eur J Immunol* 23: 761–767.
177. Schall TJ, Bacon K, Toy KJ, Goeddel DV (1990) Selective attraction of monocytes and T lymphocytes of the memory phenotype by cytokine RANTES. *Nature* 347: 669–671.
178. Randolph GJ, Furie MB (1995) A soluble gradient of endogenous monocyte chemoattractant protein-1 promotes the transendothelial migration of monocytes *in vitro*. *J Immunol* 155: 3610–3618.

179. Jose PJ, Griffiths-Johnson DA, Collins PD, Walsh DT, Moqbel R, Totty NF, Truong O, Hsuan JJ, Williams TJ (1994) Eotaxin: A potent eosinophil chemoattractant cytokine detected in a guinea pig model of allergic airways inflammation. *J Exp Med* 179: 881–887.
180. Ponath PD, Qin S, Ringler DJ, Clark-Lewis I, Wang J, Kassam N, Smith H, Shi X, Gonzalo J-A, Newman W et al. (1996) Cloning of the human eosinophil chemoattractant, eotaxin. *J Clin Invest* 97: 604–612.
181. Uguccioni-M, Loetscher P, Forssmann U, Dewald B, Li H, Lima SH, Li-Y, Kreider B, Garotta G, Thelen M et al. (1996) Monocyte chemotactic protein 4 (MCP-4), a novel structural and functional analogue of MCP-3 and eotaxin. *J Exp Med* 183: 2379–2384.
182. Daugherty BL, Siciliano SJ, DeMartino JA, Malkowitz L, Sirotina A, Springer MS (1996) Cloning, expression and characterization of the human eosinophil eotaxin receptor. *J Exp Med* 183: 2349–2354.
183. Ying S, Taborda Barata L, Meng Q, Humbert M, Kay AB (1995) The kinetics of allergen-induced transcription of messenger RNA for monocyte chemotactic protein 3 and RANTES in the skin of human atopic subjects: Relationship to eosinophil, T-cell and macrophage recruitement. *J Exp Med* 181: 2153–2159.
184. Humbert M, Ying S, Corrigan CJ, Menz G, Barkans J, Pfister R, Meng Q, Van Damme J, Opdenakker G, Durham SR et al. Bronchial mucosal expression of the genes encoding CC chemokines RANTES and MCP-3 in symptomatic atopic and non-atopic asthmatics: Relationship to the eosinophil active cytokines IL-5, GM-CSF and IL-3. *Am J Respir Crit Care Med.* In Press.
185. Sim TC, Reece LM, Hilsmeier KA, Grant JA, Alam R (1995) Secretion of chemokines and other cytokines in allergen-induced nasal late responses: Inhibition by topical steroid treatment. *Am J Respir Crit Care Med* 152: 927–933.
186. Newman-Taylor AJ, Tee RD (1989) Occupational lung disease. *Curr Opin Immunol* 1: 684–689.
187. Sears MR, Burrows B, Flannery EM, Herbison GP, Hewitt CJ, Holdaway MD (1991) Relation between airway responsiveness and serum IgE in children with asthma and in apparently normal children. *N Engl J Med* 325: 1067–1071.
188. Fabbri LM, Danieli D, Crescioli S, Bevilacqua P, Meli S, Saetta M, Mapp CE (1988) Fatal asthma in a subject sensitized to toluene diisocyanate. *Am Rev Respir Dis* 137: 1494–1498.
189. Bentley AM, Maestrelli P, Saetta M, Fabbri LM, Robinson DS, Bradley BL, Jeffery PK, Durham SR, Kay AB (1992) Activated T-lymphocytes and eosinophils in the bronchial mucosa in isocyanate-induced asthma. *J Allergy Clin Immunol* 89: 821–829.
190. Walker C, Kaegi MK, Braun P, Blaser K (1991) Activated T-cells and eosinophilia in bronchoalveolar lavages from subjects with asthma correlated with disease severity. *J Allergy Clin Immunol* 88: 935–942.
191. Humbert M, Grant JA, Taborda-Barata L, Durham SR, Pfister R, Menz G, Barkans J, Ying S, Kay AB (1996) High-affinity IgE receptor (FcεRI)-bearing cells in bronchial biopsies from atopic and nonatopic asthma. *Am J Respir Crit Care Med* 153: 1931–1937.
192. Maestrelli P, Del Prete GF, De Carli M, D'Elios MM, Saetta M, Di Stefano A, Mapp CE, Romagnani S, Fabbri LM (1994) CD8 T-cell clones producing interleukin-5 and interferon-gamma in bronchial mucosa of patients with asthma induced by toluene diisocyanate. *Scand J Work Environ Health* 20: 376–381.
193. Durham SR (1990) Late asthmatic responses. *Respir Med* 84: 263–268.
194. Cartier A, Thomson NC, Frith PA, Roberts R, Hargreave FE (1982) Allergen-induced increase in bronchial responsiveness to histamine: Relationship to the late asthmatic response and change in airway calibre. *J Allergy Clin Immunol* 70: 170–177.
195. MacIntyre D, Boyd G (1983) Site of airflow obstruction in immediate and late reactions to bronchial challenge with *Dermataphagoides pteronyssinus. Clin Allergy* 13: 213–218.
196. Bentley AM, Meng Q, Robinson DS, Hamid Q, Kay AB, Durham SR (1993) Increases in activated T lymphocytes, eosinophils and cytokine messenger RNA expression or IL-5 and GM-CSF in bronchial biopsies after allergen inhalation challenge in atopic asthmatics. *Am J Respir Cell Mol Biol* 8: 35–42.
197. Robinson DS, Hamid Q, Bentley AM, Ying S, Kay AB, Durham SR (1993) CD4+ T-cell activation, eosinophil recruitment and interleukin 4 (IL-4), IL-5 and GM-CSF messenger RNA expression in bronchoalveolar lavage after allergen inhalation challenge of atopic asthmatics. *J Allergy Clin Immunol* 92: 313–324.

198. Broide DH, Firestein GS (1991) Endobronchial allergen challenge in asthma: Demonstration of cellular source of granulocyte macrophage colony-stimulating factor by *in situ* hybridization. *J Clin Invest* 88: 1048–1053.
199. Sedgwick JB, Calhoun WJ, Gleich GJ, Kita H, Abrams JS, Schwartz LB, Volovitz B, Ben-Yaakov M, Busse W (1991) Immediate and late airway response of allergic rhinitis patients to segmental antigen challenge. *Am Rev Respir Dis* 144: 1274–1281.
200. Chand N, Harrison JE, Rooney S, Pillar J, Jkubicki R, Nolan K, Diamantis W, Sofia D (1992) Anti-IL-5 monoclonal antibody inhibits allergic late phase bronchial eosinophilia in guinea pigs: A therapeutic approach. *Eur J Pharmacol* 211: 121–123.
201. Corry DB, Folkesson HG, Warnock ML, Erle DJ, Matthay MA, Wiener-Kronish JP, Locksley RC (1996) Interleukin-4, but not interleukin-5 or eosinophils, is requied in a murine model of acute airway hyperreactivity. *J Exp Med* 183: 109–117.
202. Foster PS, Hogan SP, Ramsay AJ, Matthaei KI, Young IG (1995) IL-5 deficiency abolishes eosinophilia, airways hyperreactivity and lung damage in a mouse asthma model. *J Exp Med* 183: 195–201.
203. Drazen JM, Arm JP, Austen KF (1996) Sorting out the cytokines of asthma. *J Exp Med* 183: 1–5.
204. Hamelmann E, Oshiba A, Paluh J, Bradley K, Loader J, Potter TA, Larsen GL, Gelfand EW (1996) Requirement for CD8 T-cells in the development of airway hyperresponsiveness in a murine model of airway sensitization. *J Exp Med* 183: 1719–1729.
205. Cockcroft DW, Kalra S, Bhagat R, Swystun VA, Boulet L-P, Cote J, Laviolette M, Deschesnes F, Chapman KR, Cleland LD et al. (1996) rhuMab-E25 (E25) humanized murine monoclonal anti-IgE inhibits the allergen-induced early asthmatic response (EAR). *J Allergy Clin Immunol* 97: 315 (abstract 532).
206. Haczku A, Moqbel R, Jacobson M, Kay AB, Barnes PJ, Chung KF (1995) T-cell subsets and activation in bronchial mucosa of sensitized Brown-Norway rats after single allergen exposure. *Immunology* 85: 591–597.
207. Eidelman DH, Bellofiore S, Martin JG (1988) Late airway responses to antigen challenge in sensitized inbred rats. *Am Rev Respir Dis* 137: 1033–1037.
208. Gundel RH, Letts LG, Gleich GJ (1991) Human eosinophil major basic protein induces airway constriction and airway hyperresponsiveness in primates. *J Clin Invest* 87: 1470–1473.
209. Wegner CD, Gundel RH, Reilly P, Haynes N, Letts LG, Rothlein R (1990) Intercellular adhesion molecule-1 (ICAM-1) in the pathogenesis of asthma. *Science* 247: 456–459.
210. Mauser PJ, Pitman AM, Fernandez X, Foran SK, Adams GK, Kreutner W, Egan RW, Chapman RW (1995) Effects of an antibody to interleukin-5 in a monkey model of asthma. *Am J Respir Crit Care Med* 152: 467–472.
211. Coyle AJ, Erard F, Bertrand C, Walti S, Pircher H, Le Gros G (1995) Virus-specific CD8[+] cells can switch to interleukin-5 production and induce airway eosinophilia. *J Exp Med* 181: 1229–1233.
212. Alwan WH, Kozlowska WJ, Openshaw PJ (1994) Distinct types of lung disease caused by functional subsets of antiviral T-cells. *J Exp Med* 179: 81–89.
213. British Thoracic Society, Research Unit of the Royal College of Physicians, King's Fund Centre, National Asthma Campaign (1990) Guidelines for management of asthma in adults. *Br J Med* 310: 651–653.
214. Barnes PJ (1995) Beta-adrenergic receptors and their regulation. *Am J Respir Crit Care Med* 152: 838–860.
215. Barnes PJ, Adcock IM (1995) Transcription factors. *Clin Exp Allergy* 25 (Suppl 2): 46–49.
216. Adelroth E, Rosenhall L, Johansson SA, Linden M, Venge P (1990) Inflammatory cells and eosinophilic activity in asthmatics investigated by bronchoalveolar lavage: The effects of antiasthmatic treatment with budesonide or terbutaline. *Am Rev Respir Dis* 142: 91–99.
217. Djukanovic R, Wilson JW, Britten KM, Wilson SJ, Walls AF, Roche WR, Howarth PH, Holgate ST (1992) Effect of an inhaled corticosteroid on airway inflammation and symptoms in asthma. *Am Rev Respir Dis* 145: 669–674.
218. Bentley AM, Hamid Q, Robinson DS, Schotman E, Meng Q, Assoufi B, Kay AB, Durham SR (1996) Prednisolone treatment in asthma: Reduction in the numbers of eosinophils, T-cells, tryptase-only positive mast cells and modulation of IL-4, IL-5 and interferon-gamma cytokine gene expression within the bronchial mucosa. *Am J Respir Crit Care Med* 153: 551–556.

219. Robinson DS, Hamid Q, Ying S, Bentley AM, Assoufi B, North J, Meng Q, Durham SR, Kay AB (1993) Prednisolone treatment in asthma is associated with modulation of bronchoalveolar lavage cell interleukin-4, interleukin-5 and interferon-gamma cytokine gene expression. *Am Rev Respir Dis* 148: 401–406.
220. Goulding NJ, Godolphin JL, Sharland PR, Peers SH, Sampson M, Maddison PJ, Flower RJ (1990) Antiinflammatory lipocortin 1 production by peripheral blood leucocytes in response to hydrocortisone. *Lancet* 335: 1416–1418.
221. Payvar F, Wrange O, Carlstedt-Duke J, Okret S, Gustafsson JA, Yamamoto R (1981) Purified glucocorticoid receptors bind selectively *in vitro* to a cloned DNA fragment whose transcription is regulated by glucocorticoids *in vitro*. *Proc Natl Acad Sci USA* 78: 6628–6632.
222. Crofford LJ, Wilder RL, Ristimaki AP, Sano H, Remmers EF, Epps HR, Hla T (1994) Cyclooxygenase-1 and -2 expression in rheumatoid synovial tissues: Effects of inter-leukin-1 beta, phorbol ester and corticosteroids. *J Clin Invest* 93: 1095–1101.
223. Kharitonov SA, Yates DH, Barnes PJ (1996) Inhaled glucocorticoids decrease nitric oxide in exhaled air of asthmatic patients. *Am J Respir Crit Care Med* 153: 454–457.
224. Chung KF (1995) Leukotriene receptor antagonists and biosynthesis inhibitors: Potential breakthrough in asthma therapy. *Eur Respir J* 8: 1203–1213.
225. Spector SL, Smith LJ, Glass M (1994) Effects of 6 weeks of therapy with oral doses of ICI 204, 219, a leukotriene D4 receptor antagonist, in subjects with bronchial asthma: ACCOLATE Asthma Trialists Group. *Am J Respir Crit Care Med* 150: 618–623.
226. Sullivan P, Bekir S, Jaffar Z, Page C, Jeffery P, Costello J (1994) Anti-inflammatory effects of low-dose oral theophylline in atopic asthma. *Lancet* 343: 1006–1008.
227. Kidney J, Dominguez M, Taylor PM, Rose M, Chung KF, Barnes PJ (1995) Immuno-modulation by theophylline in asthma: Demonstration by withdrawal of therapy. *Am J Respir Crit Care Med* 151: 1907–1914.
228. Essayan DM, Huang SK, Kagey-Sobotka A, Lichtenstein LM (1995) Effects of nonselec-tive and isozyme selective cyclic nucleotide phosphodiesterase inhibitors on antigen-induced cytokine gene expression in peripheral blood mononuclear cells. *Am J Respir Cell Mol Biol* 13: 692–702.
229. Corrigan CJ, Brown PH, Barnes NC, Tsai JJ, Frew AJ, Kay AB (1991) Glucocorticoid resistance in chronic asthma: Peripheral blood T lymphocyte inhibitory effects of gluco-corticoids and cyclosporin A. *Am Rev Respir Dis* 144: 1026–1032.
230. Sher E, Leung DYM, Surs W, Kam JC, Zieg G, Kamada AK, Szefler SJ (1994) Steroid-resistant asthma: Cellular mechanisms contributing to inadequate response to gluco-corticoid therapy. *J Clin Invest* 93: 33–39.
231. Kam J, Szefler SJ, Surs W, Sher E, Leung DYM (1993) The combined effects of IL-2 and IL-4 alter the binding affinity of the glucocorticoid receptor. *J Immuol* 151: 3460–3466.
232. Adcock IM, Lane SJ, Brown CR, Lee TH, Barnes PJ (1995) Abnormal glucocorticoid recep-tor-activator protein 1 interaction in steroid resistant asthma. *J Exp Med* 182: 1951–1958.
233. Alexander AG, Barnes NC, Kay AB (1992) Trial of cyclosporin A in corticosteroid-dependent chronic severe asthma. *Lancet* 339: 324–328.
234. Lock SH, Kay AB, Barnes NC (1996) Double-blind, placebo-controlled study of cyclo-sporin A as a corticosteroid-sparing agent in corticosteroid-dependent asthma. *Am J Respir Crit Care Med* 153: 509–514.
235. Schreiber SL, Crabtree GR (1992) The mechanism of action of cyclosporin A and FK 506. *Immunol Today* 13: 136–141.
236. Sihra BS, Durham SR, Walker S, Kon OM, Barnes NC, Kay AB (1997). Inhibition of the allergen-induced late asthmatic response by cyclosporin A. *Thorax* 52: 447–452.
237. Mullarkey MF, Blumenstein BA, Andrade WP, Bailey GA, Olason I, Wetzel CE (1988) Methotrexate in the treatment of corticosteroid-dependent asthma: A double-blind cross-over study. *N Engl J Med* 318: 603–607.
238. Committee on the Safety of Medicines (1986) CSM update: Desensitizing vaccines. *Br Med J* 293: 948.
239. British Society for Allergy and Clinical Immunology (1993) Position paper on allergen immunotherapy. *Clin Exp Allergy* 23 (Suppl) 3: 1–44.
240. Varney VA, Gaga M, Frew AJ, Aber VR, Kay AB, Durham SR (1991) Usefulness of immunotherapy in patients with severe summer hayfever uncontrolled by antiallergic drugs. *Br Med J* 302: 265–269.

241. Hejjaoui A, Dhivert H, Michel FB, Bousquet J (1990) Immunotherapy with a standardized *Dermatophagoides pteronyssinus* extract. IV. Systemic reactions according to the immunotherapy schedule. *J Allergy Clin Immunol* 85: 473–479.
242. Van Metre TE Jr, Marsh DG, Adkinson NF Jr, Kagey-Sobotka A, Khattignavong A, Norman PS Jr, Rosenberg GL (1988) Immunotherapy for cat asthma. *J Allergy Clin Immunol* 82: 1055–1068.
243. Creticos PS, Reed CE, Norman PS, Khoury J, Adkinson NF Jr, Buncher CR, Busse WW, Bush RK, Gadde J, Li JT et al. (1996) Ragweed immunotherapy in adult asthma. *N Engl J Med* 334: 501–506.
244. Barnes PJ (1996) Is immunotherapy for asthma worthwhile? *N Engl J Med* 334: 531–532.
245. Briner TJ, Kuo MC, Keating KM, Rogers BL, Greenstein KL (1993) Periphral T-cell tolerance induced in naive and primed mice by subcutaneous injection of peptides from the major cat allergen Fel d I. *Proc Natl Acad Sci USA* 90: 7608–7612.

Autoimmune Aspects of Lung Disease
ed. by D. A. Isenberg and S. G. Spiro
© 1998 Birkhäuser Verlag Basel/Switzerland

CHAPTER 9
Cystic Fibrosis

Peter D. Phelan

Department of Paediatrics, Royal Children's Hospital, Parkville, Victoria, Australia

1. Introduction

Lung disease is the major manifestation of cystic fibrosis (CF). It is relentlessly progressive and is the eventual cause of death in almost all patients. However, the rate of deterioration is very variable from patient to patient for reasons that are quite unclear. The improved survival in CF seen in the last 30 years is due probably to better control of the infective component of the lung disease with antibiotics, but there have been some other unexplained changes in the clinical pattern that have contributed to improved survival.

While the lung disease in cystic fibrosis is basically the result of infection, its pathogenesis appears complex. Immunological factors certainly play a part in the progressive lung destruction that is characteristic of the disease. Susceptibility to infection is limited to the lungs, and distant infective complications are extremely rare despite the lungs, in patients with advanced disease, containing what are effectively large abscess cavities with a heavy bacterial load.

2. Initiation of Lung Disease

Much is now understood of the basic metabolic disturbance in CF. The disease results from a mutation within the CF gene which is on the long arm of chromosome 7. The gene covers approximately 250 kb of genomic DNA. It has 27 coding regions (exons) separated by non-coding regions (introns) [1]. The messenger RNA is approximately 6.2 kb in length and is capable of encoding a polypeptide of 1480 amino acids. The putative gene product protein has been called the CF transmembrane regulator (CFTR). It has five domains including two membrane-spanning domains each with six transmembrane segments. The regulatory domain has two nucleotide binding domains.

More than 500 mutations in the CF gene have been reported. The commonest is a deletion of three base pairs in exon 10, and the corresponding protein lacks the amino acid phenylalanine at position 508 (delta F 508). This amino acid is in the first nucleotide-binding fold, which is the site of a substantial number of mutations. The deletion of delta F 508 accounts for between 50 and 70% of CF gene mutations.

The highest concentration of the CFTR protein is found in the apical membrane of epithelial cells of the respiratory tract, gastrointestinal tract and sweat glands. In the respiratory tract it is more common in the submucosal glands than in the surface epithelium. CFTR is a chloride channel and is activated by a combination of phosphorylation by protein kinase A and binding of adenosine triphosphate (ATP) [2]. When activated, it allows the passage of chloride ions through the cell membrane.

Chloride secretion is absent in the respiratory epithelium of the respiratory tract because of the defective CFTR. In addition there is a threefold increase in sodium absorption [3]. The increased sodium absorption combined with the decreased chloride secretion reduces the water content of airways secretion. There continues to be debate as to the chloride level in surface epithelial fluid, with some reporting a reduction in chloride content and others an increase. The decreased water content probably results in respiratory secretions that are more viscous and difficult to clear.

There is some correlation between the genotype and phenotype, but it is not possible to predict the course of the disease in an individual patient based on the genotype. The degree of lung disease is quite different in patients with identical genotypes. Patients who are homozygous for the delta F 508 deletion tend to have more severe disease [4] than those who are heterozygous for that mutation or doubly heterozygous for other mutations [5]. Some patients who are homozygous for the delta F 508 mutation can have mild lung disease [6]. Patients with normal pancreatic function usually have mild lung disease [7], and they are almost invariably either heterozygous for the delta F 508 lesion with another mutation or have two mutations that are not delta F 508. This pattern is seen often in siblings.

There continues to be debate about what initiates lung disease in CF. The lungs appear histologically normal at birth [8]. The traditional view has been that the viscous secretions predispose to infection; however, lung infection in CF is due mainly to two microorganisms – *Staphylococcus aureus* and *Pseudomonas aeruginosa*. Occasionally *Haemophilus influenzae* contributes. It has always been difficult to explain why, if the basic problem is a mechanical one, infection should be limited to these two or three bacteria.

Recent studies of bronchoalveolar fluid obtained bronchoscopically from infants diagnosed as a result of newborn screening have added further information but with different conclusions. There is evidence which suggests that there are considerable inflammatory mediators present in the absence of infection, and it has been suggested that the basic defect results in lung inflammation and damage which then predisposes to infection [9, 10]. We have also carried out bronchoalveolar lavage in infants diagnosed as a result of screening, and our data have shown no excess of inflammatory mediators in the absence of infection [11]. The initial infecting agent is almost invariably the *S. aureus* and *P. aeruginosa* seen only after some months to years [12]. I remain strongly of the view that the initial damage to the lung is the result of infection with *S. aureus*.

Studies of surface epithelial fluid from *in vitro* cultured respiratory epithelial cells may provide an explanation for the infection. Killing of *P. aeruginosa* and *S. aureus* added to the apical surface of cultured CF airway epithelial cells has been shown to be less efficient than in normal airway epithelium [13], a result attributed to a high NaCl content in the CF surface epithelial fluid rather than the absence of bacterial factors. If this finding is confirmed *in vivo*, then the initial event in CF lung disease would be colonisation of the lower respiratory surface epithelium by *S. aureus* and, subsequently, *P. aeruginosa* because of failure of the initial defence mechanism. Secondary defences requiring the recruitment of neutrophils and other inflammatory cells would be called into play with the potential for airway damage. However, recent work from our laboratory suggests that the sodium and chloride content of surface epithelial fluid in newborn infants is not elevated in the absence of infection.

The complete explanation for the initiation of lung infection in CF thus remains unclear.

3. Progress of Lung Disease

P. aeruginosa almost certainly plays an important role in the progress of lung disease in CF. It is cultured eventually in more than 80% of patients. There is no immediate deterioration in lung function following its acquisition [14, 15]; however, one of the problems in determining its role is the inadequate predictive value of oropharyngeal cultures for lower respiratory pathogens. While the presence of *P. aeruginosa* in the pharynx is highly predictive of lower respiratory tract colonisation, it can also be present there without being cultured from the pharynx [16]. The source of *P. aeruginosa* is unknown, and cross-infection in patients does not seem to be a common phenomenon. Once infected, patients appear to have a single genotypic strain, although culture grows colonies with different morphological characteristics, serum sensitivities, serotypic profiles and antibiotic sensitivities [17].

Almost a quarter of patients will be colonised by the age of 1, and two-thirds by age 7 [18]. In families with more than one affected child, the age of acquisition is similar in the first colonised and subsequently colonised siblings.

Probably the initial epithelial injury from staphylococcal infection allows adherence of *P. aeruginosa* to the epithelial surface aided by pili, flexible filaments on the surface of smooth strains which are usually the initial coloniser. Eventually mucoid strains develop, and these are associated with more severe disease and a poor outlook [19]. Mucoid strains are unstable and rapidly revert to non-mucoid forms outside the lungs. The emergence of mucoid strains is probably contributed to by phosphate and nutrient limitation associated with high osmolality and oxygenation present in the CF airway and is seen as an adaptive response. The alginate produced predominantly by the mucoid strain imparts resistance to non-opsonic phagocytosis and intracellular killing but inhibits neutrophil chemotaxis and does not activate complement. Once *P. aeruginosa* infection is established, it can rarely be permanently eradicated. The organism presumably has local protective devices against most defences.

Even in older patients with mild lung disease, there is almost invariably bacterial infection with either *P. aeruginosa, S. aureus* or *H. influenzae* [20]. This can occur in the absence of significant symptoms of cough and sputum. Presumably in these patients there is ongoing lung damage as a consequence of the infection and the response to it.

4. Mechanism of Lung Damage

Much work has been done over recent years in elucidating the mechanism for lung damage in patients with CF who are infected with *P. aeruginosa*. There are many fewer data on the damage that results from *S. aureus*, but there may be somewhat similar mechanisms. One suggestion is that the neutrophils accompanying infection with *S. aureus* secrete elastase onto the epithelial surface which cleaves fibronectin and therefore renders the epithelial cells more amenable to *P. aeruginosa* infection [21].

Pulmonary secretions from patients with CF contain abundant neutrophils and the proinflammatory α-chemokine interleukin-8 (IL-8) present in sufficiently high concentration to overwhelm the protective anti-oxidase and anti-protease enzyme systems [22, 23]. Other inflammatory mediators such as leukotrienes, tumour necrosis factor-α and IL-1B are also present in respiratory tract secretions, and they probably contribute to the pathogenesis of CF lung disease [24, 25].

It has been hypothesised that these proinflammatory cytokines are produced by alveolar macrophages and surface epithelial cells in response to

P. aeruginosa and other bacterial infection [24, 26]. The inflammatory mediators themselves induce their further production in the epithelial cells [27].

The inflammatory mediators then recruit neutrophils into the airways. Various inflammatory mediators cause the neutrophils to release their enzymes; in particular, they produce elastase and superoxide anion through the NADPH-oxidase system in the plasma membrane of the cell [28]. Superoxide in the presence of halides and myeloperoxidase results in highly active metabolites which are very toxic to cells and cause damage to cell membranes [29]. The many enzyme cationic products from neutrophils are capable of causing extensive injury. Thus the neutrophil is a remarkable source of enzymes that can break down the major connective tissue protein of the lungs.

It appears to be the load of neutrophil elastase and other toxic neutrophil products that overwhelm the local lung defences rather than the defences themselves being impaired [28]. In fact, the levels of the elastase inhibitor, alpha-1-proteinase, is increased in the disease.

There is a systemic response to the chronic lung infection with *P. aeruginosa* and its exoproducts. The antibodies belong to immunoglobulin (Ig)A, IgM and all four subclasses of IgG [30]. These antibodies form immune complexes with the antigens. While in general there is a relationship between high levels of circulating immune complexes and deteriorating pulmonary function, this is not always the case. Certainly the levels are higher in chronically infected patients. These immune complexes may contribute to some of the less common manifestations of CF such as the characteristic migratory polyarthritis.

There is no evidence of any defect in local or systemic defences to infection in patients with CF. The lung damage seems to be due to the direct effect of bacterial infection and the immunological response to it. The infection does not spread beyond the airways and lung tissues. Pleural involvement is extremely rare even with advanced disease; septicaemia and other distant infections are not seen.

5. Lung Pathology

The initial lung pathology is suppurative bronchiolitis and bronchitis. Again, for reasons which are not clear, the upper lobes of the lung seem to be predominantly affected in the early stages. However, eventually the changes become widespread.

Bronchiolectasis and bronchiectasis are invariable consequences of suppurative bronchitis. There is substantial peribronchial and peribronchiolar inflammation. Segmental or lobar collapse is common and is almost certainly the consequence of the purulent endobronchial secretions.

Segmental or lobar pneumonia is rare, and when it occurs, it seems to follow the course for a typical lobar pneumonia with rapid clearing in the absence of severe underlying disease. Recurrent pneumonia is not a true manifestation of CF. Rather repeated exacerbations of the suppurative bronchitis and bronchiolitis characterise the course of the disease.

In the lungs the alveoli are dilated due to air trapping, but destruction of alveolar walls characteristic of emphysema is not a prominent feature. Occasionally localised regions of emphysema secondary to necrotising infection may be seen in older patients. Emphysematous blebs are commonly seen, particularly at the apical pleural surface. They are the source of pneumothorax, which can be a particular problem in older patients.

Eventually there is widespread bronchiectasis involving both lungs. The dilated bronchi are filled with thick purulent material. Haemoptysis is common, with bleeding usually from bronchiectatic lesions or from dilated bronchial arteries or bronchopulmonary arterial anastomoses in granulomas around bronchi.

With progressive pulmonary involvement, the primary divisions of the pulmonary artery become dilated, and there is hypertrophy of the arterial muscular walls. There is pruning of pre-acinar arteries at the terminal bronchiolar level. Eventually the pulmonary artery pressure becomes elevated but falls with the administration of 100% oxygen, suggesting that the elevated pressure is partly secondary to muscular spasm rather than destruction of small vessels in the alveolar walls [31]. Right ventricular hypertrophy and terminal cor pulmonale are characteristic.

6. Clinical Features

The characteristic symptoms of the lung disease of CF are a loose cough and, in older patients, the expectoration of purulent sputum. In the early years of life the cough may be intermittent, and there may be prolonged periods of total freedom from symptoms. Exacerbations occur from time to time and often appear to be triggered by intercurrent viral infection. Eventually all patients develop a persistent productive cough, but the age at which this occurs is extremely variable. Some have a loose cough from soon after birth which never clears completely. Others may have no more than three or four episodes of bronchitis lasting several weeks until mid- to late teenage years. However, by the second decade of life the majority of patients will produce purulent sputum on a daily basis. Despite the production of a small amount of purulent sputum, most patients remain systemically very well provided malabsorption, which occurs in 90% of patients, is well controlled. They may remain very active and enjoy an essentially normal lifestyle for many years.

Wheezing is commonly seen in younger children and is probably a reflection of suppurative bronchitis characteristic of the disease. Asthma occurs in between 10 and 20% and can be difficult to diagnose and to control. Some patients develop allergic bronchopulmonary aspergillosis, though this seems to be less commonly seen now than 10 to 20 years ago.

Haemoptysis occurs with more advanced disease, as does pneumothorax. With extensive bronchiectasis, large amounts of purulent sputum are expectorated every day. There is progressive impairment of general health, and exercise tolerance becomes limited. Most patients die of respiratory failure, right heart failure being a terminal event.

At present, major clinics are reporting a predicted survival of about 50% by age 30, with the survival of males being superior to that of females for unexplained reasons. This is a marked improvement on the 50% survival to age 10 seen 30 years ago. Many factors have contributed to this improvement, probably the major one being the establishment of specialised multidisciplinary clinics for CF in major paediatric and more recently in major adult medical centres. There have, however, been changes in the pattern of CF. Twenty years ago it was common to see young infants presenting in the first few months of life with very extensive lung disease and dying soon after [32]. This is now a rare event and was so even before the introduction of newborn screening. In fact, survival from age 5 is only marginally better now than it was 20 years ago.

7. Monitoring the Progress of Lung Disease

The progress of lung disease is monitored using a combination of clinical featues, lung function measurements and chest radiographs. The presence of cough and the amount of sputum produced are the best indicators of the activity of the lung disease. There is progressive loss of lung function, and studies of large groups of patients indicate an annual loss of about 2% of FEV_1 [5]. However, again in an individual patient the rate of loss is very variable. FEV_1 remains the best objective monitor for the progress of lung disease. Radiological changes are very variable and initially occur in the upper lobes. There is peribronchial inflammation progressing to bronchiectasis and widespread peribronchial infiltration.

8. Control of Lung Disease

The management of CF lung disease has been extensively discussed elsewhere [33] and will not be repeated in detail here. The principles will, however, be mentioned, with particular emphasis on current efforts to control the immunopathological component of the disease.

The mainstays of treatment of lung disease in CF are the use of antibiotics to control bacterial infection and mechanisms to clear respiratory secretion. Most of the regimes used to treat bacterial infection have never been subject to proper double-blind controlled trials, and there have been no adequate controlled trials showing the value of continuous antibiotics in those with mild lung disease. Nonetheless, with increasing understanding of the pathogenesis of the lung disease, there is a move to more prolonged and intensive use of antibiotics. The drugs used, however, must be effective against both *S. aureus* and *P. aeruginosa* even if the former organism is not grown from sputum culture, since *S. aureus* may be overwhelmed by *P. aeruginosa* and difficult to detect. Milder exacerbations can be treated with oral antibiotics; the more troublesome ones will usually require a period of intravenous therapy. This can be given either in hospital or at home. Inhaled antibiotics may also have a place in therapy.

Removal of mucopurulent bronchial secretions seems to be very important. The most effective form of physiotherapy in this disease remains an area of considerable contention. There are increasing data to suggest that at least in some patients postural drainage may exacerbate gastro-oesophageal reflux [34], which is probably more frequent in patients with CF than in other patients. Presumably, subsequent aspiration may exacerbate lung disease. Forced expiration techniques with physiotherapy are probably more effective.

Regular physical activity is probably vitally important to encourage the removal of pulmonary secretions and maintain general health. It is certainly a widespread belief that patients with CF who are physically very active maintain better health than those who do not.

Attempts at controlling the immunopathological components of lung disease have included trials of the use of regular corticosteroids, but the results have been conflicting [35]. In general, this form of therapy has not received widespread acceptance. A recent study of the anti-inflammatory drug ibuprofen suggested that it may be useful in slowing the progress of mild lung disease [36] by reducing the inflammatory response. Further trials with it are necessary to determine its precise role.

Attempts at thinning bronchial secretions may be effective, and there is widespread use of synthetic DNase. Regrettably, this drug has received very widespread acceptance based on little scientific evidence for it being a cost-effective form of treatment. The lack of rigorous scientific evaluation of therapy for CF remains a major problem.

Attempts to alter the basic defect by gene therapy or to alter the local environment in the lung are likely to be more effective. But to date use of these forms of therapy have been very limited and are not yet a realistic option.

9. Conclusion

The mechanism of lung disease in CF is complex, but its pathogenesis is gradually being elucidated. The defective CF gene seems to alter the local environment in the lung, which predisposes it to infection initially with

S. aureus and subsequently with *P. aeruginosa*. Bacterial infection and the immunological response to it then leads to progressive lung disease with the enzyme products of neutrophils being a major factor in the lung damage.

In the present state of knowledge, lung disease in CF is relentlessly progressive and eventually leads to respiratory failure and cor pulmonale. While the use of antibiotics probably retards the progress of lung disease, the place of agents to alter the immunological component remains less clear. Ultimately, effective therapy is likely to be a pharmacological approach to restore to normality the lung environment.

References

1. Riordan JR, Rommens JM, Kerem B, Alon N, Rozmahel R, Grzelczak Z, Zielinski J, Lok S, Plavsic N, Chou JL, et al. (1989) Identification of the cystic fibrosis gene: Cloning and characterisation of complementary DNA. *Science* 245: 1066–1073.
2. Collins FS (1992) The CF gene: Perceptions, puzzles and promises. *Pediat Pulmonol* (Suppl) 8: 63–64.
3. Knowles M, Gazty J, Boucher RC (1981) Increased bioelectric potential difference across respiratory epithelia in cystic fibrosis. *N Engl J Med* 305: 1489–1495.
4. Kerem E, Corey M, Kerem B, Rommens J, Markiewicz D, Levison H, Tsui L-C, Durie P (1990) The relationship between genotype and phenotype in cystic fibrosis: Analysis of the most common mutation (delta F508). *N Engl J Med* 323: 1517–1522.
5. Johansen HK, Nir M, Holby N, Koch C, Schwartz M (1991) Severity of cystic fibrosis in patients homozygous and heterozygous for delta F508 mutation. *Lancet* 337: 631–634.
6. Santis G, Osborne L, Knight RA, Hodson ME (1990) Independent genetic determinants of pancreatic and pulmonary status in cystic fibrosis. *Lancet* 336: 1081–1084.
7. Gaskin K, Gurwitz D, Durie P, Corey M, Levison H, Forstner G (1982) Improved respiratory prognosis in patients with cystic fibrosis and normal fat absorption. *J Pediat* 100: 857–862.
8. Chow CW, Landau LI, Taussig LM (1982) Bronchial mucus glands in the newborn with cystic fibrosis. *Eur J Paediatr* 139: 240–243.
9. Khan TZ, Wagener J, Bost T, Martinez J, Accurso FJ, Riches DWH (1995) Early pulmonary inflammation in infants with cystic fibrosis. *Am J Respir Crit Care Med* 151: 1075–1082.
10. Balough K, McCubbin M, Weinberger M, Smits W, Ahrens R, Fick R (1995) The relationship between infection and inflammation in the early stages of lung disease from cystic fibrosis. *Pediat Pulmonol* 20: 63–70.
11. Armstrong D, Grimwood K, Guiterrez J, Carzino R, Carlin A, Olinsky A et al. (1996) Lower respiratory infection and inflammation in infants and young children with cystic fibrosis. *Am J Respir Crit Care Med* 153: A777.
12. Armstrong DS, Krimwood K, Carzino R, Carlin JB, Olinsky A, Phelan PD (1995) Lower respiratory infection and inflammation in infants with newly diagnosed cystic fibrosis. *Br Med J* 310: 1571–1572.
13. Smith JJ, Travis SM, Greenberg EP, Welsh MJ (1996) Cystic fibrosis airway epithelial cells fail to kill bacteria because of abnormal airway surface fluid. *Cell* 89: 229–236.
14. Kerem E, Corey M, Gold R, Levison H (1990) Pulmonary function and clinical course in patients with cystic fibrosis after pulmonary colonisation with *Pseudomonas aeruginosa*. *J Pediatr* 116: 714–719.
15. Phelan PD (1996) Pulmonary infection in cystic fibrosis: The Australian approach. In: Bauernfeind A, Marks MI, Strandvik B (eds). *Cystic fibrosis pulmonary infections: Lessons from around the world*. Basel: Birkhäuser, 149–159.
16. Ramsey BW, Weiss KR, Smith AL, Richardson M, Williams Warren J, Hodges DL, Gibson R, Redding GJS, Lent K, Harris K (1991) Predictive value of oropharyngeal cultures for identifying lower respiratory bacteria in cystic fibrosis patients. *Am Rev Respir Dis* 144: 331–337.

17. Ogle JW, Janda JM, Woods DE (1987) Characterisation and use of a DNA probe as an epidemiological marker for *Pseudomonas aeruginosa. J Infect Dis* 115: 119–126.
18. Kerem E, Corey M, Stein R, Gold R, Levison H (1990) Risk factors for *Pseudomonas* colonisation in cystic fibrosis patients. *Pediatr Infect Dis J* 9: 494–498.
19. Henry RK, Mellis CM, Petrovic L (1992) Mucoid *Pseudomonas aeruginosa* as a marker of poor survival in cystic fibrosis. *Pediat Pulmonol* 12: 158–161.
20. Konstan MW, Hilliard KA, Norwell TM, Berger M (1994) Bronchoalveolar lavage findings in cystic fibrosis patients with stable, clinically mild lung disease suggest ongoing infection and inflammation. *Am J Respir Crit Care Med* 150: 448–454.
21. Birrer P, McElvaney NG, Rudeberg A, Wiaz Sommer C, Liechti-Gallati S, Kraemer R, Hubbard R, Crystal RG (1994) Protease-antiprotease inbalance in the lungs of children with cystic fibrosis. *Am J Respir Crit Care Med* 150: 207–213.
22. Richman-Eisenstat JB, Jorens PG, Hebert CA, Ueki I, Nadel JA (1993) Interleukin-8: An important chemoattractant in sputum of patients with chronic inflammatory airway diseases. *Am J Physiol* 264 (Lung Cell Mol Physiol 8): L413–418.
23. Richman-Eisenstat J (1996) Cytokine soap: Making sense of inflammation in cystic fibrosis. *Pediat Pulmonol* 21: 3–5.
24. Bonfield TL, Panuska JR, Konstan MW, Hilliard KA, Hilliard JB, Ghnaim H, Berger M (1995) Inflammatory cytokines in cystic fibrosis lungs. *Am J Respir Crit Care Med* 152: 2111–2118.
25. Salva PS, Doyle NA, Graham L, Eigen H, Doerschuk CM (1996) TNF-α, IL-8 soluble ICAM-1 and neutrophils in sputum of cystic fibrosis patients. *Pediat Pulmonol* 21: 9–11.
26. Massion PD, Inoue H, Richman-Eisenstat J, Grunberger D, Jorens PG, Housset B et al. (1994) Novel *Pseudomonas* product stimulates interleukin-8 production in airway epithelial cells *in vitro. J Clin Invest* 93: 26–32.
27. Levine SJ (1995) Bronchial epithelial cell-cytokine interactions in airway inflammation. *J Invest Med* 43: 241–249.
28. O'Connor CM, Gaffney K, Keane J, Southey A, Byrne N, O'Mahoney S, Fitzgerald MX (1993) α_1-Proteinase inhibitors, elastase activity and lung disease in cystic fibrosis. *Am R Respir Dis* 148: 1665–1670.
29. Meyer KC, Zimmerman J (1993) Neutrophil mediators, *Pseudomonas* and pulmonary dysfunction in cystic fibrosis. *J Lab Clin Med* 121: 654–661.
30. Kronborg G (1995) Lipopolysaccharide (LPS), LPS immune complexes and cytokines as inducers of pulmonary inflammation in patients with cystic fibrosis and chronic *Pseudomonas aeruginosa* lung infection. *Apmis* (Suppl) 5: 1–30.
31. Goldring RM, Fishman AP, Turino GM, Cohen HI, Denning CR, Andersen DH (1964) Pulmonary hypertension and cor pulmonale in cystic fibrosis of the pancreas. *J Pediat* 65: 501–524.
32. Hudson I, Phelan PD (1987) Are sex, age at diagnosis or mode of presentation prognostic factors for cystic fibrosis? *Pediat Pulmonol* 3: 288–297.
33. Phelan PD, Olinsky A, Robertson CF (1994) *Respiratory illness in children*. Oxford: Blackwell Scientific Publications, 207–251.
34. Button BM, Heine RG, Catto-Smith AG, Phelan PD, Olinsky A (1995) Effect of postural drainage chest physiotherapy on gastroesophageal reflux in infants with cystic fibrosis. *Am J Respir Crit Care Med* 151: A738.
35. Eigen H, Rosenstein BJ, Fitzsimmons S, Schidlow DV (1995) A multicentre study of alternate-day therapy in patients with cystic fibrosis. *J Pediat* 126: 515–523.
36. Konstan MW, Byard PJ, Hoppel CL, Davis P (1995) Effect of high-dose ibuprofen in patients with cystic fibrosis. *N Engl Med J* 332: 848–854.

Autoimmune Aspects of Lung Disease
ed. by D.A. Isenberg and S.G. Spiro
© 1998 Birkhäuser Verlag Basel/Switzerland

CHAPTER 10
Role of the Immune System in the Pathogenesis of Cryptogenic Fibrosing Alveolitis

Helen Booth and Geoffrey J. Laurent

Centre for Cardiopulmonary Biochemistry and Respiratory Medicine, University College London Medical School and Royal Free Hospital School of Medicine, London, UK

1. Introduction

Pulmonary fibrosis is the "final common pathway" of a number of known insults. However, in the majority of cases no obvious cause can be identified, and these are classified as cases of cryptogenic fibrosing alveolitis (CFA) or idiopathic pulmonary fibrosis (IPF). This condition is the main focus of this chapter. Although immunological factors have, for a long time, been thought to be important in the pathogenesis of pulmonary fibrosis, there is little direct evidence to support this. What is clear is that there is non-specific activation of the humoral immune response and evidence for impaired cell-mediated immunity. Whether these immunological changes are the cause or result of pulmonary fibrosis are discussed. Another concept we explore is that an inflammatory/immune response *per se* may be a "normal" reaction, and it is an inappropriate fibrotic response, with lack of normal homeostatic controls, which is particularly damaging. Such losses in control, either in the immune response or regulation of matrix production, are proposed as key events to explain the wide ranges in susceptibility of individuals to fibrogenic stimuli and the variable clinical course in patients with CFA.

2. Causes of Pulmonary Fibrosis

A number of known insults may result in chronic pulmonary inflammation and fibrosis. These insults may be inhaled, direct physical, delivered systemically or associated with known autoimmune conditions. Some are listed in Table 1 along with the approximate proportion of patients who, when exposed to a particular agent, will develop pulmonary fibrosis. Many of these are dealt with in more detail in other chapters of this book, but are considered in general below.

A major route of exposure to fibrogenic insults is by inhalation. In this group fibrosis usually progresses slowly and is dose-dependent [1]. For example, the latency period between exposure and detection of asbestosis is 15 years or more [2]. The lung is usually the only organ involved, although a unique association has been established between silica exposure and autoimmune diseases, particularly systemic sclerosis [3]. The direct pulmonary damage which results from thoracic radiation therapy is also dose-dependent [4] but develops relatively quickly, within 2 to 3 months. Circulating toxins or drugs, either ingested (e.g. paraquat) or administered intravenously (e.g. bleomycin), can result in selective fibrosis of the lung, which develops within days to months [5]. In contrast, the autoimmune connective tissue diseases are often associated with fibrosis of multiple organs, including the lung.

Why only a proportion of people exposed to these insults develop fibrosis is unknown. However, certain potentiating factors have been identified: administration of oxygen or ionising radiation increases the risk of antineoplastic drug-induced lung damage [5], and smoking has been shown to increase the risk and severity of asbestosis [6]. Many workers over the last 20 years have tried to identify an immunogenetic factor involved in the pathogenesis of pulmonary fibrosis. Most have concentrated on trying to find an association with a human leucocyte antigen (HLA) type. The results of these studies have been inconclusive [7, 8]. However, Briggs et al. [9] have reported that the presence of DR3/DRw52a haplotype or anti-Scl-70 autoantibodies confers a relative risk of 16.7 for the development of pulmonary fibrosis in patients with scleroderma. Further studies to investigate the molecular basis of genetic susceptibility are urgently needed.

2.1. Cryptogenic Fibrosing Alveolitis

In most cases, the aetiology of pulmonary fibrosis is unknown, and cases are classified as CFA. CFA shares some clinical characteristics with asbestosis; it occurs in the elderly (mean age of onset is approximately 60 years), it is associated with finger clubbing, the fibrosis is predominately at the lung bases and the disease process is limited to the lung [10].

Table 1. Known causes of pulmonary fibrosis

Cause	Examples	% exposed population or patients with underlying disease who develop pulmonary fibrosis	Comments
Inhaled/directly acting agent			
Extrinsic allergic alveolitis	farmer's lung bird fancier's lung	0.5–7.5%	depends on immunogenicity of organic dust and exposure level
Pneumoconiosis	asbestosis	7–21%	depends on cumulative exposure level, duration of exposure and fibre type
Thoracic external beam radiation		50%	with 1000 units estimated lung dose
Systemic diseases/causes			
Autoimmune rheumatic disease associated fibrosing alveolitis	rheumatoid arthritis systemic sclerosis	5% 10–50% 30–60% 100%	symptomatic pulmonary fibrosis subclinical pulmonary fibrosis symptomatic pulmonary fibrosis subclinical pulmonary fibrosis
Drug-induced	methotrexate amiodarone gold salts	8% 1–6% <1%	

It is of note, therefore, that Hubbard et al. [11] estimate that 20% of cases of CFA are attributable to previous occupational exposure to wood or metal dust. Although a rare familial form of CFA has been reported [12], no linkage with an HLA type has been consistently established [13]. A viral aetiology for CFA has been suspected for some time, but there is little data to support this. Epstein-Barr virus (EBV) replication in type II pulmonary epithelial cells has been demonstrated in a high proportion of patients with CFA [14], but data to the contrary were reported recently [15]. The involvement of viruses in CFA needs to be explored further, as incorporation of viral sequences can clearly have profound effects on cell function and lead to disease states. In the context of CFA it is possible that viral genes could be incorporated into the genome and enhance the promoter activity of genes that regulate the production of the extracellular matrix [16] or influence the activity of cytokines and growth factors which promote inflammation and fibrosis. Alternatively, immune cross-reactivity between EBV and host antigens may occur, a mechanism that has been postulated to explain the role of cytomegalovirus in graft rejections [17].

It is likely that under the clinical label of CFA there are a number of different factors, either alone or in combination, responsible for the development of pulmonary fibrosis. This may in part explain the wide individual variation in response to treatment and the rate of disease progression; the mean length of survival is 3–5 years, but 25% of patients are alive at 10 years [18].

3. Pathogenesis of Pulmonary Fibrosis

Pulmonary fibrosis is a general term which describes disorders in which there is excessive deposition of a host of matrix proteins, including collagens, laminins, fibronectins and elastin in the pulmonary interstitium – the extracellular space between the alveoli epithelium, the vascular endothelium and the pleural mesothelium [19, 20]. Most abundant is collagen, which represents 10–20% of total lung protein. An outline of collagen metabolism and how this is altered in pulmonary fibrosis follows.

3.1 Collagen Metabolism

The collagens are a family of at least 18 closely related proteins which have different structural and metabolic characteristics. They are coded for by over 25 genes on several chromosomes [21]. In the adult human lung approximately 90% of collagens are types I and III in a ratio of 2:1. Fibroblasts account for 37% of all lung parenchymal cells [10] and are the major producers of types I and III collagen.

Collagen synthesis involves at least eight steps; transcription of collagen genes, translation of messenger RNA (mRNA) to precursor molecules (pre-procollagens) followed by a number of intracellular and extracellular modifications. The latter includes cleavage of C- and N-terminal propeptides converting procollagens to collagen. The formation of covalent cross-links between the triple-helical collagen chains results in the assembly of mature fibrils in the extracellular space. A significant proportion of procollagen is degraded intracellularly within minutes of its production, whilst mature collagen can be broken down by a family of tissue metalloproteinases [22].

It is now recognised that collagens are not as inert as once thought and that fibroblasts are metabolically active cells continuously synthesising and degrading collagens. For example, in the lungs of young rodents it has been estimated that one-tenth of total lung collagen is synthesised and degraded per day [23], although this rate diminishes with age [24]. This concept of the lung as a metabolically dynamic organ is important in modelling approaches to prevent excess scar tissue accumulating in response to the constant exposure of the lungs to inhaled particulates and antigens. For example, a subtle imbalance between collagen production and/or degradation could result in the excessive collagen deposition which characterises CFA. Likewise, shifts in these processes, induced by drugs, could underpin novel forms of therapy.

3.2. Collagen Metabolism in Pulmonary Fibrosis

Progressive pulmonary fibrosis results from the excessive and disordered deposition of predominately type I and III collagen, although increased expression of other collagen types also occurs [25]. This may result from increased collagen synthesis rates, which have been reported in several animal models of pulmonary fibrosis [26]. An increase in collagen synthesis rates in humans is suggested by increased levels of N-terminal propeptide of type III collagen (PIIINP) in bronchoalveolar lavage (BAL) fluid [27]. However, interpretation of these studies is difficult. Measurement of BAL protein levels is complicated by the complex flux of fluid and solutes which occurs between the vascular and the BAL compartment during the bronchoscopic procedure [28], and these may be altered in patients with interstitial lung disease [29]. Further, total estimation of BAL PIIINP may detect different PIIINP-related antigens which reflect processes other than collagen synthesis [30]. However, type I collagen gene expression, when assessed by in situ hybridisation, has been shown to be increased [31] and provides supporting evidence that fibroblasts of patients with fibrosis are activated to produce more collagen.

Increased collagen deposition may also result from changes in the fibroblast population, either by migration or local proliferation. Fibroblasts with an enhanced migratory phenotype [32] and a high replication rate [33] have been reported in patients with fibrotic lung disease. Additionally, cells which do not normally synthesise specific extracellular matrix proteins may become activated to do so. For example, Matsui et al. [16] have recently reported that type II alveolar cells can be induced to secrete type I collagen.

The above discussion highlights the need to identify an *in vivo* marker which accurately reflects active lung collagen synthesis/degradation in humans and which can be used to follow disease progression and monitor the effect of treatment. Procollagen III peptide levels are currently used to assess rates of collagen synthesis, but their validity has been questioned [34]. There is no established index of the rate of lung collagen degradation. However, there is active research into identifying reliable indices of collagen turnover in general. This is illustrated by the demonstration that urinary excretion of pyridinoline and deoxypyridinoline, cross-linking amino acids of collagen found mainly in bone and cartilage, appears to be a useful marker of collagen degradation in metabolic bone disease and arthritic disorders [35].

3.3. Role of the Immune System in the Pathogenesis of CFA

3.3.1. Pathological changes: The histology of CFA varies between a predominately cellular pattern, where the interstitium is infiltrated with inflammatory cells, to a predominately fibrotic pattern in which there are very few inflammatory cells present. A more cellular pattern is associated with a better prognosis [36]. This has led to the widely held belief that inflammation, in response to an endothelial or epithelial injury, occurs early in the natural history of the disease and that the production of a variety of mediators from inflammatory/immune or injured resident cells then results in the activation of fibroblasts or other collagen-producing cells (Figure 1). However, the concept that alveolitis always precedes fibrosis is not supported by the study by Harrison et al. [37], which showed that the ultrastructural features of open lung biopsies from patients with systemic sclerosis and CFA were indistinguishable from each other and that the early features were characterised by interstitial oedema and fibrosis accompanied by endothelial and epithelial cell damage but not necessarily inflammation. Further, although subclinical interstitial pulmonary inflammation is a frequent accompaniment of many autoimmune rheumatic diseases, only a small proportion of cases develop clinically significant fibrotic lung disease [38].

Many of the events leading to fibrosis are seen during normal wound-healing, but the progressive deposition of extracellular matrix proteins suggests that the wound-healing response lacks the normal controls. This may be due to the continued presence of the initiating stimulus, for example the

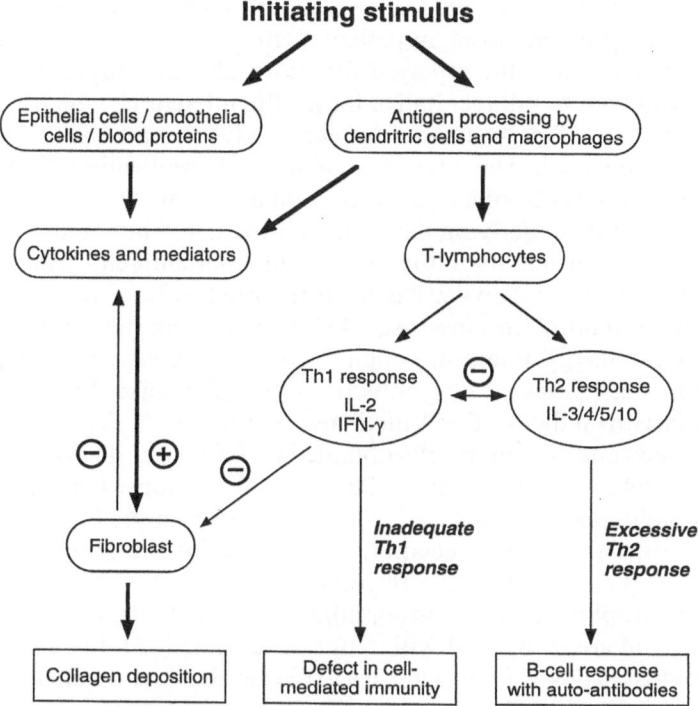

Features of Cryptogenic Fibrosing Alveolitis

Figure 1. Role of the immune system in CFA. This diagram presents the hypothesis that defects in the immune response and/or the interaction of immune cells with interstitial fibroblasts may be vital to the development of pulmonary fibrosis in patients with CFA. The initiating stimulus, which, for CFA, is currently unknown, promotes release of cytokines from resident cells and/or flux of polypeptide mediators from blood. Antigens (host or foreign) are presented to dendritic cells or pulmonary macrophages leading to an immune response which in this disease is predominantly of the Th2 type. This promotes a B-cell response with the production of autoantibodies. Reciprocal suppression of the Th1 immune response results in defects in cell-mediated immunity found in CFA (see Section 3.3.2) and reduced production of antifibrotic cytokines (e.g. interferon-γ). Fibroblasts may also have impaired homeostasis with defects in their release of autocrine factors (e.g. PGE$_2$), impaired production of cytokines which inhibit fibrosis from Th1 cells, and an excess of profibrotic cytokines and mediators derived from cells and blood (see Table 2).

expression of viral genes [39]. Alternatively, there may be loss of normal homeostasis, with perpetuation of the inflammatory/immune response itself or loss of inhibitory control of the regulation of collagen deposition (see Figure 1).

3.3.2. Immune dysregulation/dysfunction: Clinical conditions associated with CFA suggest that patients may have an underlying defect of cell-mediated immunity (Figure 1). Ten percent of patients with CFA die of lung cancer, a relative risk 14 times that of the normal population [40].

There is also a higher incidence of common bacterial respiratory infections, including tuberculosis, in patients with pulmonary fibrosis [41]. Of note in this context is the reported failure of alveolar macrophages from patients with CFA to kill facultative intracellular bacteria, which seemed to reflect a defect in T-cell function impairing alveolar macrophage recruitment/activation [42]. The presence of actively replicating EBV in the alveolar epithelial cells of a high proportion of patients with CFA [14] may further suggest an underlying defect in cell-mediated immunity.

However, skin reactivity to tuberculin and other antigens, which reflects delayed-type hypersensitivity, has been reported to be normal in patients with CFA but reduced in asbestosis [43]. This is in contrast to the high rate of peripheral anergy found in patients with sarcoidosis [44], who do not have an increased risk of lung infections or malignancy. In this group of patients *in vitro* indices of cell-mediated immunity are depressed in peripheral blood cells but not in cells obtained by BAL [45]. This has led to the concept of compartmentalisation of the immune response between the lung and extrapulmonary compartment. This suggests that the local pulmonary immune response is more accurately reflected by sampling solutes and cells obtained by BAL than peripheral blood/skin tests.

BAL neutrophilia and/or eosinophilia are the usual findings in patients with CFA and are associated with reduced survival [46]. In contrast, BAL lymphocytosis is associated with less fibrotic disease, a better prognosis and a greater likelihood of steroid responsiveness [47], especially in those with activated cytolytic lymphocytes [48]. BAL lymphocytosis is the usual finding in other interstitial lung diseases, such as sarcoid and extrinsic allergic alveolitis in which only a minority of cases progress to fibrosis (Table 1). In these conditions BAL lymphocytosis does not predict deteriorating lung function or a poor prognosis [49, 50]. Further, impairment of lavage T-lymphocyte proliferation characterises the more chronic active phase of pulmonary sarcoid, whereas those who present with Löfgrens syndrome, which has a good prognosis, have increased proliferative responses [51]. That lymphocytes may be important in suppressing the development of fibrosis is further supported by the lack of parenchymal abnormalities (on transbronchial biopsy and high-resolution CT scan) in patients with Sjögren's syndrome and BAL lymphocytosis [52]. Similarly, Garcia et al. [53] reported no evidence of clinical fibrosing alveolitis in patients with rheumatoid arthritis and BAL lymphocytosis.

To investigate directly the role of cell-mediated immunity in pulmonary fibrosis, Corsini et al. [54] examined the inflammatory and fibrotic response in BAL and lung histology of normal immunocompetent mice, T-cell deficient mice and immune-reconstituted mice after exposure to asbestos. The immunodeficient mice had a more intense and prolonged inflammatory cell response, mainly neutrophils, and increased incidence and severity of collagen deposition. Lymphocyte reconstitution resulted in the reduction of a number of these excessive pulmonary responses. In humans, a case of rapidly progressing fibrosing alveolitis after administration of antithymocyte globulin therapy has been reported [55]. Taken together, these results suggest that T lymphocytes may have a protective role in pulmonary fibrosis and that reduced or defective cell-mediated immunity may be directly involved in the pathogenesis rather than merely a result of pulmonary fibrosis.

In contrast to cell-mediated immunity, the humoral immune response appears to be activated in CFA (Figure 1). Hypergammaglobulinaemia, positive autoantibodies (antinuclear antibodies and rheumatoid factors) and circulating immune complexes are present in about one-third of patients with CFA. There is an increase in B-lymphocyte growth factor activity [56] and immunoglobulin levels in BAL from patients with CFA compared with normal subjects. In the pulmonary parenchyma the predominant lymphoid cell is the B lymphocyte [57], and immune complexes are deposited at sites of disease activity. Recent studies have shown that patients with CFA have a high incidence of serum autoantibodies to endogenous lung protein(s) associated with alveolar lining cells [58] and to collagen [59]. Whether these autoantibodies are an epiphenomenon or are important in the pathogenesis of CFA remains uncertain.

3.3.3. Cytokines and inflammatory mediators: The immune response can be divided into two by the production of different cytokine profiles by immune cells. A Th1 immune response promotes a delayed-type hypersensitivity/granulomatous reaction and is defined by the production of IL-2 and interferon-gamma (IFN-γ). A Th2 reaction favours the development of a humoral or antibody-mediated immune response and is associated with the IL-4, IL-5, IL-6 and IL-10 cytokines. It is of little surprise, given the immunological abnormalities in CFA described above, that a Th2 pattern of immune response appears to predominate (Figure 1). Wallace et al. [60] reported that most infiltrating mononuclear cells in human lung biopsies from patients with CFA stained positive for IL-4 and IL-5 but only a minority for IFN-γ. Using the technique of mRNA *in situ* hybridisation, it appeared that cells were transcribing IFN-γ mRNA but not producing the cytokine. That impaired IFN-γ production may be important aetiologically in CFA is suggested by the report that patients with the highest serum IFN-γ levels responded to corticosteroids, whereas a higher proportion of patients with impaired IFN-γ production from peripheral blood mononuclear cells showed disease progression [61]. Further, procollagen III peptide levels in BAL have been reported to be inversely correlated with IFN-γ levels in patients with progressive CFA [62].

IFN-γ is a cytokine produced by antigen-activated T-cells and natural killer cells. It has antiviral, some antitumour and a wide range of immunoregulatory actions [63]. It preferentially inhibits the proliferation of Th2 cells and may be involved in self-tolerance mechanisms [64]. IFN-γ also has inhibitory effects on collagen synthesis (Figure 1). *In vitro*, it inhibits human lung fibroblast proliferation and collagen production [65]. Intramuscular IFN-γ reduced lung procollagen 1 and hydroxyproline levels in a bleomycin mouse model of lung fibrosis [66]. In summary, in patients with CFA there is evidence of impaired IFN-γ production, which may induce the immunological abnormalities observed (see above) and reduce the antifibrotic cytokine balance in the lungs.

Much of our research has been directed at identifying profibrotic cytokines which may be active in CFA. Transforming growth factor-β_1 (TGF-β_1) is one such cytokine. TGF-β_1 has actions at different levels of collagen metabolism which result in a net increase in the amount of collagen produced. It stimulates procollagen gene transcription, increases mRNA stability [67], decreases intracellular degradation [68] and limits extracellular degradation [69]. Increased levels have been found in animal models of pulmonary fibrosis. TGF-β_1 genes have been reported to be activated [31], and the levels of the peptide present in increased amounts at sites of extracellular matrix deposition in patients with CFA [70]. Recently, antibodies to TGF-β_1 and TGF-β_2 have been shown to partially attenuate collagen deposition in bleomycin-induced pulmonary fibrosis in mice [71]. This cytokine fulfils the criteria we have established for a profibrotic cytokine, which are that

1. it should stimulate fibroblast replication/procollagen synthesis, or reduce collagen degradation *in vitro*.
2. it should be present in increased amounts in the lungs (BAL/lung biopsies) of patients with pulmonary fibrosis.
3. inhibitors (including antibodies and receptor antagonists) should attenuate fibrosis in animal models.

Table 2 lists other potential profibrotic cytokines and indicates to what extent they are known to fulfil these criteria [71–78].

Macrophages and monocytes are felt to be the primary source of inflammatory and fibrotic mediators, but it is now apparent that other cells such as epithelial and endothelial cells and even fibroblasts themselves contribute to the local cytokine milieu (Figure 1). Cytokines which are considered to be primarily profibrotic may also have immunoregulatory actions [79]. The regulation of inflammation and fibrosis is therefore complex, with the effect of any one cytokine depending on a number of factors which include:

1. the presence of other cytokines. For example, IL-1 and tumour necrosis factor (TNF) individually stimulate but in combination inhibit fibroblast proliferation and collagen synthesis *in vitro* [80].
2. the state of activation/phenotype of the fibroblasts. For example, TGF-β induces immature but not mature cartilage cells to produce collagen [81, 82].
3. the presence of different cytokine receptors with different affinities for the cytokine [83].

Table 2. Putative profibrotic cytokines

Cytokine	Source	Effect on fibroblasts	Levels increased in BAL/ biopsies in CFA patients	Inhibitors attenuate lung fibrosis in animal models	Suggested references
Endothelin 1 ET-1	endo/epithelial cells fibroblasts macrophages	↑ proliferation chemoattractant	yes	?	[72, 73]
Insulin-like growth factor-1 IGF-1	fibroblasts macrophages smooth muscle cells	↑ collagen synthesis ↑ proliferation	yes	?	[74, 75]
Platelet-derived growth factor B PDGF-B	endothelial cells smooth muscle cells macrophages platelets	↑ proliferation chemoattractant	yes	?	[76]
Transforming growth factor β TGF-β	endo/epithelial cells fibroblasts platelets macrophages	↑ collagen synthesis ↓ collagen degradation	yes	yes	[67–71]
Tumour necrosis factor TNF	endothelial cells T lymphocytes macrophages	↑/↓ proliferation ↑ collagen synthesis	yes	yes	[77, 78]
Interleukin-1 (IL-1)	macrophages mast cells	↑/↓ collagen synthesis ↑ proliferation	yes	?	[77, 78]

↑ increased; ↓ decreased.

It is possible that fibrogenic mediators may be generated independent of inflammatory/immune cells. There is evidence of endothelial cell injury in pulmonary fibrosis [38] which allows an influx of proteins and inflammatory cells from the circulation into the pulmonary interstitium and alveolar space. Not only may the presence of serum affect the actions of cytokines [80], but recent evidence from our laboratory suggests that products of the coagulation cascade, including thrombin and cleavage products of fibrinogen, may themselves be potent fibroblast growth factors [84, 85].

3.3.4. Response to immunosuppressive treatment: The mainstay of treatment of CFA is high-dose oral corticosteroids. But though these drugs have a variety of anti-inflammatory effects and reduce collagen synthesis rates *in vitro*, only 15–30% of patients show clinical improvement with corticosteroids [86]. The survival curve of untreated patients falls between that of steroid-unresponsive and steroid-responsive patients [18]. This is probably because those with more severe or progressive disease were treated, but conversely it may be that reducing cell-mediated immunity with corticosteroids may have worsened the prognosis in some patients. Interestingly, in this context, corticosteroids have been shown to actually increase Platelet-derived growth factor (B) (PDGF(B)) mRNA in alveolar macrophages [87].

Second-line immunosuppressive treatment in patients with CFA is often with oral cyclophosphamide. This depletes lymphocytes and has been shown to cause a greater suppression of neutrophil alveolitis compared with corticosteroids [88], but the response rate is still low [86] and appears to be limited to those who show an initial improvement on corticosteroids [89]. It is of note, given the hypothesis (see above) that T lymphocytes may have a protective role in pulmonary fibrosis, that cyclophosphamide treatment has been reported to exacerbate bleomycin-induced pulmonary disease in a mouse model, an action which was negated by lymphocyte reconstitution [90]. Cyclophosphamide has significant acute and long-term toxicity; the latter includes a high rate of malignancies [91], which limits its use.

Azathioprine therapy suppresses lymphocyte and natural killer cell function, antibody production and antibody-dependent cell cytotoxicity. Small trials suggest that it is not as effective in CFA as cyclophosphamide [92] but that in general it has fewer significant adverse reactions. Other immunosuppressive treatments, such as cyclosporin [93] and methotrexate, have been used in patients with CFA, but they have been uncontrolled, anecdotal and/or have shown little extra clinical benefit.

In summary, a response to immunosuppressive treatments occurs in only a small minority of patients with CFA. This suggests that although immune mechanisms may be important in the pathogenesis of pulmonary fibrosis of some patients with CFA, in the majority, who usually present late in the natural history of their disease, additional or completely different factors are responsible for ongoing interstitial fibrosis.

4. Conclusions

CFA may result from a variety of initiating stimuli and has a variable natural history, suggesting that its pathogenesis is likely to be multifactorial. It is often suggested that inflammation precedes and is responsible for disease progression to fibrosis. In the minority of cases which respond to anti-inflammatory therapies this appears to be the case. In the remainder, however, fibrosis continues despite broad-spectrum immunosuppressive or anti-inflammatory therapy. In this chapter we have explored the possibility that the inflammatory/immune reaction is a "normal" response to injury and that an intact cell-mediated immune response protects against the development of pulmonary fibrosis. A defect in this immune response could result in a switch from a healing inflammatory response to fibrogenesis and progressive matrix deposition. One possibility is the inappropriate selection of a Th2 rather than a Th1 immune response. The resulting loss of antifibrotic activity of IFN-γ, defects in cell-mediated immunity and activated humoral immune response may be important in the switch to fibrogenesis. This raises the possibility that targeting immunomodulators, which enhance a Th1 and suppress the Th2 immune response, may be an alternative approach to developing new treatments for CFA.

Whatever the initiating factor, progressive pulmonary fibrosis is the "final common pathway". Inappropriate control of the processes regulating matrix turnover is another potential site for dysregulation. It is logical, therefore, that new treatments should be directed at influencing matrix synthetic and degradative processes. There has been recent intensive research into the regulation of collagen gene activation, the biochemical pathways of collagen metabolism and mediators of fibrogenesis. This has identified targets for potential new antifibrotic therapeutic strategies; thus, future treatment of CFA may see a combination of immunomodulator and antifibrotic therapy.

References

1. Ng TP, Chan SL, Lee J (1991) Predictors of mortality in silicosis. *Respir Med* 86: 115–119.
2. Becklake MR (1991) Asbestos and other fiber-related disease of the lungs and pleura. *Chest* 100: 248–254.
3. Silicosis and Silicate Disease Committee. Diseases associated with exposure to silica and non-fibrous silicate minerals. *Arch Pathol Lab Med* 1988; 112: 673–720.
4. Mah K, van Dyk J, Keane T, Poon PY (1987) Acute radiation-induced pulmonary damage: A clinical study on the response to fractionated radiation therapy. *Int J Radiat Oncol Biol Phys* 13: 179–188.
5. Cooper JAD, White DA, Mathay RA (1986) Drug-induced pulmonary disease. Part 1. Cytotoxic drugs. *Am Rev Respir Dis* 133: 321–340.
6. McMilan GHG, Pethybridge RJ, Sheers G (1980) Effect of smoking on attack rates of pulmonary and pleural lesions related to exposure to asbestos dust. *Br J Ind Med* 37: 268.
7. Hillarby MC, McMahon MJ, Grennan DM, Cooper RG, Clarkson RW, Davies EJ, Sanders PA, Chattopadhyay C, Swinson D (1993) HLA associations in subjects with rheumatoid arthritis and bronchiectasis but not with other pulmonary complications in rheumatoid disease. *Br J Rheumatol* 32: 794–797.

8. Shih JF, Hunninghake GW, Goeken NE, Galvin JR, Merchant JA, Schwartz DA (1993) The relationship between HLA-A, B, DQ and DR antigens and asbestos-induced lung disease. *Chest* 104: 26–31.
9. Briggs DC, Vaughan RW, Welsh KI, Myers A, duBois RM, Black CM (1991) Immuno-genetic prediction of pulmonary fibrosis in systemic sclerosis. *Lancet* 338: 661–662.
10. Crystal RG, Bitterman PB, Rennard SI, Hance AJ, Keogh BA (1984) Interstitial lung disease of unknown cause: Disorders characterised by chronic inflammation of the lower respiratory tract. *NEJM* 310: 154–166.
11. Hubbard R, Lewis S, Richards K, Johnston I, Britton J (1996) Occupational exposure to metal or wood dust and aetiology of cryptogenic fibrosing alveolitis. *Lancet* 347: 284–289.
12. Bitterman PB, Rennard SI, Keogh BA, Wewers MD, Adelberg S, Crystal RG (1986) Familial idiopathic pulmonary fibrosis: Evidence of lung inflammation in unaffected family members. *N Engl J Med* 314: 1343–1347.
13. Musk AW, Zilko PJ, Manners P, Kay PH, Kamboh MI (1986) Genetic studies in familial fibrosing alveolitis: Possible linkage with immunoglobulin allotypes (Gm). *Chest* 89: 206–210.
14. Egan JJ, Stewart JP, Hasleton PS, Arrand JR, Carroll KB, Woodcock AA (1995) Epstein-Barr virus replication within pulmonary epithelial cells in cryptogenic fibrosing alveolitis. *Thorax* 50: 1234–1239.
15. Wangoo A, Nicholson AG, Diss TC, Farrell PJ, duBois RM, Shaw RJ (1996) Cryptogenic fibrosing alveolitis does not appear associated with Epstein-Barr virus infection. *Thorax* 51: A11.
16. Matsui R, Goldstein RH, Mihal K, Brody JS, Steele MP, Fine A (1994) Type I collagen formation in rat type II alveolar cells immortalised by viral gene products. *Thorax* 49: 201–206.
17. Fulinami RS, Nelson JA, Walker L, Oldstone MA (1988) Sequence homology and im-munologic cross-reactivity of human cytomegalovirus and HLA-DR B chain: A means for graft rejection and immunosuppression. *J Virol* 62: 100–105.
18. Turner-Warwick M, Burrows B, Johnson A (1980) Cryptogenic fibrosing alveolitis: Response to corticosteroid treatment and its effect on survival. *Thorax* 35: 593–599.
19. Kirk JME, DaCosta PE, Turner-Warwick M, Littleton RJ, Laurent GJ (1986) Biochemical evidence for an increased and progressive deposition of collagen in lungs of patients with pulmonary fibrosis. *Clin Sci* 70: 39–45.
20. Selaman M, Montano M, Ramos C, Chapale R (1986) Concentration, bio-synthesis and degradation of collagen in idiopathic pulmonary fibrosis. *Thorax* 41: 355–359.
21. Mays PK, Laurent GJ (1994) The regulation of collagen and elastin gene expression in normal lung and during pulmonary disease. In: PJ Barnes, RA Stockley (eds.). *Molecular biology of lung disease*. Oxford, Blackwell, pp 216–260.
22. Murphy G, Docherty JP (1992) The matrix metalloproteinase and their inhibitors. *Am J Respir Cell Mol Biol* 7: 120–125.
23. McAnulty RJ, Laurent GJ (1987) Collagen synthesis and degradation *in vivo*: Evidence for rapid rates of collagen turnover with extensive degradation of newly synthesized collagen in tissues of the adult rat. *Collagen Rel Res* 7: 93–104.
24. Mays PK, McAnulty RJ, Laurent GJ (1989) Age-related changes in lung collagen meta-bolism: A role for degradation in regulating lung collagen production. *Am Rev Respir Dis* 140: 410–416.
25. Specks U, Nerlich A, Colby TV, Wiest I, Timpl R (1995) Increased expression of type IV collagen in lung fibrosis. *Am J Respir Crit Care Med* 151: 1956–1964.
26. McAnulty RJ, Moores SR, Talbot RJ, Bishop JE, Mays PK, Laurent GJ (1991) Long-term changes in mouse lung following inhalation of a fibrosis-inducing dose of $^{239}PuO_2$: Changes in collagen synthesis and degradation rates. *Int J Radiat Biol* 59: 229–238.
27. Low RB, Giancola MS, King TE, Chapitis J, Vacek P, Davis GS (1992) Serum and broncho-alveolar lavage of N-terminal type III procollagen peptides in idiopathic pulmonary fibro-sis. *Am Rev Respir Dis* 146: 701–706.
28. Walters EH, Gardiner PV (1991) Bronchoalveolar lavage as a research tool. *Thorax* 46: 613–618.
29. Ward C, Fenwick J, Weddle A, Booth H, Walters EH (1997) Albumin is not suitable as a marker of bronchoalveolar lavage (BAL) dilution in interstitial lung disease. *Eur Respir J; in press.*

30. Harrison NK, McAnulty RJ, Kimpton WG, Fraser JRE, Laurent TC, Laurent GJ (1993) Heterogeneity of type III procollagen N-terminal peptides in BAL fluid from normal and fibrotic lungs. *Eur Respir J* 6: 1443–1448.
31. Broekelmann TJ, Limper AH, Colby TV, McDonald JA (1991) Transforming growth factor β_1 is present at sites of extracellular matrix gene expression in human pulmonary fibrosis. *Proc Natl Acad Sci USA* 88: 6642–6646.
32. Suganuma H, Sato A, Tamura R, Chida K (1995) Enhanced migration of fibroblasts derived from lungs with fibrotic lesions. *Thorax* 50: 984–989.
33. Jordana M, Schulman J, McSharry C, Irving LB, Newhouse MT, Jordana G, Gauldie J (1988) Heterogeneous proliferative characteristics of human adult lung fibroblast lines and clonally derived fibroblasts from control and fibrotic lung tissue. *Am Rev Respir Dis* 137: 579–584.
34. Risteli L, Risteli J (1986) Radioimmunoassays for monitoring connective tissue metabolism. *Rheumatology* 10: 216–245.
35. McLaren AM, Isdale AH, Whiting PH, Bird HA, Robins SP (1993) Physiological variations in the urinary excretion of pyridinium crosslinks of collagen. *Br J Rheumatol* 32: 307–312.
36. Wright PH, Heard BE, Steel SJ, Turner-Warwick M (1981) Cryptogenic fibrosing alveolitis: Assessment by graded trephine lung biopsy histology compared with clinical, radiographic and physiologic features. *Br J Dis Chest* 75: 61–70.
37. Harrison NK, Myers AR, Corrin B, Soosay G, Dewar A, Black CM et al. (1991) Structural features of interstitial lung disease in systemic sclerosis. *Am Rev Respir Dis* 144: 706–713.
38. Lynch JP, Hunninghake GW (1992) Pulmonary complications of collagen vascular disease. *Ann Rev Med* 43: 17–35.
39. Jimenez SA (1994) New insights into the pathogenesis of interstitial pulmonary fibrosis. *Thorax* 49: 193–195.
40. Panos RJ, Mortenson RL, Niccoli SA, King TE (1990) Clinical deterioration in patients with idiopathic pulmonary fibrosis: Causes and assessment. *Am J Med* 88: 396–403.
41. Sachor Y, Schindler D, Siegal A, Lieberman D, Mikulski Y, Bruderman I (1989) Increased incidence of pulmonary tuberculosis in chronic interstitial lung disease. *Thorax* 44: 151–153.
42. Savici D, Campbell PA, King TE (1989) Bronchoalveolar macrophages from patients with idiopathic pulmonary fibrosis are unable to kill facultative intracellular bacteria. *Am Rev Respir Dis* 139: 22–27.
43. Pierce R, Turner-Warwick M (1980) Skin tests with tuberculin (PPD) *Candida albicans* and *Trichophyton* spp. in cryptogenic fibrosing alveolitis and asbestos-related lung disease. *Clin Allergy* 10: 229–237.
44. Scadding JG (1956) Insensitivity to tuberculin in pulmonary tuberculosis. *Tubercle* 37: 371.
45. Hudspith BN, Flint KC, Geraint-James D, Brostoff J, Johnson NM (1987) Lack of immune deficiency in sarcoidosis: Compartmentalisation of the immune response. *Thorax* 42: 250–255.
46. Boomars KA, Wagenaar SS, Mulder PG, van-Velzen-Blad H, van der Bosch JM (1995) Relationship between cells obtained by bronchoalveolar lavage and survival in idiopathic pulmonary fibrosis. *Thorax* 50: 1087–1092.
47. Watters LC, Schwarz MI, Cherniack RM, Waldron JA, Dunn TL, Stanford RE, King TE (1987) Idiopathic pulmonary fibrosis: Pretreatment bronchoalveolar lavage cellular constituents and their relationship with lung histopathology and clinical response to therapy. *Am Rev Respir Dis* 135: 696–704.
48. Karpel JP, Norin AJ (1989) Association of activated cytolytic lung lymphocytes with response to prednisone therapy in patients with idiopathic pulmonary fibrosis. *Chest* 96: 794–798.
49. Cormier Y, Belanger J, Laviolette M (1987) Prognostic significance of bronchoalveolar lymphocytosis in farmer's lung. *Am Rev Respir Dis* 135: 692–695.
50. Laviolette M, La Forge J, Tennina S, Boulet L-P (1911) Prognostic value of bronchoalveolar lavage lymphocyte count in recently diagnosed pulmonary sarcoidosis. *Chest* 100: 380–384.
51. Lecossier D, Valeyre D, Loiseau A, Cadranel J, Tazi A, Battesti JP, Hance AJ (1991) Antigen-induced proliferative response of lavage and blood T lymphocytes. *Am Rev Respir Dis* 144: 860–866.

52. Gardiner PV, Ward C, Allison A, Ashcroft T, Simpson W, Walters H et al. (1993) Pleuro-pulmonary abnormalities in primary Sjögren's syndrome. *J Rheum* 20: 831–837.
53. Garcia JG, James HL, Zinkgraf S, Perlman MB, Keogh BA (1987) Lower respiratory tract abnormalities in rheumatoid interstitial lung disease: Potential role for neutrophils in lung injury. *Am Rev Respir Dis* 136: 811–817.
54. Corsini E, Luster MI, Mahler J, Craig WA, Blazka ME, Rosenthal GJ (1994) A protective role for T lymphocytes in asbestos-induced pulmonary inflammation and collagen deposition. *Am J Respir Cell Mol Biol* 11: 531–539.
55. Zomas A, Marsh JC, Harrison NK, Hyer SL, Nussey SS, Knee G, Wilson AG, Lakhani A, Gordon-Smith EC (1995) Rapid progression of fibrosing alveolitis and thyrotoxicosis after antithymocyte globulin therapy for aplastic anaemia. *Ann Hematol* 71: 49–51.
56. Emura M, Nagi S, Takeuchi M, Kitaichi M, Izumi T (1990) *In vitro* production of B-cell growth factors and B-cell differentiation factors by peripheral blood mononuclear cells and bronchoalveolar lavage T lymphocytes from patients with idiopathic pulmonary fibrosis. *Clin Exp Immunol* 82: 133–139.
57. Campbell DA, Poulter LW, Janossy G, du Bois RM (1985) Immunohistological analysis of lung tissue from patients with cryptogenic fibrosing alveolitis suggesting local expression of immune hypersensitivity. *Thorax* 40: 405–411.
58. Wallace WAH, Roberts SN, Caldwell H, Thornton E, Greening AP, Lamb D, Howie SEM (1994) Circulating antibodies to lung protein(s) in patients with cryptogenic fibrosing alveolitis. *Thorax* 49: 218–224.
59. Nakos G, Adams A, Andriopoulos N (1993) Antibodies to collagen in patients with idiopathic pulmonary fibrosis. *Chest* 103: 1051–1058.
60. Wallace WAH, Ramage EA, Lamb D, Howie SEM (1995) A type 2 (TH2-like) pattern of immune response predominates in the pulmonary interstitium of patients with cryptogenic fibrosing alveolitis. *Clin Exp Immunol* 101: 436–441.
61. Prior C, Haslam PL (1992) *In vivo* levels and *in vitro* production of interferon gamma in fibrosing interstitial lung diseases. *Clin Exp Immunol* 88: 280–287.
62. Kuroki S, Ohta N, Sueoka N, Katoh O, Yamada H, Yamaguchi M (1995) Determination of various cytokines and type III procollagen aminopeptide levels in bronchoalveolar lavage fluid of the patients with pulmonary fibrosis: Inverse correlation between type III procollagen aminopeptide and interferon-γ in progressive patients. *Br J Rheum* 34: 31–36.
63. de Maeyer E, de Maeyer-Guignard J (1992) Interferon-γ. *Curr Opin Immunol* 4: 321–326.
64. Liu Y, Janeway C (1990) Interferon-γ plays a critical role in the induced cell death of effector T-cell: A possible third mechanism of self-tolerance. *J Exp Med* 172: 1735–1739.
65. Narayanan AS, Whitehey BA, Souza A, Raghu G (1992) Effect of γ-interferon on collagen synthesis by normal and fibrotic human lung fibroblasts. *Chest* 101: 1326–1331.
66. Gurujeyalakshmi G, Giri SN (1995) Molecular mechanisms of antifibrotic effect of interferon gamma in bleomycin-mouse model of lung fibrosis: Downregulation of TGF-beta and procollagen I and III gene expression. *Exp Lung Res* 21: 791–808.
67. Pentinnen RP, Kobayashi S, Bornstein P (1988) Transforming growth factor β increases mRNA for matrix proteins both in the presence and in the absence of changes in mRNA stability. *Proc Natl Acad Sci USA* 85: 1105–1108.
68. McAnulty RJ, Campa JS, Cambrey AD, Laurent GJ (1991) The effect of transforming growth factor β on rates of procollagen synthesis and degradation *in vitro*. *Biochem Biophys Acta* 1091: 231–235.
69. Edwards DR, Murphy G, Reynolds JJ, Whitham SE, Docherty AJP, Angel P, Heath JK (1987) Transforming growth factor beta modulates the expression of collagenase and metalloproteinase inhibitor. *EMBO J* 6: 1899–1904.
70. Corrin B, Butcher D, McAnulty RJ, duBois RM, Black CM, Laurent GJ, Harrison NK (1994) Immunohistochemical localisation of transforming growth factor-β1 in the lungs of patients with systemic sclerosis, cryptogenic fibrosing alveolitis and other lung disorders. *Histopathology* 24: 145–150.
71. Giri SN, Hyde DM, Hollinger MA (1993) Effect of antibody to transforming growth factor β on bleomycin-induced accumulation of lung collagen in mice. *Thorax* 48: 959–966.
72. Peacock AJ, Dawes KE, Shock A, Gray AJ, Reeves JT, Laurent GJ (1992) Endothelin 1 and endothelin 3 induce chemotaxis and replication of pulmonary artery fibroblasts. *Am J Respir Cell Mol Biol* 7: 492–499.

73. Giaid A, Michel RP, Stewart DJ, Sheppard M, Corrin B, Hamid Q (1993) Expression of endothelin-1 in lungs of patients with cryptogenic fibrosing alveolitis. *Lancet* 341: 1550–1554.
74. Goldstein RH, Poliks CF, Pilch PF, Smith BD, Fine A (1989) Stimulation of collagen formation by insulin and insulin-like growth factor I in cultures of human lung fibroblasts. *Endocrinology* 124: 964–970.
75. Harrison NK, Cambrey AD, Myers AR, Southcott AM, Black CM, duBois RM, Laurent GJ, McAnulty RJ (1994) Insulin-like growth factor-1 is partially responsible for fibroblast proliferation induced by bronchoalveolar lavage fluid from patients with systemic sclerosis. *Clin Sci Colch* 86: 141–148.
76. Heldin CH, Westermark B (1990) Platelet-derived growth factor: Mechanism of action and possible *in vivo* function. *Cell Reg* 1: 555–566.
77. Zhang Y, Lee TC, Guillemin B, Yu MC, Rom WM (1993) Enhanced IL-1β and tumour necrosis factor-α release and messenger RNA expression in macrophages from idiopathic pulmonary fibrosis or after asbestos exposure. *J Immunol* 150: 4188–4196.
78. Diaz A, Munoz E, Johnston R, Korn JH, Jimenez SA (1993) Regulation of human lung fibroblast $\alpha 1$(I) procollagen gene expression by tumor necrosis factor α, interleukin-1β and prostaglandin E_2. *J Biol Chem* 268: 10364–10371.
79. Bermudez LE (1993) Production of transforming growth factor-β by *Mycobacterium avium*-infected human macrophages is associated with unresponsiveness to IFN-γ. *J Immunol* 150: 1838–1845.
80. Elias JA, Freundlich B, Kern JA, Rosenbloom (1990) Cytokine networks in the regulation of inflammation and fibrosis in the lung. *Chest* 97: 1439–1445.
81. Seyedin SM, Thompson AY, Bentz H, Rosen DM, McPherson JM, Conti A, Siegel NR, Galluppi GR, Piez KA (1986) Cartilage-inducing factor A: Apparent identity to transforming growth factor beta. *J Biol Chem* 261: 5693–5695.
82. Harrison NK, Argent AC, McAnulty RJ, Black CM, Corrin B, Laurent GJ (1991) Collagen synthesis and degradation by systemic sclerosis lung fibroblasts: Response to transforming growth factor β. *Chest* 99: 71 S.
83. Massague J, Andres J, Attisano L, Cheifetz S, Lopez-Casillas F, Ohtsuki M, Wrana JL (1992) TGFβ receptors. *Mol Reprod Dev* 32: 99–104.
84. Gray AJ, Bishop JE, Reeves JT, Mecham RP, Laurent GJ (1995) Partially degraded fibrin(ogen) stimulates fibroblast proliferation. *Am J Resp Mol Biol* 12: 684–690.
85. Hernandez-Rodriguez NA, Cambrey AD, Harrison MD, Chambers RC, Gray AJ, Southcott AM, duBois RM, Black CM, Scully MF, McAnulty RJ et al. (1995) Role of thrombin in pulmonary fibrosis. *Lancet* 346: 1071–1073.
86. Johnson MA, Kwan S, Snell NJC, Nunn AJ, Darbyshire JH, Turner-Warwick M (1989) Randomised controlled trial comparing prednisolone with cyclophosphamide and low-dose prednisolone in combination in cryptogenic fibrosing alveolitis. *Thorax* 44: 280–288.
87. Haynes AR, Shaw RJ (1992) Dexamethasone-induced increase in platelet-derived growth factor (B) mRNA in human alveolar macrophages and myelomonocytic HL60 macrophage-like cells. *Am J Respir Cell Mol Biol* 7: 198–206.
88. O'Donnell K, Keogh B, Cantin A, Crystal R (1987) Pharmacological suppression of the neutrophil component of the alveolitis in idiopathic pulmonary fibrosis. *Am Rev Respir Dis* 136: 288–292.
89. van-Oortegem K, Wallaert B, Marquette CH, Ramon P, Perez T, Lafitte JJ, Tonnel AB (1994) Determinants of response to immunosuppressive therapy in idiopathic pulmonary fibrosis. *Eur Respir J* 7: 1950–1957.
90. Schrier DJ, Phan SH (1984) Modulation of bleomycin-induced pulmonary fibrosis in the BALB/c mouse by cyclophosphamide-sensitive T-cells. *Am J Pathol* 116: 270–278.
91. Hoffman GS, Kerr GS, Leavitt RY et al. (1992) Wegener granulomatosis: An analysis of 158 patients. *Ann Intern Med* 6: 488–498.
92. Raghu G, Depaso WJ, Cain K, Hammar SP, Wetzel CE, Dreis DF, Hutchinson J, Pardee NE, Winterbauer RH (1991) Azathioprine combined with prednisolone in the treatment of idiopathic pulmonary fibrosis: A prospective double-blind, randomized, placebo-controlled clinical trial. *Am Rev Respir Dis* 144: 291–296.
93. Moolman JA, Bardin PG, Rossouw DY, Joubet JR (1991) Cyclosporin as a treatment for interstitial lung disease of unknown aetiology. *Thorax* 46: 592–595.

Autoimmune Aspects of Lung Disease
ed. by D. A. Isenberg and S. G. Spiro
© 1998 Birkhäuser Verlag Basel/Switzerland

CHAPTER 11
Drugs and Other Factors

Robert M. Bernstein

Rheumatology Department, Manchester Royal Infirmary, Manchester, UK

1. Introduction

Toxic substances can reach the lungs by inhalation or via the bloodstream. Most of the reactions discussed in this chapter involve drugs and toxins arriving by the bloodborne route, but the great burden of lung disease is caused by the inhalation of microorganisms, allergens, dusts and cigarette smoke. About one-tenth of an acre of internal surface is exposed to inhaled gases, and there are several lines of defence: physical (cough, mucociliary

clearance), secretions containing antibacterial proteins (lysozyme, lactoferrin, secretory immunoglobulins, complement), and cellular defences
(lymphocytes, macrophages, plasma cells and granulocytes).

This chapter is concerned with what may be immunologically mediated
reactions to drugs and toxins, although evidence for a classical immune
response to the inciting agent may not always be certain. First, the reaction
may be rare; second, the response may not be immune (e.g. byssinosis and
asbestosis); third, the immune response may be directed at an unknown
metabolite of the parent compound. The justification for inclusion here
depends on the presence of lymphocytes or antibody, or on similarity to a
reaction seen in the autoimmune rheumatic diseases. It is possible that
immune effector mechanisms such as complement activation take part
without the need for a prior specific immune trigger.

Once a drug reaction is suspected, support may be adduced by finding
improvement after the suspect drug is withdrawn. This approach is not
always straightforward. First, stopping the drug may have an appreciable
morbidity and even mortality of its own (e.g. amiodarone or cytotoxic
chemotherapy). Second, one of several agents given concurrently may be
responsible. Third, it may be difficult to distinguish between an exacerbation of the underlying disease and a reaction to a drug (e.g. pneumonitis in
a patient with an autoimmune rheumatic disease being treated with a cytotoxic drug). Fourth, it is also essential to exclude intercurrent illness,
particularly infection. All this requires careful clinical assessment, which
may include bronchoalveolar lavage (BAL) and transbronchial or open
lung biopsy. In difficult cases, the best source of lung tissue for histology
remains open lung biopsy, as specimens obtained by transbronchial biopsy
are usually inadequate.

The reactions to be considered below include drug-induced lupus,
pulmonary hpyertension, anaphylaxis, asthma, granulomatous diseases
such as extrinsic allergic alveolitis, pneumonitis (non-infective interstitial
shadowing), pulmonary eosinophilia and pulmonary fibrosis, organising
pneumonia and pleural effusion. Some of the more common examples are
shown in Table 1.

2. Pulmonary Vascular Disease

2.1 Pulmonary Hypertension

Pulmonary hypertension unexplained by parenchymal lung disease, and
without evidence of pulmonary embolism, has developed during and also
after administration of several therapeutic agents. The anorectic drugs
aminorex (no longer available) and fenfluramine have both been implicated. The odds ratio of a true association with fenfluramine may be as high
as 10−20 [1].

Table 1. Some drug reactions in the lung

	Pneumonitis	PIE	Fibrosis	BOOP	LE	Pulm. vasc.
Amiodarone	+		+	+		
Ampicillin	+					
Azathioprine	+					
Beta blockers	+			+		
Barbiturates				+		
Bleomycin	+		+	+		+
Busulphan			+			+
Captopril	+					
Carbamazepine	+				+	
Chlorambucil	+					
Chlorpromazine		+				+
Chlorpropamide		+				
Dothiepin	+		+			
Hydralazine	+				+	
Isoniazed					+	
Melphelan			+			
Methotrexate	+					
Minocycline		+			+	
Mitomycin			+			
NSAID's and aspirin		+				
Oestrogen					*	+
Penicillamine	+	+	+	+	+	
Penicillin		+				
Procainamide	+				+	
Quinidine	+	+				
Sulphasalazine	+	+		+	+	
Sulphonamides	+	+			*	+
Tetracyclines		+				
Vasopressin	+					

* May trigger idiopathic SLE.
  PIE: Pulmonary infiltrates with eosinophilia; BOOP: Bronchiolitis obliterans with organizing pneumonia; LE: Lupus erythematosus; Pulm. vasc.: Pulmonary vascular disease.

Pulmonary hypertension of primary type occurs with an overall annual incidence between one and five cases per million. It generally progresses relentlessly, even in those few cases when an inciting drug has been recognised and withdrawn. The overall mean survival remains under 5 years despite new approaches to treatment [2]. Calcium antagonists may sometimes slow down or even halt progression in the earlier stages, supporting the idea that vasospasm leads to obliteration of the arterial lumen. Only about a quarter of patients show a significant reduction in pulmonary artery pressure and pulmonary vascular resistance with high doses of nifedipine (such as 240 mg/day), and there is a danger of reducing cardiac output if systemic vasodilation embarrasses venous return [3].

Continuous infusion of prostacyclin has been successful in stabilising the disease in a few cases over many months [4], and there is some hope that the new oral analogue of prostacyclin will prove useful once this becomes available. Lung and heart-lung transplantation have been employed only rarely because of the shortage of donors and the rapid terminal course of pulmonary hypertension.

In future, inhaled nitric oxide may have a place in the treatment of pulmonary hypertension, since selective pulmonary vasodilatation avoids the problems of systemic vasodilatation (hypotension and reduced venous return) that can occur with calcium antagonists and prostacyclin therapy. Nitric oxide appears to have vasodilator and bronchodilator effects in the lung, but may also have proinflammatory effects that may need to be overcome [5]. Moreover, nitric oxide has a very short biological half-life and has to be inhaled continuously.

2.2. Pulmonary Thromboembolism

Pulmonary thromboembolism appears to be a rare complication of the drug-induced lupus syndrome but may be underestimated. Two case reports have implicated procainamide and chlorprozamine in generating lupus anticoagulant and anticardiolipin antibodies in patients presenting with thrombosis. In both cases the syndrome resolved and the antibodies disappeared, once the offending drug had been withdrawn [6].

Oestrogen therapy given as the oral contraceptive pill or hormone replacement therapy has been associated with a threefold increase in the incidence of venous thrombosis and pulmonary embolism [7]. The risk appears to be very small except, presumably, in the presence of some other condition promoting coagulation, such as the lupus anticoagulant. Hence, there may be a need for caution in prescribing hormone replacement therapy in elderly patients with systemic lupus erythematosus (SLE) even though oestrogens in low dose probably do not often exacerbate the underlying autoimmune disease.

2.3. Drug-Induced Lupus

Drug-induced lupus is quite uncommon compared with idiopathic SLE, but it responds so well to the withdrawal of the offending drug that the diagnosis must not be missed. The salient features of the syndrome are listed and compared with idiopathic SLE in Table 2.

The pulmonary manifestations of drug-induced lupus include pleurisy, pleural effusion and pulmonary infiltrates [8]. Published series suggest quite high frequencies for pleuropulmonary involvement (25% with hydralazine-induced lupus and over 30% with procainamide lupus), but involvement is probably rather less frequent now that the diagnosis is often made at an earlier stage [9]. The patient is likely also to have arthralgia,

Table 2. Clinical and laboratory manifestations of idiopathic SLE and drug-induced lupus

Manifestations	Proportion positive (%)		
	SLE	Hydralazine lupus	Procainamide lupus
Arthralgia	90	90	90
Arthritis		50	18
Fever	84	5	45
Rash	72	25	5–18
Lymphadenopathy	59	14	0–9
Myalgia	48	2–34	20–50
Pleurisy	45		
Pleural effusion	33	25–30	33
Pulmonary infiltrate	8		30
Pericarditis	31	2	16
Hepatosplenomegaly	5–10		20–33
CNS/seizures	16–25	0	1
Raynaud's phenomenon	23	rare	5
Joint deformities	10–26	0	0
Renal involvement	46	2–20	0–5
Anaemia (Hb < 11.5 g/dl)	57	30	9–21
Leucopaenia (< 4×10^9/l)	43	26	2–32
LE cells	76	66	76
ANA	95	100	100
Rheumatoid factor	50	22	32–50
False positive test for syphilis	11	5–18	rare
Coombs' test	25	rare	33
Anti-native DNA antibody	60*	rare	rare
Anti-poly (ADP-ribose) antibody	60*	100*	not known
Anti-histone antibody	60*	100*	100*

Adapted from a review of several series by Harmon and Portanova (1982) [8].
* Approximate percentages.

myalgia, elevated erythrocyte sedimentation rate, and antinuclear antibody in high titre and homogenous pattern without antibody to double-stranded DNA. Drug-induced antinuclear antibodies are much more common than symptomatic illness [10] and generally react against histones and poly(adenosine diphosphate-ribose) [11]. There may also be antibodies to a neutrophil cytoplasmic antigen, myeloperoxidase [12], but glomerulo-nephritis and vasculitis are uncommon in drug-induced lupus [13].

The list of drugs suspected of causing drug-induced lupus grows longer; the more important examples are shown in Table 3. Most research has centered on hydralazine and procainamide [14], neither of which is now in common use. In the 1950s, Perry [15] recognised that up to 10% of patients treated with large doses of hydralazine developed a lupus syndrome, whereas with modern smaller doses the risk is 1–2% [10]. The risk factors are clear (Table 4). A modest dose must be taken for 1–2 years or a larger dose for several months. The patient almost always is a slow acetylator [14, 16], implying that less drug is acetylated on first pass through the liver. The

Table 3. Drugs reported to induce a lupus syndrome

Definite	hydralazine
	isoniazid
	procainamide
Probable	penicillamine
	sulphasalazine
	minocycline
	acebutalol
	labetalol
	methyldopa
	captopril
	phenytoin
	carbamazepine
	chlorpromazine
	lithium
	prophylthiouracyl
	quinidine
	psoralen/ultraviolet A (PUVA)
	venocuran

Table 4. Risk factors for hydralazine lupus

	Hydralazine-treated controls	Hydralazine lupus	Odds ratio
Mean hydralazine intake	65 g	150 g	
Female	31%	81%	9.9
White	63%	96%	8.2
Slow acetylator	55%	96%	8.2
HLA-DR4	25%	73%	8.1
C4-null	43%*	76%	4.3

* Healthy controls not hydralazine treated.

other factors important in the case of hydralazine-induced lupus are female gender, carriage of the human leucocyte antigen HLA-DR4 [16] and a C4-null allele in the major histocompatibility (MHC) locus [17]. Inhibition of the function of the complement C4 component by a drug metabolite may be a factor in pathogenesis [18].

2.4. Blackfat Tobacco Disease

In Guyana the smoking of poor quality tobacco adulterated with mineral oils to improve the flavour has led to cases of pulmonary vasculitis and pneumonitis progressing to pulmonary hypertension and fibrosis, and eventually to *cor pulmonale* and death [19].

2.5. *Goodpasture's Syndrome*

Some cases of acute glomerulonephritis are caused by the development of autoantibodies reacting with the basement membrane of the kidney and lung. Immunoglobulin G eluted from affected kidneys and lungs can bind to alveolar basement membrane. Pulmonary haemorrhage appears in only a proportion of cases and is largely restricted to cigarette smokers (an environmental toxin influencing the course of an immunologically mediated disease) [20].

D-penicillamine, sometimes used in the treatment of rheumatoid arthritis, systemic sclerosis and Wilson's disease, can itself induce an interesting range of autoimmune diseases, including myasthenia gravis, myositis, lupus, pemphigus and Goodpasture's syndrome. The relevant autoantibodies develop just as they do in the idiopathic diseases. Goodpasture's syndrome induced by penicillamine is rare; alveolar haemorrhage and renal failure develop, and the prognosis is improved by removing the antibodies to basement membrane through immunosuppression and plasmapheresis, just as in the idiopathic disease [21].

3. Asthma and Anaphylaxis

The exacerbation of asthma by drugs such as beta-blockers and non-steroidal anti-inflammatory drugs (NSAIDs) appears to have a pharmacological mechanism. However, some drugs have an idiosyncratic effect on the airways involving immediate hypersensitivity, such as the acute anaphylactic reactions to penicillin or intravenous iron-dextran.

Non-steroidal anti-inflammatory drugs, as a class, may cause asthma in about 2% of people and can exacerbate the condition in up 20% of known asthmatics. Urticaria and rhinitis may also occur. The mechanism is not certain, but it is thought that inhibition of cyclo-oxygenase results in the shunting of arachidonate metabolism from prostaglandin production to the 5-lipoxygenase pathway, leading to increased generation of leucotrienes. Sulphidopeptide leucotrienes (LTC4, LTD4 and LTE4) may be most important. Inhibitors of 5-lipoxygenase may counteract this adverse effect of aspirin and NSAID's, and such inhibitors may offer a new therapeutic approach to asthma in general [22].

4. Granuloma Formation

Granulomas may form around particles of inert material such as talc or silica; these foreign body granulomas contain mainly macrophages. By contrast, some substances such as salts of beryllium cause the formation of immune, hypersensitivity granulomas, which contain both macrophages and activated lymphocytes. Hypersensitivity granulomas occur classically in tuberculosis, sarcoidosis, Wegener's granulomatosis and Churg-Strauss vasculitis, but also in extrinsic allergic alveolitis (such as farmer's lung). Mediastinal lymph node enlargement with giant cell granulomas giving a sarcoidosis-like picture has been attributed on rare occasions to treatment with penicillin, phenytoin or methotrexate.

4.1. Beryllium Disease

Beryllium disease occurs in workers exposed to inhalation of beryllium salts. It is a multi-system disease with granuloma formation essentially indistinguishable from sarcoidosis apart from the occupational history. Beryllium may act as an immunogenic hapten. BAL reveals increased numbers of T lymphocytes and increased CD4:CD8 ratio; the BAL lymphocytes express activation markers (HLA Class II and IL-2 receptor), and release IL-2. The T-lymphocyte response to beryllium is antigen-specific, IL-2 dependent, MHC class II-restricted and polyclonal [23]. This is in keeping with a classical cellular immune response. Both lung and blood T-cells from patients with the disease transform in response to beryllium in vitro, and cells obtained by BAL express the CD45R0 phenotype of primed T lymphocytes [24].

4.2. Extrinsic Allergic Alveolitis

This is a granulomatous disease probably caused by the inhalation of specific antigens and largely mediated by T lymphocytes. There are also humoral immune phenomena that were recognised 30 years ago by Pepys [25]. The condition is less common among cigarette smokers [26].

Fluid obtained by BAL contains increased numbers of lymphocytes and a slight excess of CD8 suppressor cytotoxic cells over CD4 helper cells. These changes may be seen in healthy farmers exposed to mouldy hay who have not developed farmer's lung, but in pigeon fancier's lung a defect in antigen-specific immunosuppression has been found in those with the disease [27].

Precipitating antibodies present in the serum of patients with extrinsic allergic alveolitis are thought to react with antigens in the inhaled material leading to the activation of complement within the lung. In farmer's lung antibodies can be detected in the lung 36 h after inhalation of the mould [28]. The interplay between the humoral and cellular immune processes needs more study.

4.3. Caplan's Syndrome

Typical rheumatoid nodules are seen occasionally in the lungs of patients with rheumatoid arthritis. Caplan noted massive shadows on the chest radiographs of coalminers with rheumatoid arthritis [29]. These were much larger than rheumatoid nodules and occurred more frequently. They are believed to represent an irritative response to coal dust particles, an example of an idiopathic disease process exacerbated by an environmental factor.

5. Interstitial Pneumonitis

A large number of drugs can cause breathlessness with an interstitial infiltrative process evident as widespread shadowing on the chest X-ray [30]. Usually, the condition occurs during therapy with a drug that has been taken for a considerable time but may also occur early. In the case of a drug such as amiodarone that persists in the tissues, pneumonitis may develop weeks after the drug has been stopped.

The onset of pneumonitis is unpredictable and can be acute or subacute. Dry cough and breathlessness are the first symptoms. The chest radiograph shows infiltrates, which vary in size and location but are more common in the lower than in the upper zones. Lung function tests show a restrictive defect and often a disproportionate fall in the single-breath carbon monoxide transfer factor.

BAL usually reveals lymphocytes. These are often predominantly CD8 positive, but in methotrexate pneumonitis they are mainly CD4 positive [31]. In the case of interferon-α therapy, a proliferative response of lymphocytes to the drug has been demonstrated [32].

5.1. Differential Diagnosis of Interstitial Pneumonitis

When considering a possible drug-induced pneumonitis, one must also consider progression of an underlying disease (e.g. fibrosing alveolitis, pulmonary oedema or infiltrating malignancy), and an infective pneumonia (perhaps caused by an opportunistic infection such as *Pneumocystis carinii*, fungus or cytomegalovirus if the patient is receiving immunosuppressive therapy). The overall clinical picture and course of the illness may give clues. Examination of the sputum is essential, and BAL is often recommended to exclude infection especially in patients who are immunocompromised.

Lung biopsy should be considered before embarking on high-dose steroid therapy or cytotoxic therapy, when there is serious concern about the possibility of an infection such as tuberculosis. In an interstitial pneumonitis there is usually a dense mononuclear infiltrate and sometimes desquamation of inflammatory cells into the alveolar spaces; granulomas are rare, and there is no significant fibrosis. Recovery from interstitial pneumonitis may take days or weeks and is probably hastened by steroid therapy. The overall mortality is low, but very severe or advanced cases may be fatal despite intensive care.

5.2. Specific Drugs Causing Pneumonitis

5.2.1. Amiodarone: Amiodarone is commonly prescribed, as it is effective in both ventricular and supraventricular arrhythmias. It has a long half-life and tends to accumulate in the tissues. Amiodarone has a partic-ular propensity to cause interstitial pneumonitis and is now one of the commonest causes of this reaction. It may cause particular problems in management for two reasons. First, the differential diagnosis of pulmonary oedema arises in patients with impaired left ventricular function. Second, stopping amiodarone may lead to the recurrence of a potentially fatal arrhythmia.

The development of pneumonitis depends on the dose and duration of treatment [33]. The frequency increases from about 2% with daily doses of 200 mg up to 50% with daily doses over 1200 mg. The dura-tion of treatment prior to onset of pneumonitis is variable but tends to be about 3 years with low doses and less than 1 year with higher doses. Most patients developing pneumonitis will have had cumulative intakes of over 200 g.

There is increasing breathlessness, often accompanied by fever, weight loss and high erythrocyte sedimentation rate. The pattern of shadowing on the chest X-ray is variable, usually showing bilateral asymmetrical shadows, but occasionally there is a unilateral segmental or lobar opacity, and a pleural effusion may occur as well. The extent of the damage may be assessed by computed tomography (CT scanning), and small foci invisible on the chest X-ray may be seen in asymptomatic patients taking amiodarone [34]. BAL may show excess lymphocytes or neutrophils [35], and the histo-logical findings include excess lipid, thickening of the alveolar walls and sometimes fibrosis, but these investigations are not usually required in clinical practice.

Once amiodarone therapy has been withdrawn, pneumonitis resolves in most cases (except for any fibrosis), but the combined pulmonary and cardiac mortality may reach 20%. Deposits of amiodarone are leeched out of the lungs over months, so even after the drug has been stopped, it may be helpful to prescribe steroid therapy to retard the development of fibrosis. Rechallenge with amiodarone usually leads to a recurrence of pneumonitis, but it may be possible to continue treatment with low-dose amiodarone under steroid cover when use of the drug is essential.

5.2.2. Cytotoxic drugs: Several cytotoxic agents can cause interstitial pneumonitis. Bleomycin is the best-known example, but other drugs include cyclophosphamide, chlorambucil, azathioprine and methotrexate. Daily dose and total intake are poor guides to the risk of pneumonitis. Concurrent steroid therapy may not protect the lungs.

There may be particular difficulty in distinguishing a drug reaction from atypical pneumonia or a manifestation of the underlying disease (fibrosing alveolitis or lymphangitis carcinomatosa, for instance). BAL is useful in excluding *P. carinii* and other opportunistic infections.

5.2.3. Methotrexate: Low-dose methotrexate is often used in rheumatoid arthritis, where it causes pneumonitis in 2–3% of cases. The condition often develops within the first 6 months of treatment, with the total consumption ranging from 60–250 mg [36]. However, it may not begin until the drug has been taken for 3 years or longer. Pre-existing lung disease (fibrosing alveolitis) may predispose to the development of methotrexate pneumonitis. Obstructive airways disease is probably not a risk factor, but care is still needed, as such patients may be less able to tolerate additional lung damage. (see also p 134 for further description).

Methotrexate pneumonitis generally presents with breathlessness, dry cough and pulmonary crackles. It may be mild, responding rapidly to withdrawal of the drug and to the use of high-dose steroid therapy, but some cases require intensive therapy with mechanical ventilation and even then may be fatal.

6. Fibrotic Reactions

6.1. Pulmonary Fibrosis

Pulmonary fibrosis can develop insidiously during treatment with some cytotoxic drugs, gold, sulphasalazine and nitrofurantoin. It is associated with breathlessness, cough and sometimes a low-grade fever. Shadowing on the chest X-ray may be restricted to the lower zones or may be diffuse, often with a ground-glass appearance. Lung function tests show a restrictive lung defect, with a reduced gas transfer factor. BAL may show neutrophilia. Biopsy shows fibrosis with some mononuclear cells and dysplastic alveolar type II cells [35]. Corticosteroid therapy may retard the fibrosis, which tends to progress even after the offending drug has been withdrawn.

6.2. Systemic Sclerosis

Scleroderma-like disease with the typical microvascular and fibrotic changes can follow exposure to a variety of agents. Bleomycin-induced scleroderma is well recognised and often associated with pulmonary fibrosis. Rats treated with bleomycin developed skin thickening associated with increased collagen synthesis [37]. More controversial are reports of scleroderma associated with drugs including carbidopa, pentazocine, penicillamine and various appetite suppressants such as mazindol. There are also numerous reports of systemic sclerosis developing after even very brief exposure to various volatile organic chemicals, but there is concern about ascertainment bias, as epidemiological evidence is lacking [38, 39]. There is no convincing evidence for claims of an association between silicone implants and the development of autoimmune rheumatic diseases such as systemic sclerosis [40].

6.3. Silicosis

In the absence of adequate dust control, intense exposure to silica dust, such as in miners and stonemasons, can cause pulmonary fibrosis. Rounded opacities are seen on the chest X-ray, and hilar node enlargement is common. Histology of the lung lesions shows discrete nodules made of concentric layers of dense collagen tissue with a core containing birefringent quartz particles. After many years the nodules may develop a calcified shell. Not only is there an increased risk of tuberculosis developing on a background of silicosis, but it is said that the risk of systemic sclerosis is 3-fold greater among East German coal miners than among the normal male population and 155-fold greater in those with established silicosis [38]. A recent study of 14 patients with silica-associated systemic sclerosis (including pulmonary fibrosis in all cases) found antibody to topoisomerase I (Scl-70) in nine cases, as well as one with antibody to centromere and two with antibodies to Ro and La, about the same frequency as found in idiopathic systemic sclerosis [41].

6.4. Vinyl Chloride Disease

Workers exposed to vinyl chloride for prolonged periods in the manufacture of polyvinyl chloride were liable to an illness characterized by breathlessness, Raynaud's phenomenon and contracture of the hands with thickening of the skin. Pulmonary fibrosis developed in some of the more severe cases (whereas the more usual finding of obstructive airways disease may have been due to coincidental cigarette smoking). Deposits of complement and fibrinogen were found in blood vessel walls, emphasising that like systemic sclerosis this is a disease of the microvasculature as well as fibrosis. Anticentromere and anti-Scl-70 antibodies are absent. It is suggested that HLA-DR5 influences susceptibility, and DR3 the severity of vinyl chloride disease [42].

7. Pulmonary Eosinophilia

7.1. Pulmonary Infiltrates with Eosinophilia

A patient with cough, wheeze, malaise and fever may have pulmonary infiltrates evident on the chest radiograph and eosinophilia in the blood and BAL. The syndrome may be idiopathic or associated with systemic conditions such as Churg-Strauss vasculitis and inflammatory bowel disease. Pulmonary infiltrates with eosinophilia (PIE) can be a drug reaction, notably to several antibiotics and many NSAIDs. PIE usually responds quickly to withdrawal of the drug, and recovery may be hastened by steroid therapy [43, 44].

7.2. Eosinophilia-Myalgia Syndrome

An illness with acute pneumonitis, myalgias, fever and blood eosinophilia occurred as an epidemic in the United States in the late 1980s. The condition was attributed to a contaminant in the manufacture of L-tryptophan, possibly in just one factory. The acute illness often resolved but in some cases progressed to pulmonary hypertension and chronic changes in liver, heart and nervous system [45].

7.3. Spanish Toxic Oil Syndrome

In 1981 over 20,000 people were poisoned by ingestion of contaminated cooking oil. The initial picture was of fever with interstitial pneumonitis, myalgia, arthralgia, rash and blood eosinophilia. A few patients died of respiratory failure, but the early acute pulmonary changes generally resolved without fibrosis. Most patients recovered, but some went on to a chronic phase of neuromuscular atrophy and scleroderma [46].

8. Bronchiolitis Obliterans

In rheumatoid arthritis there have been a few reports of severe and fatally progressive small airways obstruction with the forced expiratory volume in 1 s falling to very low levels. The airways are said to be narrowed by granulation tissue and endobronchial fibrosis [21]. Most cases have been associated with penicillamine therapy and a few with the use of gold. However, the association remains unproven, and airways obstruction progresses even when the drug is discontinued (except, perhaps, in the earliest stages).

9. Organising Pneumonia and "BOOP"

A further type of pulmonary parenchymal reaction to drugs can be distinguished from pneumonitis and pulmonary fibrosis on the basis of radiological and histological findings. The condition occurs also occasionally in rheumatoid arthritis and with inflammatory bowel disease. When there is an element of bronchiolitis obliterans (BO) with the organising pneumonia (OP), the condition is known as BOOP. The patient may have breathlessness, fever, crackles and occasionally chest pain with a pleural rub. The chest X-ray shows patches of consolidation, which may be migratory. Histology shows proliferating buds of connective tissue. The condition generally responds to withdrawal of the drug and to corticosteroid therapy [47].

10. Pleural Effusion

Pleural effusion can occur as a rather infrequent feature of drug-induced pneumonitis and organising pneumonia and in about 5–30% of cases in drug-induced lupus syndrome (the higher rate in older series with more advanced disease). Pleural thickening in plaques is well recognised in relation to asbestos exposure but is also reported with the use of various ergot derivatives [30].

11. Conclusion

Toxic reactions, and particularly reactions to drugs, can mimic underlying lung diseases and infection. The differential diagnosis may include pulmonary oedema, fibrosing alveolitis, lymphangitis carcinomatosa and pneumonia. There is good evidence for an immunological basis to anaphylaxis, extrinsic allergic alveolitis and beryllium disease. Elsewhere the evidence comes from the presence of excess lymphocytes in BAL fluid or similarity with an effect of a systemic autoimmune disease (such as pulmonary hypertension).

The most common reaction is pneumonitis. This usually resolves upon withdrawal of the offending agent and recurs with rechallenge, but the time course may not be typical of an immune reaction. Further insight into pathogenesis may require a greater understanding of the metabolism of drugs and toxins within the lung and within each type of pulmonary cell. The important environmental lung diseases related to cigarette smoking, asbestosis and pneumoconiosis appear not to have an immunological basis.

References

1. Abenhaim L, Moride Y, Brenot F, Rich S, Benichou J, Kurz X, Higenbottam T, Oakley C, Wouters E, Aubier M et al. (1996) Appetite-suppressant drugs and the risk of primary pulmonary hypertension. *N Engl J Med* 335: 609–616.
2. Bishop A, Oldershaw P (1996) Thromboembolism in primary pulmonary hypertension. *Br Med J* 313: 1418–1419.
3. Rich S, Kaufmann E, Levey P (1992) The effects of high doses of calcium channel blockers on survival in primary pulmonary hypertension. *N Engl J Med* 328: 76–81.
4. Higenbottam T, Wheeldon D, Wells F, Wallwork J (1984) Long-term treatment of primary pulmonary hypertension with intravenous eprostanol (prostacyclin). *Lancet* i: 1046–1047.
5. Barnes PJ, Belvisi MG (1993) Nitric oxide and lung disease. *Thorax* 48: 1034–1043.
6. Asherson RA, Zulman J, Hughes GRV (1989) Pulmonary thromboembolism associated with procainamide-induced lupus syndrome and anticardiolipin antibodies. *Ann Rheum Dis* 48: 232–235.
7. Daly E, Vessey MP, Hawkins MM, Carson JL, Gough P, Marsh S (1996) Risk of venous thromboembolism among users of postmenopausal oestrogens. *Lancet* 348: 977–980.
8. Harmon CE, Portanova JP (1982) Drug-induced lupus: clinical and serological studies. *Clin Rheum Dis* 8: 121–135.
9. Bernstein RM (1993) Rheumatic complications of drugs and toxins. In: Maddison PJ, Isenberg DA, Woo P, Glass DN (eds). *Oxford textbook of rheumatology*. Oxford University Press, Oxford, pp. 1089–1095.
10. Mansilla-Tinoco R, Harland SJ, Ryan PFJ, Bernstein RM, Dollery CT, Hughes GRV, Bulpitt CJ, Morgan A, Jones JM (1982) Hydralazine, antinuclear antibodies and the lupus syndrome. *Br Med J* 284: 936–939.
11. Hobbs RN, Clayton A-L, Bernstein RM (1987) Antibodies to the five histones and poly(adenosine diphosphate-ribose) in drug-induced lupus: Implications for pathogenesis. *Ann Rheum Dis* 46: 408–416.
12. Cambridge G, Wallace H, Bernstein RM, Leaker B (1994) Autoantibodies to myeloperoxidase in idiopathic and drug-induced systemic lupus erythematosus and vasculitis. *Br J Rheumatol* 33: 109–114.
13. Bernstein RM, Egerton-Vernon J, Webster J (1980) Hydralazine induced cutaneous vasculitis. *Br Med J* 1: 156–157.
14. Woosley RL, Dryer DE, Riedenberg MM, Nies AS, Carr K, Oates JA (1978) Effects of acetylator phenotype on the rate at which procainamide induces antinuclear antibodies and the lupus syndrome. *N Engl J Med* 298: 1157–1160.
15. Perry HM Jr, Schroeder HA (1954) Syndrome simulating collagen disease caused by hydralazine (Apresoline). *J Amer Med Ass* 154: 670–673.
16. Batchelor JR, Welsh KI, Tinoco RM, Dollery CT, Bernstein RM, Hughes GRV, Ryan P, Naish PF, Aber GM, Bing RF et al. (1980) Hydralazine-induced systemic lupus erythematosus: The influence of HLA-DR and sex upon susceptibility. *Lancet* i: 1107–1109.
17. Speirs C, Fielder AHL, Chapel H, Davey NJ, Batchelor JR (1989) Complement system protein C4 and susceptibility to hydralazine-induced systemic lupus erythematosus. *Lancet* i: 922–924.
18. Sim E, Gill EW, Sim RB (1984) Drugs that induce systemic lupus erythematosus inhibit complement component C4. *Lancet* ii: 422–424.
19. Miller GJ, Ashcroft MT, Beadnell HM, Wagner JC, Pepys J (1971) The lipoid pneumonia of Blackfat tobacco smokers in Guyana. *Q J Med* 40: 457–470.
20. Donaghy M, Rees AJ (1983) Cigarette smoking and lung haemorrhage and glomerulonephritis caused by autoantibodies to glomerular basement membrane. *Lancet* ii: 1390–1392.
21. Zitnik RJ, Cooper AJ (1990) Pulmonary disease due to antirheumatic agents. *Clin Chest Med* 11: 139–150.
22. Lee TH, Christie PE (1993) Leukotrienes and aspirin-induced asthma. *Thorax* 48: 1189–1190.
23. Saltini C, Winestock K, Kirby M, Pinkston P, Crystal RG (1989) Maintenance of the alveolitis in patients with chronic beryllium disease by beryllium-specific helper T-cells. *J Exp Med* 320: 1103–1109.

24. Saltini C, Dirby M, Trapnell BC, Tamura N, Crystal RG (1990) Biased accumulation of T lymphocytes with "memory-type" CD45 leucocyte common antigen gene expression on the epithelial surface of the human lung. *J Exp Med* 171: 1123–1140.
25. Pepys J, Turner-Warwick M, Dawson PC, Hinson KFW (1968) Arthus (type 3) skin test reactions in man: Clinical and immunopathological features. In: Rose B, Richer M, Seahon A, Frankland SW (eds). *Allergology*. Amsterdam: Excerpta Medica, 221–235.
26. Warren CPW (1977) Extrinsic allergic alveolitis: A disease commoner in nonsmokers. *Thorax* 32: 567–569.
27. Keller RH, Swartz S, Schlueter DP, Bar-Sela S, Fink JN (1984) Immunoregulation in hypersensitivity pneumonitis: Phenotypic and function studies of bronchoalveolar lavage lymphocytes. *Am Rev Respir Dis* 130: 766–771.
28. Ghose T, Landrigan P, Killeem R, Dill J (1974) Immunopathological studies in patients with farmer's lung. *Clin Allergy* 4: 119–129.
29. Caplan A (1953) Certain unusual radiological appearances in the chest of coal-miners suffering from rheumatoid arthritis. *Thorax* 8: 29–37.
30. Camus P, Gibson GJ (1995) Adverse pulmonary effects of drugs and radiation. In: Brewis RAL, Corrin B, Geddes DM, Gibson GJ (eds). *Respiratory Medicine*, 2nd ed. London: WB Saunders, pp. 630–657.
31. White DA, Rankin JA, Stover DE, Gellene RA, Gupta S (1989) Methotrexate pneumonitis: Bronchoalveolar lavage findings suggest an immunologic disorder. *Am Rev Respir Dis* 139: 18–21.
32. Kamisako T, Adachi Y, Chihara J, Yamamoto T (1993) Interstitial pneumonitis and inter-feron-alpha. *Br Med J* 306: 896.
33. Coudert B, Bailly F, Andre F, Lombard JN, Camus P (1992) Amiodarone pneumonitis: Bronchoalveolar lavage findings in 15 patients and review of the literature. *Chest* 102: 1005–1012.
34. Kuhlman JE (1991) The role of chest computed tomography in the diagnosis of drug-related reactions. *J Thorac Imaging* 6: 52–61.
35. Huang MS, Colby TV, Goellner JR, Martin WJ Jr (1989) Utility of bronchoalveolar lavage in the diagnosis of drug-induced pulmonary toxicity. *Acta Cytol* 33: 533–538.
36. Hilliquin P, Renoux M, Perrot S, Puechal X, Menkes CJ (1996) Occurrence of pulmonary complications during methotrexate therapy in rheumatoid arthritis. *J Rheumatol* 35: 441–445.
37. Bourgeois P, Aeschlimann A (1991) Drug-induced scleroderma. *Clin Rheum* 5: 13–20.
38. Haustein UF, Herrmann K (1994) Environmental scleroderma. *Clin Dermatol* 12: 467–473.
39. Silman A, Jannini S, Symmons D, Bacon P (1988) An epidemiological study of sclero-derma in the West Midlands. *Br J Rheumatol* 27: 286–290.
40. Sanchez-Guerrero J, Schur PH, Sergent JS, Liang MH (1994) Silicone breast implants and rheumatic disease: Clinical, immunologic and epidemiologic studies. *Arthritis Rheum* 37: 158–168.
41. McHugh MJ, Whyte J, Harvey G, Haustein UF (1994) Anti-topoisomerase 1 antibodies in silica-associated systemic sclerosis: A model for autoimmunity. *Arthritis Rheum* 37: 1198–1205.
42. Black CM, Walker AE, Welsh KI, Bernstein RM, Catoggio LJ, McGregor AR, Jones JK (1983) Genetic susceptibility to scleroderma-like syndrome induced by vinyl chloride. *Lancet* i: 53–55.
43. Sitbon O, Bidel N, Dussopt C, Azarian R, Braud ML, Lebargy F, Fourme T, de Blay F, Piard F, Camus P (1994) Minocycline pneumonitis and eosinophilia: A report on eight patients. *Arch Intern Med* 154: 1633–1640.
44. Goodwin SD, Glenny RW (1992) Nonsteroidal anti-inflammatory drug-associated pulmonary infiltrates with eosinophilia: Review of the literature and Food and Drug Administration Adverse Reaction reports. *Arch Intern Med* 152: 1521–1524.
45. Campagna AC, Blanc PD, Criswell LA, Clarke D, Sack KE, Gold WM, Golden JA (1992) Pulmonary manifestations of the eosinophilia-myalgia syndrome associated with trypto-phan ingestion. *Chest* 101: 1274–1281.
46. Phelps RG, Fleischmajer R (1988) Clinical, pathologic and immunopathologic manifestati-ons of the toxic oil syndrome: Analysis of fourteen cases. *J Am Acad Dermatol* 18: 313–324.
47. Rosenow EC, Myers JL, Swensen SJ, Pisani RJ (1992) Drug-induced pulmonary disease: An update. *Chest* 102: 239–250.

Autoimmune Aspects of Lung Disease
ed. by D. A. Isenberg and S. G. Spiro
© 1998 Birkhäuser Verlag Basel/Switzerland

CHAPTER 12
Overview

David A. Isenberg[1] and Stephen G. Spiro[2]

[1] Centre for Rheumatology/Bloomsbury Rheumatology Unit, Department of Medicine,
University College London, London, UK
[2] Department of Thoracic Medicine, University College London Hospitals, London, UK

Traditional teaching in respiratory medicine has focused on histopathology and physiology to explain disease and its mechanisms. Whilst physiology remains essential for the understanding of many functional disorders in the lung and the airways, the explosion of information that is occurring at the cellular levels is becoming apparent. Cell function, mediators released by cells, their role in pathogenesis, disease modulation and, perhaps, treatment is knowledge that now needs to be assimilated in the understanding of many lung disorders. The lungs are especially vulnerable as they are constantly exposed to inhaled foreign particles, including allergens, microbes, viruses, protozoa, fungi and also toxins. They have the largest blood supply of any organ within the body and this mechanism can also be a source of delivering harmful substances.

The earlier chapters of the book have confirmed the wide range of conditions that affect the lungs. In order to determine a diagnosis, a detailed history is still paramount, to help identify an intrinsic or environmental cause, e.g. asbestos, a drug – often an important contributor to pulmonary pathology, or an external allergen. We still rely on clinical patterns to make a diagnosis now aided by the use of tests such as high resolution CT. Nevertheless, histopathology must remain the gold standard for disease classification.

It is clear from this book that immunological mechanisms play a very important part in the development of most of the major lung diseases, particularly those affecting the parenchyma.

As Catterall and Sheffield have described in Chapter 1, the mechanisms by which lymphocytes are recruited from the circulation into the lungs, their interaction with other cells and the regulation of a pulmonary immune response are increasingly understood at the molecular level. The existence of bronchus-associated lymphoid tissue as part of the more general mucosal associated lymphoid tissue (MALT) is now well established. These lymphocytes are likely to provide an integral part of the immune defence system that is focused on the lungs. These lymphocytes are thought to be a mixture of naive and memory cells, whereas most of the lymphocytes in the alveoli and interstitium are of the memory variety (presumably having already been exposed to antigens).

Major developments in our understanding of the homing mechanisms by which lymphocytes are attracted to the pulmonary endothelium have taken place in the past five years. Certain key molecules, including L-selectin, the β-2 integrin LFA-1 and the β-2 integrin CLA-4 appear to be critical. Equally important are antigen presenting cells, including dendritic cells, alveolar macrophages and the Langerhans's cells. Dendritic cells in particular are widely distributed in the normal lung, and these cells and the Langerhans' cells are almost certainly the most important with respect to presenting antigen to lymphocytes in the first instance. Since pulmonary T-cells carry the CD4 or CD8 antigens, cellular interactions are likely to be MCH-restricted. A great deal of interest is also focusing at present on the additional co-stimulatory signals which are required to facilitate interaction between antigen presenting cells and lymphocytes. As discussed in Chapter 1, these signals are likely to be provided by the B-7 molecules, CD-86 and CD-80 on the antigen presenting cells and their respective ligands, CD-28 and CTLA-4 and lymphocytes.

Lymphocyte effects are clearly mediated by cytokines, which are many and varied! Unfortunately, the rapid pace of discovery compounds the difficulty in trying to keep up with both the number of these cytokines and the precise roles they might be playing in the development of lung disorders as well as other diseases. Furthermore, the relatively recent suggestion that there were two distinct types of T-helper cells, TH_1 and TH_2, with different patterns of lymphokine production (TH_1 secreting IL-2 and IL-12 and γ interferon; TH_2 secreting IL-4, IL-5, IL-6 and IL-10) and that these different subsets were associated with different diseases, has even more recently been challenged and is evidently not as clear-cut as it was once thought. Nevertheless, the key to our understanding of many diseases of the lungs will almost certainly ultimately depend upon a detailed knowledge of how cytokines act locally. By analogy, the recent demonstration that monoclonal antibodies to $TNF\alpha$ can have a remarkable, albeit transient, effect on Crohn's disease and rheumatoid arthritis, leads to some perhaps guarded optimism that other monoclonal antibodies may yet prove to be of value in the treatment of some lung conditions.

As many of the chapters in this book have demonstrated, there are very clearly immunological perturbations and in some cases overt autoimmunological mechanisms underlying many diseases of the lungs. However, interstitial fibrosis is the common end-point of a battery of insults and stimuli to the immune system. The classification of fibrosing alveolitis into cryptogenic, that associated with systemic autoimmune rheumatic disorders, those associated with a particular immune reaction, e.g., bronchiolitis obliterans organising pneumonia, or caused by an external pathogen such as extrinsic allergic alveolitis provide good examples of this dilemma.

Immunological investigation clearly provides us with considerably greater knowledge about the mechanisms of an illness – but with the exception of a few conditions, e.g., C-ANCA in Wegener's granulomatosis, rarely identifies a specific process or substance that will determine aetiology, outcome or provide a guide for therapy. Nevertheless, it is inevitable that the better the understanding of the evolution of a disease, the greater the chance is of improving its management. Treatment certainly of the autoimmune-mediated lung disease remains unsatisfactory. Thus, steroids and other immunosuppressive or cytoxic agents, while sometimes effective, have a high toll in side-effects, principally infection, and their efficacy varies considerably. This approach still dominates the treatment of pulmonary infiltrative illnesses, but airway diseases, such as asthma, have benefited greatly from topical applications of inhaled corticosteroids, and newer compounds such as leukotrine antagonists may hold further promise.

The wide range of lung involvement in rheumatic diseases highlights the fact that the airways, bronchial cartilages, parenchyma and blood vessels themselves can all be involved at different times. Sophisticated diagnostic investigation remains elusive. Broncho-alveolar lavage, whilst providing information on cellular activity in disease, and some data on mediators, is still rarely diagnostic. Open lung biopsy remains the final arbiter for interstitial problems, and yet it too can still provide non-specific data. The distinguishing between disease, super-added infection and possible drug-related reactions is dealt with in considerable detail.

Much of the rapid increase in our understanding of the abnormalities that cause asthma also come from specific investigations aimed at increasing knowledge rather than affecting management directly. The role of BAL and, more recently, fibre-optic bronchial biopsy in patients with asthma is summarised in chapter 8. The same can be said for BAL in patients who are HIV positive. These studies have identified the spread of the HIV into the lung parenchyma, the appearance of local HIV-specific immune responses which attempt to eradicate the virus from the respiratory tract.

The concept of host resistance appears extremely important, both in HIV disease and in malignancy. Immunological competence and surveillance plays a part in controlling tumour growth, and the malaise and debility present when the immune system begins to fail seems disproportionate to the patient's tumour burden. Whilst immune function can be shown to be impaired in most suffers of lung cancer, therapy based on improving the immune response has not yet been successful.

In conclusion, this book summarises what is known about normal functioning of the immune system in the lungs, the perturbations to this system, and a wide variety of pulmonary diseases and the therapeutic approaches that are currently in vogue. The rapid pace of progress in our understanding of the mechanisms that lead to lung diseases are now opening the door to the realistic promise of newer and more specific modalities of treatment based upon more accurate comprehension of aetiopathogenesis. Such innovations should be widely welcomed.

Index

274

leprosy 89
liver 11 β-hydroxydsteroid dehydrogen-
    ase type 1 (11 β HSD-1) 103
L-tryptophan 263
lung CD4+ T-cell in human immunodefi-
    ciency virus (HIV) infection 144
lung CD8+ T-cell in human immunodefi-
    ciency virus (HIV) infection 144
lung function test 30
lung haemorrhage, ANCA-associated 72
lung lymphocyte 88
lung parenchyma 25
lupus anticoagulant 254
lupus erythematosus cell 42
lupus pneumonitis 28
Lyme disease 89
lymph node 2
lymphocyte 95
lymphocyte activation 8
lymphocyte circulation 5
lymphocyte in lung of human immuno-
    deficiency virus (HIV) infected
    patient 143
lymphocyte in the immune response to
    lung cancer 174
lymphocyte, γ/δ T cell in human immuno-
    deficiencyvirus (HIV) infection 145
lymphocyte, human immunodeficiency
    virus (HIV)- specific CTL 144
lymphocyte, interstitial pool 88
lymphocytic interstitial pneumonitis 28
lymphoid tissue, organization 142
lymphokine killer cell 176
lymphoma 33
lymphomatoid granulomatosis 77

major histocompatibility (MHC) class II
    antigen 178
major histocompatibility antigen class 1
    target molecule 178
macrophage in the immune response to
    lung cancer 172
mast cell 188, 190, 195-197
mediastinal node 93
Melphelan 253
methotrexate 134, 253
methotrexate pneumonitis 261
microscopic polyangiitis 59, 72, 73
microscopic polyangiitis, antibody to
    myeloperoxidase 71, 72

microscopic polyangiitis, antibody to
    proteinase 3 71, 72
microscopic polyangiitis, clinical fin-
    dings 61, 71, 72
microscopic polyangiitis, diagnosis 71,
    72
microscopic polyangiitis, histological
    findings 71, 72
microscopic polyangiitis, survival 73
microscopic polyangiitis, therapy 72, 73
Minocycline 253
Mitomycin 253
mixed connective tissue disease (MCTD)
    31, 78
mixed cryoglobulinaemia 78
model of autoimmune disease 90
monocyte chemotactic factor (MCF) 95
monocyte migration inhibition factor
    (MIF) 95
mononeuritis multiplex 61
mucosal and systemic immunisation 88
myasthenia gravis 31, 116
mycobacteria 91, 100
mycoplasma 120
myeloperoxidase (MPO) 59

natural killer cell 174
necrotising sarcoid granulomatosis 99
nephritis, , ANCA-associated 72
neutrophil elastase 227
nitric oxide 254
nocardia 126
nodular necrotizing sarcoidosis 78
non-steroidal anti-inflammatory drug
    (NSAID) 257
non-steroidal anti-inflammatory drug
    (NSAID) and aspirin 253

obliterative bronchiolitis (OB) 26
Oestrogen 253
open lung biopsy 29, 269
opportunistic infection 27
organising pneumonia 264

p53 170
paraneoplastic syndrome 169
patchy alveolar infiltrate 28
pathergic necrosis 68
PDGF β 102
Penicillamine 253
Penicillin 253

D. Raeburn, *Rhône-Poulenc Rorer Ltd, Dagenham, UK*
M.A. Giembycz, *Royal Brompton National Heart and Lung Institute, London, UK (Eds)*

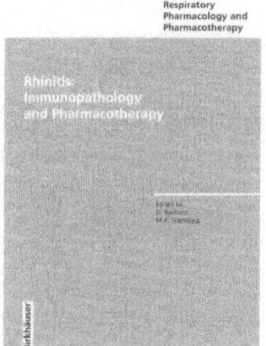

Respiratory
Pharmacology and
Pharmacotherapy

Rhinitis:
Immunopathology
and Pharmacotherapy

Rhinitis: Immunopathology and Pharmacotherapy

1997. 248 pages. Hardcover • ISBN 3-7643-5301-5

Continuing the Respiratory Pharmacology and Pharmacotherapy series, this volume explores the pathophysiology and therapy of rhinitis. The volume is introduced by a chapter describing the normal anatomy and physiology of the nose and sinuses. Against this background the contributing authors describe and discuss the immunological and pathological changes which occur in rhinitis. The various causes and the types of rhinitis – such as allergic, vasomotor, and infectious – are considered as are the treatments available (pharmacotherapy, immuno-therapy, surgery). The book concludes with a description of the animal models of rhinitis which are now available. This book will be indispensable to bench scientists and clinicians alike.

From the contents:
V. Lund: Anatomy and Physiology of the Nasal Cavity and Paranasal Sinuses
J.G. Widdicombe: Pathophysiology of the Nose in Rhinitis
G.K. Scadding: Immunology of the Nose
M. Andersson, C. Svensson, L. Greiff, I. Erjefält and C.G.A. Persson: Inflammation in Rhinitis
R.J. Davies and M.A. Calderon: Allergic Rhinitis
J. Krasnick and R. Patterson: Vasomotor Rhinitis
S. Criscione and E. Porro: Infectious agent-induced Rhinitis
J. Bousquet, P. Demoly and F.-B. Michel: Specific Immunotherapy in Allergic Rhinitis
J.A. Cook: Surgery of Rhinitis
K.L.S. Chen: Animal models of Rhinitis

For detailed information please see
http://www.birkhauser.ch
or mail to
sales@birkhauser.ch

Birkhäuser Verlag • Basel • Boston • Berlin

D.F. Rogers, National Heart and Lung Institute, London, UK /
M.I. Lethem, Univ. of Brighton, UK (Eds)

Airway Mucus: Basic Mechanisms and Clinical Perspectives

1997. 400 pages. Hardcover. ISBN 3-7643-5691-X
(Respiratory Pharmacology and Pharmacotherapy)

Conceptually unsavoury, airway mucus is nevertheless vital to homeostasis in the respiratory tract. In contrast, when abnormal, mucus contributes significantly to the pathophysiology of a number of severe bronchial diseases, including asthma, chronic bronchitis and cystic fibrosis. This volume provides wide-ranging and in depth coverage of the scientific and clinical aspects of airway mucus.

Discussion of the scientific aspects of airway mucus commences with chapters which address the biochemical and molecular biological basis of airway mucus and is extended by chapters which provide comprehensive coverage of the various physiological and rheological aspects of respiratory secretions. The clinical aspects of the topic are then considered in chapters discussing the involvement of mucus secretions in bacterial infections and the role of mucus in hypersecretory diseases of the airway. The volume concludes with a discussion of the therapeutic aspects of the topic, both in terms of the possible approaches to the treatment of mucus hypersecretion and of the interaction of drugs used in respiratory disease with airway mucus.

Contents:
1. Airway Surface Liquid: Concepts and Measurements
2. Structure and Biochemistry of Human Respiratory Mucins
3. Airway Mucin Genes and Gene Products
4. The Microanatomy of Airway Mucus Secretion
5. Mechanisms Controlling Airway Ciliary Activity
6. Rheological Properties and Hydration of Airway Mucus
7. Goblet Cells: Physiology and Pharmacology
8. Airway Submucosal Glands: Physiology and Pharmacology
9. Mucus–Bacteria Interactions
10. Experimental Induction of Goblet Cell Hyperplasia *In Vivo*
11. Mucus Hypersecretion and Its Role in the Airway Obstruction of Asthma and Chronic Obstructive Pulmonary Disease
12. Mucus and Airway Epithelium Alterations in Cystic Fibrosis
13. Drug–Mucus Interactions
14. Therapeutic Approaches to the Lung Problems in Cystic Fibrosis
15. Therapeutic Approaches to Airway Mucous Hypersecretion

For detailed information please see
http://www.birkhauser.ch
or mail to
sales@birkhauser.ch

Birkhäuser Verlag • Basel • Boston • Berlin

R.W. Wilmott,
Children's Hospital Medical Center, Cincinnati, OH, USA (Ed.)

The Pediatric Lung

1997. 352 pages. Hardcover • ISBN 3-7643-5703-7
Respiratory Pharmacology and Pharmacotherapy (RPP)

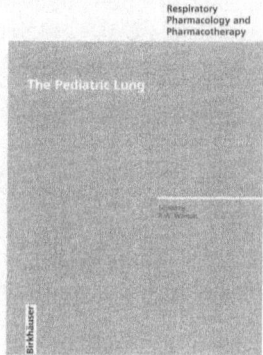

Focussed specifically on children and pediatric respiratory diseases, *The Pediatric Lung* reviews the current status of pharmacological therapy for asthma, viral pneumonia, cystic fibrosis, bronchopulmonary dysplasia and acute respiratory failure. A review of aerosol delivery systems in children and an up-to-date treatise on mucolytic agents is also included.

The chapters are written by leading specialists in the field and summarize the latest developments in pediatric pulmonology, as well as covering a comprehensive range of respiratory diseases in children.

Pediatric pulmonologists, allergologists, intensivists, neonatologists and general pediatricians will find *The Pediatric Lung* an invaluable source of reference. Clinicians will be particularly interested in the new information concerning aerosol delivery systems, gene therapy for cystic fibrosis, new modalities of therapy for asthma, the emerging role of nitric oxide and a treatise on modern mycolytic agents.

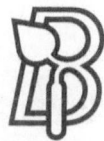

Birkhäuser Verlag • Basel • Boston • Berlin

Y. Martinet, Brabois Hospital, Vandoeuvre, France / F.R. Hirsch, Copenhagen University Hospital, Denmark / N. Martinet, INSERM U14, Vandoeuvre, France / J.-M. Vignaud, Nancy Central Hospital, France / J.L. Mulshine, National Cancer Institute, Rockville, MD, USA (Eds)

Clinical and Biological Basis of Lung Cancer Prevention

1997. Approx. 350 pages. Hardcover
ISBN 3-7643-5778-9
(Respiratory Pharmacology and Pharmacotherapy)

Lung cancer is a disease with pandemic public health implications as it is now the leading cause of cancer mortality throughout the world. This book results from two recent International Association for the Study of Lung Cancer (IASLC) Workshops on lung cancer prevention. It strikes a balance between considering public health approaches to tobacco control and population-based screening, advances in clinical evaluation of chemoprevention approaches, and the biology of lung carcinogenesis.

Indeed, while the science of smoking cessation is evolving as new pharmacological tools are moving into clinical evaluation, the current impact of molecular diagnostics is profound. The rapidly-evolving diagnostic technologies are revolutionizing basic scientific investigation of cancer, and this trend is expected to soon spill over into the clinical practice of medicine. The evolution of economical diagnostic platforms to allow for direct bronchial epithelial evaluation in high-risk populations promises to improve the diagnostic lead-time for this disease. The hope is that enough progress will occur to permit lung cancer detection in advance of clinical cancer so that the disease can be addressed early on, while it is still confined to the site of origin.

Chemoprevention, which is designed to intervene in the early phase of carcinogenesis prior to any subjective clinical manifestation of a cancer, is also generating greater research interest. Moreover, the benefit of aerosolized administration of chemoprevention agents over conventional oral administration has strong appeal and may result in the reduction of the incidence of cancer when combined with new diagnostic technologies.

For detailed information please see
http://www.birkhauser.ch
or mail to
sales@birkhauser.ch

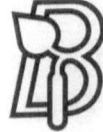

Birkhäuser Verlag • Basel • Boston • Berlin